D1478716

Social Neuroscience

Social Neuroscience

Brain, Mind, and Society

EDITED BY

Russell K. Schutt

Larry J. Seidman

AND

Matcheri S. Keshavan

Harvard University Press

Cambridge, Massachusetts
London, England
2015

First Printing

Library of Congress Cataloging-in-Publication Data

Social neuroscience : brain, mind, and society / edited by Russell K. Schutt,
Larry J. Seidman, Matcheri S. Keshavan.
pages   cm
Includes bibliographical references and index.
ISBN 978-0-674-72897-4 (hardcover : alk. paper)
1. Cognitive neuroscience.   2. Neuroscience—Social aspects.
3. Neuropsychology.   4. Social psychology.   I. Schutt, Russell K., 1951–
II. Seidman, Larry J., 1950–   III. Keshavan, Matcheri S., 1953–
QP360.S592   2015
612.8'233—dc23
2014040690

To our families

Contents

THE SOCIAL WORLD

Color Plates follow page 148

Preface

The development of social neuroscience at the end of the twentieth century is engaging the disciplines of psychiatry, psychology, and neuroscience with the concerns about social relations on which sociologists have traditionally focused, while it is also starting to reengage the discipline of sociology with the field of biology after a hiatus of one hundred years. As it does so, social neuroscience is also creating a basis for connecting these disciplines and the other social and clinical sciences within a common paradigm for understanding human sociality. The result has been an avalanche of articles, a profusion of books, and the funding of interdisciplinary research projects of breathtaking scope.

We have observed these developments from the complementary vantage points of our respective core disciplines—psychiatry (Keshavan), psychology (Seidman), and sociology (Schutt)—and have found that social neuroscience allows us to overcome the polarities that have so often driven our disciplines apart: reductionism or emergence, biology or society, free will or determinism. We have participated in and contributed to these developments with research agendas that increasingly intersect: the emergence of psychosis in young people (Seidman and Keshavan); the neurobiology of the brain (Keshavan and Seidman); the impact of the social environment (Schutt, Seidman, and Keshavan). We have learned that social neuroscience is improving our understanding of people and their social world as well as generating more effective treatments for psychiatric illness and more promising directions for social policy. Paradoxically, the deepening impact of the molecular biological revolution on psychiatry has increased appreciation of nonbiological psychosocial treatment by demonstrating the impact of such treatment on the brain and illuminating how environmental factors interact with genetic susceptibilities.

It is not that major controversies have been resolved or that the most important research has been completed. Rather, it is time for taking stock of what has been learned, how our disciplines can best collaborate, and where research should next focus. It was for these purposes that we organized an interdisciplinary seminar at Harvard's Radcliffe Institute for Advanced Study in March 2011. With generous funding from Radcliffe, we were able to bring together some of the leading researchers in our disciplines who are building the knowledge base of social neuroscience. This book emerged from presentations at the Radcliffe seminar and the inspiration it provided to reexamine progress to date.

Social neuroscience is growing so rapidly and reaching into so many disciplines that we could include only a small fraction of the leading researchers and a few of the key disciplines in our Radcliffe seminar. We have maintained a similar focused approach in this book, drawing attention to research in our own three disciplines. We have centered most applications on understanding schizophrenia—an illness in which social malfunction is a profound characteristic and that has been investigated for many years by the laboratories directed by Drs. Keshavan and Seidman. Although we do give attention to some other major mental health problems, including depression and psychosocial deprivation, a full coverage of psychosocial aspects across the areas of psychiatry is beyond the scope of this work. We have likewise not attempted to include in our history of the emergence of social neuroscience (Chapters 1, 2, 6, and 10) the bases for our differences with sociobiology and evolutionary psychology or an analysis of the controversy between those approaches and the multilevel (group) selection theory that we favor. We also have not included contributions from the cognate fields of neuroanthropology, neuropolitics, or neuroeconomics, although neurosociology is well represented in Jonathan H. Turner's chapter. From our perspective, social neuroscience can best be understood as a broad interdisciplinary approach that encompasses all of these "neuro" specialties.

Although we cannot claim to represent the full scope of social neuroscience in this volume, we have tried to chart a direction for increasing cross-disciplinary fertilization and conceptual integration. We hope thereby to reignite the excitement that greeted Darwin's theory of evolution by national selection, even as it faced unstinting criticism in the late nineteenth century from those rooted in the paradigms of the past, and to encourage reconsideration of the role of human neurobiology as both cause and consequence of human sociality. We hope also to exemplify the value of scientific methods for understanding human propensities and human pathologies, while taking full account of the complexities of human subjectivity, the challenges of perceptual limitations, and the vagaries of self-interest.

An important motivation for our work in psychiatry, psychology, and sociology has been to improve care for persons with serious mental illness and to stimulate more effective social policies within the larger community. Just as our species' survival odds were multiplied by our ability to cooperate in groups, so our current functioning and future achievements are enhanced when we can reap the rewards of our inherent sociality. The clinical programs our chapter authors have investigated and the social policies they have suggested represent only a few of the many potential practical implications of social neuroscience.

We invite our colleagues throughout social science, neuroscience, and medicine to consider the interdisciplinary framework of social neuroscience, the discoveries that it has generated, and its potential for identifying new solutions to age-old problems of the human condition. We invite students to reap the intellectual and career benefits of starting to master this exciting new area of investigation and practice.

It is inevitable that the boundaries between our disciplines continue to erode as knowledge about human sociality expands. It is predictable that the connections between medical care and community processes will increase as psychiatry takes greater account of the social context for the progression of and recovery from serious mental illness. It is time to recognize just how far we have come and to envision what is still to be accomplished.

Russell K. Schutt
Larry J. Seidman
Matcheri S. Keshavan
Boston, Massachusetts

1.

Changing Perspectives in Three Disciplines

Russell K. Schutt, Larry J. Seidman,
and Matcheri S. Keshavan

Human beings are social animals: we evolved in the company of
others, we develop through relations with others, and we flourish in
proportion to our positive social ties. There is no more certain impediment
to normal physical and mental development than social deprivation; there
is no more common a correlate of impaired functioning than social isolation. We cannot understand the operation of our brains or the content of
our minds without taking into account the society around us, nor can we
understand that society without considering how the individuals who comprise it are shaped by their brains and minds.

At the extremes of pathology, the reciprocal effects of individual and
social dysfunction are impossible to ignore. The "not guilty by reason of
insanity" plea by James Holmes—the twenty-four year old who dressed up
as "The Joker" and then killed twelve people in a Colorado movie theater—
attempts to explain this attack on his social world as a result of his personal mental dysfunction (Healey, 2013a). The stunted physical and psychological growth of children in Romanian orphanages reflected the
Ceausescu dictatorship's policy of neglecting meaningful emotional attachments in children's social environments (Behen & Chugani, chapter 12;
Nelson, 2014; Perlez, 1996). At the extremes of achievement, the reciprocal
benefits of individual and social accomplishment are no less evident. Einstein's unusual brain has been credited for some of his outsized impact on
society (Healey, 2013b), while the most socially connected communities

provide a considerable mental health advantage to their residents (McCulloch, 2001).

But between these extremes, in relation to the experiences that are the focus of the daily lives of most individuals and societies—and of most academic research and even clinical practice—the connection between brain, mind, and society is much less evident and the direction of influence much more in dispute. Despite an interdisciplinary consensus that humans are social animals, the disciplines of psychiatry, psychology, and sociology have taken markedly different stances toward the practical salience and the causal direction of the brain-mind-society link; at times during the past century, each discipline has even rejected the need to investigate this connection.

Disciplinary divergence never seemed greater than when President George H. W. Bush declared the 1990s to be "The Decade of the Brain." His July 17, 1990, proclamation of this interagency initiative focused only on the internal workings of the brain and the illnesses presumed to ensue from its malfunction; it did not mention the social environment or draw any connection to the social sciences (www.loc.gov/loc/brain/proclaim .html). Yet as research on the brain accelerated, it became increasingly clear that internal examination alone was insufficient for understanding the development and functioning of this "3-pound mass of interwoven nerve cells that controls our activity" (Bush, 1990). What was most remarkable about the brain was its ability to process information from the environment, adapt to the environment, and effect change in the environment. And describing social relations was central to understanding this reciprocal process. It was time for a new intellectual paradigm (Kandel, 1998, 1999).

A biopsychosocial paradigm (Engel, 1977, 1980) is now becoming a dominant perspective in medicine, psychiatry, and psychology, as discoveries in neuroscience identify connections between neurological and social processes and highlight the value of psychosocial treatments for mental illness (Garland & Howard, 2009). The term *social neuroscience,* first proposed in 1992 (Cacioppo & Berntson, 1992), has since become a recognized subdiscipline with its own journal and professional association (Rose & Abi-Rached, 2013); "social cognition"—as recently as 1991 a topic within psychology conceived as needing no attention to neuroscience (Fiske & Taylor, 1991)—has been reconceptualized as linking "brains to culture" (Fiske & Taylor, 2013); "neurosociology" has gained adherents within its parent discipline (Franks & Turner, 2013; Smith & Franks, 1999). Recent books and conferences have begun to connect social neuroscience to broader social processes and social problems (Lieberman, 2013; Rose & Abi-Rached, 2013; Social Brain Conference, 2008).

After twenty-five years of rapid scientific progress, we are thus at a uniquely fertile moment in the development of the biopsychosocial paradigm. However, despite this progress, the potential of social neuroscience for interdisciplinary integration has yet to be achieved. Many psychiatrists remain focused solely on psychopharmacological solutions to serious mental illness, some psychologists typically conceive of social neuroscience as extending "upward" only to topics in social psychology (discussed by Cacioppo & Berntson, 1992; Ochsner & Lieberman, 2001), social cognition as developed by psychologists has had little impact on sociologists who study social interaction, and while a few sociologists conceive of neurosociology as "the nexus between neuroscience and social psychology" (Franks, 2010; Franks, 2013; Franks & Smith, 1999/2008), most remain "in the position of being the last to know about how our very biological brain is simultaneously social in nature" (Franks, 2010, p. 2).

Social Neuroscience: Brain, Mind, and Society seeks to build the interdisciplinary foundation for social neuroscience by presenting research that illustrates its potential within each of our disciplines and by critiquing the assumptions that have lessened interest in cross-disciplinary engagement. Our chapter authors have maintained a common focus on understanding mental illness in order to facilitate cross-disciplinary comparison. We give particular attention to contributions by sociologists so that our book helps broaden the conception of social neuroscience to encompass social processes at the community, national, and cultural levels. We seek, in other words, to chart a course for further progress in psychiatry, psychology, and sociology that is grounded in a truly interdisciplinary social neuroscience and that can guide development of more effective treatments for serious mental illness. We also connect our approach to related developments in anthropology, economics, and political science, although these disciplines are not represented among our chapter authors.

We find support for our approach in three developments. First is the recent explosion of discoveries in neuroscience and related fields that has identified many points of intersection between the brain and the social world (Cacioppo, Visser, & Pickett, 2006; Lieberman, 2013; Rose & Abi-Rached, 2013; Chapter 2 by Keshavan, this volume). This research has made it clear that the human brain was sculpted by the social world in which our species evolved and that its daily functioning can be understood only in relation to the social world in which we live. Social influence on the evolution of our species is replicated by the ontogenetic development of the brain: the brain is exquisitely shaped by the caretaking environment on a daily basis, and this in turn has profound effects on society (Conti &

Heckman, 2012). It is only when we recognize this fundamental social character of the human brain that we can understand the unique features of the human mind. This book is first and foremost an effort to present leading examples from this large body of recent research, with a particular focus on its implications for our understanding of serious mental illnesses—particularly schizophrenia—that involve social difficulties.

We also find support for our approach in the nascent efforts within sociology to engage with the biologically based understanding of human sociality that has emerged from neuroscience research, although our primary motivation for making this connection is the evidence of how much remains to be done rather than what has been achieved. As British sociologist Nikolas Rose comments in his recent book with Joelle Abi-Rached (2013), most sociologists continue to reject the relevance of biology and neuroscience for understanding larger social processes (p. 160) and remain unaware that the "most sophisticated" perspective in the new brain services is that "the biological and the social are not distinct but intertwined" (p. 3). Although this resistance is more than a century old and has at times served a positive function (Degler, 1991), we believe it has become an anachronism: psychiatry and psychology have recognized the importance for their disciplines of taking account of the social world, and the costs of failing to do so are increasingly evident. Our introduction to the book's section on the influence of the social world reviews the origins of this disjuncture in sociology, while the chapters that follow identify ways to engage the field in productive interdisciplinary collaboration.

Perhaps the strongest evidence in support of our interdisciplinary effort at this time is the fact that we have much distinguished company. Science is by design a collaborative enterprise, and so scientific advances always emerge from a process of sharing discoveries, reviewing evidence, and identifying gaps in understanding. We therefore are more confident in the importance of our own effort because it joins a panoply of outstanding books and distinguished authors, including Eric R. Kandel's (2005) *Psychiatry, Psychoanalysis, and the New Biology of Mind;* John T. Cacioppo, Penny S. Visser, and Cynthia L. Pickett's (2006) *Social Neuroscience: People Thinking about People;* Matthew D. Lieberman's (2013) *Social: Why Our Brains Are Wired to Connect;* Jonathan H. Turner's (2007) *Human Emotions: A Sociological Theory;* Douglas S. Massey's *Strangers in a Strange Land: Humans in an Urbanizing World* (2005); and David D. Franks's (2010) *Neurosociology: The Nexus between Neuroscience and Social Psychology.* It is definitely a fertile time for advancing the perspective of social neuroscience and developing a truly interdisciplinary understanding of sociality.

What most distinguishes our approach from these earlier contributions is the disciplinary and thus explanatory reach of our chapters, from the brain's neurobiology to the mind's psychology to social factors at the family, neighborhood, and societal levels. By contrast, psychiatrist Eric Kandel's (2005) "new intellectual framework for psychiatry" highlights the implications of neurobiology for psychiatry but does not make connections to the disciplines of psychology or sociology. Psychologists John T. Cacioppo and colleagues (2006) focus squarely on the points of intersection between neuroscience and psychology but without engaging sociology. While chapters in their book contribute to "wiping off the cobwebs of twentieth-century simplicities about human nature and human nurture" (Banaji, 2006, p. x), we believe that the value of the new field of social neuroscience will not be realized until it includes attention to the macro level of the social world on which most sociologists focus. Douglas S. Massey's 2001 American Sociological Association presidential address outlined for sociologists the new approach to understanding human evolution that we also endorse (Massey, 2002), but both that address and his subsequent related book (Massey, 2005) did not attempt to connect to the understanding of mental illness and social cognition that has been developed in psychiatry and psychology. As recently as 1999, sociologists David Franks and Thomas Smith (1999/2008) edited a volume about the sociology of emotions without examples from the large body of related research in psychology, neuroscience, or psychiatry.

The most recent contributions in this genre reflect the growing recognition "that integrative multilevel analysis can contribute to the development of more comprehensive models of complex social behavior" (Norman et al., 2013, p. 77) and hence the broader perspective that has also informed this book (Decety & Cacioppo, 2011). Both psychologist Matthew D. Lieberman (2013) and sociologist Nikolas Rose and Joelle M. Abi-Rached (2013) connect research on the brain to group behavior and social processes, while contributions in an American Psychological Association volume edited by Mario Mikulincer and Philip R. Shaver (2014) span the same range—even though they include no sociologists. The latest books by neurosociologists David D. Franks (2010) and Warren D. TenHouten (2013) are consciously interdisciplinary, as is the new *Handbook of Neurosociology* by Franks and Turner (2013). Although somewhat older and oriented to anthropology, the volume by Sussman and Chapman (2004) on human sociality is also quite consciously interdisciplinary.

Historically, the crux of disciplinary divergence has been the role of the mind in the relation between brain, mind, and society (Degler, 1991, pp. 330–333; Mead, 1913), while the impetus for recent disciplinary convergence has been the ability to connect mental states to both neural and social processes (Lieberman, 2013). It is in our minds that we harbor our sense of ourselves as unique individuals, and in which we have the ability to review our past, engage the present, and plan the future. It is our minds that allow us to believe that we are quite unlike other animals in our knowledge of ourselves and in our ability to shape the world in which we live into something markedly different from the world in which we evolved. Yet despite its marvelous capacities, we cannot put our hands on our mind, nor can we find our mind in the world around us. There is no unimpeachable answer to the question of what the human mind "is."

From a purely biological perspective, the mind is the product of the unique organ that is the human brain. It can be understood in terms of the neurological structure from which it emerges and the neural connections with which it functions:

> there are no questions concerning the physical basis of consciousness that differ in principle from other ordinary problems about the physical and functional basis of genes, inheritance, or solidity and liquidity. (Bownds, 1999, n.p.)

From a strictly sociological perspective, the mind is created by engagement in the social world—from the myriad interactions that help us understand who we are in relation to others.

> If failure or disgrace arrives, if one suddenly finds that the faces of men [sic] show coldness or contempt instead of the kindliness and deference that he is used to, he will perceive from the shock, the fear, the sense of being outcast and helpless, that *he was living in the minds of others without knowing it,* just as we daily walk the solid ground without thinking how it bears us up. (Cooley, 1922, p. 208)

Modern social neuroscience is founded on the belief that it is no longer either necessary or appropriate to choose between purely biologically and sociologically based understandings of the human mind. A leading example of how neuroscience now provides the foundation for this more inclusive perspective is provided by neurologist Antonio Damasio's (2010) book, *Self Comes to Mind: Constructing the Conscious Brain.* A self that has both feelings and conscious awareness emerges from specific neural processes in the brain that allow both monitoring and managing the body in which it resides as well as understanding and reacting to the social world in which that body lives. It is this understanding of the mind as reflecting in its very essence both neural and social processes that guides our own approach to connecting brain, mind, and society. We elaborate on this understanding in this chapter and return to it when we introduce the other chapters in our volume. The entire book shows how to understand the human mind as enabled by biological structures and processes that evolved to allow the brain to enhance the fitness of the entire human organism in its natural, highly social, environment. We return to this point in Chapter 16.

We use this introductory chapter to review the history of efforts in each of our disciplines to understand the connection between the biological and the social. We then identify the recent developments that require reconsideration of this connection, including scientific advances in neuroscience, evolutionary biology, anthropology, infant development, and neighborhood effects. We end the chapter by reviewing the key themes and research questions that have guided the authors of our chapters in the three areas of brain, mind, and society.

Simply put, our overall approach is to demonstrate that it is not possible to understand the functioning of the human brain, the course of human development, or the operation of human society without taking into account both biological processes and social ties and the bidirectional link between these different levels of investigation. Neuroscience and psychiatry, psychology and sociology each require the insights of the other if they are to explain adequately the processes that are their primary focus. There is no alternative if we are to explain recent research findings and no better way to enrich our disciplines.

Biology and Society in the Development of Three Disciplines

The Scientific Revolution of the seventeenth and eighteenth centuries transformed human understanding of the physical world and natural processes within it (Tarnas, 1991, pp. 248–271). In the next century, Darwin's (1871) theory of natural selection provided an encompassing framework for the explanation of species' characteristics, their interrelations, and their engagement with the natural world. The resulting paradigm shift diminished the importance of our species in the cosmos: the earth was just one planet in one solar system in a vast universe; *Homo sapiens* had evolved over millennia from less complex species; natural laws constrained physical processes irrespective of human will.

One result was a revolution in human understanding of and responses to health and illness. After systematic observation and careful experimentation, bacterial and viral infections replaced imbalances of "phlegms" or "humors" as the putative sources of much disease (Weatherall et al., 2006). Elimination of infectious agents through sanitation, prevention of illness

through inoculation, and destruction of pathogens through medication replaced bleeding, purging, flagellating and other such nonspecific and use-
less responses (e.g., Ward & Warren, 2007). The prevalence of infectious
diseases began to plummet, the rate of infant mortality began to drop, and
human longevity began a steady climb.

For a time, as the twentieth century approached, those leading the
emerging sciences devoted to brain, mind, and society anticipated that a
comparable revolution was imminent in the understanding and treatment
of mental illness. Phrenologists such as Franz Joseph Gall in the nineteenth
century believed that careful measurement of head shapes would capture
the outward manifestations of brain differences (Kosik, 2003). Early neu-
rologists, including the young Sigmund Freud in the late nineteenth century,
presumed that they would find in the organ of the brain the explanation for
mental illness and the means for its cure (Galbis-Reig, 2004; Schore, 1997).
Surgeons in the early twentieth century presumed that scalpels, yielded
skillfully by psychosurgeons, would provide the ultimate cure for serious
mental illness (Valenstein, 1986). Herbert Spencer (1873, p. 321) argued
in his *The Study of Sociology* (in its twenty-first edition by the time of his
death in 1903) that the pressure for "survival of the fittest"—the centerpiece of Darwin's (1871) theory of natural selection but first proposed by
Spencer—would lead to an average improvement of the species, since "only
those who do advance under it eventually survive." The "social Darwinism"
that developed from this perspective was widely accepted (Hawkins,
1997, p. 82).

But this time of naïve optimism about mental illness was short lived, for
clinical outcomes called into question its underlying assumptions. The brain
was far too complex and its structure much too microscopic for its secrets
to be revealed by the relatively primitive instruments available in the nineteenth century. Although many soon recognized the foolhardiness of phrenology, the crudeness and harmfulness of psychosurgery, and the inadequacy
of social Darwinism, there were no good alternatives for extending understanding of mental processes with neuroscientific research. From the standpoint of explaining mind and society, the brain was relegated to the status
of the proverbial causal "black box": important for the transmission of
thought into action, but in a way that was not understood and seemingly
could not be understood at the time.

Freud had, by the turn of the twentieth century, uncovered evidence of
unconscious mental processes that seemed to explain problems in engagement in the social world. Such processes, Freud concluded, were shaped by
early experiences and disordered thinking (Schore, 1997, p. 811). Although
Freud never entirely abandoned the goal of his Project for a Scientific Psy-

chology to develop a neuroscience of the mind, he recognized that the technology and knowledge of his day precluded a satisfactory model of the brain-mind linkage (Freud, 1895/1953). He turned his attention to intrapsychic and interpersonal processes, with psychoanalysis providing a means for exposing these unconscious processes and then using the analyst's relation to the analysand to turn him or her in a less troubled direction. From the standpoint of most psychoanalysts after Freud, it was not necessary to understand either neural wiring or chemical balancing in order to explain or treat psychiatric disorder (Crews, 1996).

In the United States, many psychologists in the early to mid-twentieth century turned away from neuroscience in favor of a more optimistic perspective that learning ("conditioning") could explain all behavior. B. F. Skinner's (1987) behaviorist psychology thus encouraged his followers in the discipline to turn their backs on the mind as well as on the brain. If the science of psychology could best be advanced by learning how adjustments in the environment change individual behavior, there was no need for understanding how the mind makes sense of human experience, much less how the brain enables the process of sense-making (Degler, 1991, pp. 152–165). Manipulating rewards to change behavior was a mechanical process that could work as effectively in people as in pigeons, irrespective of the differences in their brains. Although the "air crib" that Skinner designed for his second daughter was falsely accused of being just another "Skinner box" like those he used for experiments on pigeons, his ideal of a controlled environment with reduced noise and other outside interference is a far cry from the constant mother-infant contact that characterized childrearing in primitive human societies (Joyce & Faye, 2010). To his credit, Skinner relied on systematic scientific methodologies to test his ideas, rather than the largely anecdotal case reports that underlie theorizing in the Freudian tradition, but those methods did not attempt to investigate neural processes.

Sociology as a discipline quickly turned away from the crude efforts of its earliest leaders to ground understanding of social processes in the basic premises of Darwin's evolutionary biology. When sociologist William Graham Sumner, Spencer's American acolyte, claimed that the only alternative to the "survival of the fittest" was the "survival of the unfittest," the *New York Times* (1883) editorialized against "The Selfish Sciences," and Sumner grew silent on the topic (Bannister, 1973; Keller, 1910). In the early twentieth century, W. I. Thomas (American Sociological Association president, 1927) and other American sociologists adopted environmental rather than biological explanations of racial differences (Degler, 1991, pp. 87–90). Friedrich Adolf Julius von Bernhardi's militaristic, biologically based rhetoric in support of Germany in World War I and Adolf Hitler's distorted

biological logic in justification of the Third Reich's murderous racism ensured that sociologists kept social Darwinism's coffin securely sealed (Bannister, 1973; Black, 2003). Émile Durkheim and Max Weber, the two theo-
rists who became sociology's most highly regarded founders, avoided the
difficulties of relating neural to social processes at that time by placing
them outside the field's concerns. Durkheim (1893/1984, pp. 144–145) rejected explicitly Spencer's individualist "theory that places egoism as the
point of departure for humanity" and instead declared "everywhere that
societies exist there is altruism," rejecting at the same time any disciplinary
connection to biology or psychology. The sociological method was to rest
"wholly on the basic principle that social facts must be studied as things,
that is, as realities *external* to the individual" (Durkheim, 1951/1997,
pp. 37–38, emphasis added). Durkheim (1912/1915, pp. 15–16) acknowledged that people as individuals are biological beings "whose sphere of
action is strictly limited by this fact," but because "man [*sic*] is double,"
"that which is in the individual but surpasses him" (p. 448) and "represents within us the highest reality in the intellectual and moral realm"
should be understood as due to societal forces that have no connection to
that individual biological being. Individual factors that may affect the incli-
nation to suicide belong "to psychology alone" (Durkheim, 1951/1997, p. 46),
while social forces that create societal variation in suicide rates "act upon
men from without" (p. 325).

The hubris about the impact of the social environment that accompanied the rejection of mind and brain as significant sources of disordered
behavior played a key role in both the rise and decline of state psychiatric
institutions. When nineteenth-century social reformer Dorothea Dix recognized the harm wrought by the decrepit conditions for severely mentally
ill persons in jails and poorhouses, she assumed that a well-ordered social
and physical environment—the asylum—would be sufficient as a cure

(Grob, 1994). Other social reformers joined Dix in touting a "well-ordered institution" as the solution to insanity in what they perceived as an increasingly chaotic, disorganized society (Rothman, 1990, p. 138). When a century later sociologist Erving Goffman (1961) discovered that these large psychiatric institutions had themselves become sites for social degradation, his call for their abolition still echoed Dorothea Dix by assuming that the social environment was the key to patients' mental illness.

What emerged from this early history, in the post–World War II era, was a thoroughly sociological perspective on human behavior that was shared by many in the disciplines of psychology and psychiatry. The National Institute of Mental Health (NIMH) focused attention on understanding the value of the community environment in mental health services and on psychosocial rehabilitation as a primary response to mental illness (Grob, 1994, pp. 211–215; Segal & Aviram, 1978). "Organic syndromes" were distinguished categorically from mental illness and resources were focused more on the amelioration of maladies such as depression with its many plausible social origins rather than on less tractable illnesses like schizophrenia (Grob, 1994). Eric Kandel (2006) described his experience in the early 1960s as a psychiatry resident at Harvard Medical School's Massachusetts Mental Health Center (where we each now have faculty appointments):

> Most of our supervisors were heavily oriented toward psychoanalytic theory and practice . . . a number of psychoanalysts took a far more radical stance— biology, they argued, is irrelevant to psychoanalysis. (pp. 154, 366)

In fact, Kandel (2006, p. 336) recalled, "Most psychiatrists thought that the social determinants of behavior were completely independent of the biological determinants." Schizophrenia and other illnesses for which no changes in brain anatomy had yet been consistently identified were "functional," perhaps the fault of parental suggestion or for other reasons "'in a patient's mind,'" but certainly not biological.

The sociological perspective on biology and society in this period rested on four propositions (cf. Barkow, Cosmides, & Tooby, 1992):

(1) Evolutionary displacement. The development of biological capacities that supported sociality was a key aspect of the evolution of *Homo sapiens*. Once the species emerged, however, these prosocial biological capacities are no longer subject to environmental influence (Barkow, 2006; Degler, 1991, p. 209). Once evolved, the influence of the human genome is both fixed and universal. Biology has a unidirectional influence; individuals' human biology would not vary in response to the environment. Of course at that time,

twenty-first-century concepts of genetic malleability through gene
expression, proteins, and epigenetics were not known.

(2) Human malleability. Because normal variation among humans is
not subject to biological influence, variation among individuals
must be explained entirely by social influence. The almost infinite
malleability of humans means that individual behavior can be
shaped by society in almost any direction. The environment is the
important factor, and so it is through environmental manipulation
that mental illness can be cured and human potential achieved
(Mirowsky & Ross, 2003).

(3) Societal rationalization. The development of modern society was
associated with the rise of a rational social order that has largely
expunged the influence of emotional bonds that were so evident
in "primitive" and traditional societies (Weber, 1947). Similarly,
modern childrearing means assisting an infant ruled almost exclusively by emotion to become an adult who has little need for and
no necessary engagement with emotion. Action guided by reason
is the pinnacle of societal and human development alike; its full
exercise requires that emotions be expunged. Emotions arose from
the visceral system that human bodies share with animals, while
reason is what distinguishes humans from these lesser beings and
can be used to prevent the influence of emotion (Damasio, 1994).

(4) Social construction. Human consciousness allows us to create a
social world that is fundamentally distinct from the biological and
physical world. What is important is what we think, what we
create, and what we communicate, not the neural processes that
make this possible. Meaning is what matters, and meaning is a
social construction (Horwitz, 2002, p. 2).

One exception, and a very disturbing one, to this disciplinary divorce
from biological influence was the ongoing efforts of a small minority of
scientists to establish the premise that the black "race" was inherently (i.e.,
biologically) inferior to the white "race" (Ritter, 2007). This racist expression
in the United States paralleled continuing European currents of anti-Semitism
that were similarly based on the pseudoscience of eugenics (Gould, 1981),
although it had been rejected by many sociologists and psychologists (and
anthropologists) early in the century (Degler, 1991, pp. 167–186). This sub-
current in social science relied on specious reasoning and spurious correlations, as well as self-serving inattention to overwhelming evidence of racial
mixing throughout human history. Unfortunately, a side effect of this mali-
cious biology led most sociologists and others to warn against the potential

for including biology in explanations of human behavior and to encourage avoidance of any disciplinary connections to genetics or any other aspect of biology, for fear of being associated with the racist, pseudoscientific theories (Templeton, 1998). This caution, while a reasonable stance in the post–World War II era, as victims of misguided social policies were often blamed for their own difficulties (Ryan, 1971), also hampered integrative sciences from evolving.

Biology Reconsidered

Interest in biological influence had continued among some social scientists in the post-war years (Degler, 1991, pp. 215–244), but it was not until the 1970s and 1980s that interdisciplinary anti-biological consensus began rapidly to break down for psychiatry and psychology with the advent of neuroimaging techniques, including computerized axial tomography (CAT) scans and magnetic resonance imaging (MRI). The ability to visualize and safely measure the human brain in vivo was an enormous advance, with an outpouring of studies demonstrating brain abnormalities in psychiatric disorders, especially schizophrenia. Empirical findings replaced speculation, and a connection of mental illness to biological features could not be denied. Another area of rapid advance was in the area of psychotropic medications, with neurobiological mechanisms identified for their effects. Some experiments and clinical trials (cf. Mays & Franks, 1980) were interpreted to show that psychotherapy and any related learning processes were ineffective; only pharmacotherapy held out hope of a cure for schizophrenia. Although we now know this to be a gross oversimplification, these simplistic explanations dominated the field.

The American Psychiatric Association (APA) task force that developed the third edition of the *Diagnostic and Statistical Manual for Mental Disorders* (*DSM-III;* APA, 1980) also sanctified the identification of clusters of symptoms in a way that paralleled medical diagnoses. With the launch of the Human Genome Project in the early twenty-first century (National Institutes of Health [NIH], 2012), the foundation for a basically biological understanding of mental illness in psychiatry seemed established. Identifying specific genes and neurotransmitters for specific mental illnesses appeared to be the key to both understanding and treatment.

Few sociologists of mental health followed the biological turn (Pearlin, Avison, & Fazio, 2007). Rejection of biological influence had become part of the very definition of sociology for some and an unspoken assumption for most (and a spoken assumption for some like-minded psychiatrists)

(Szasz, 1974). Sociologists who studied severe mental illness did so from a standpoint that stood in stark contrast to the position adopted by most psychiatric researchers and clinical psychologists (Mirowsky & Ross, 2003). First, sociologists emphasized the role of external causation, while psychiatrists looked inward. For sociologists, severe mental illness was most likely to reflect problems in the social world, while psychiatrists suspected biological aberrations. Second, the sociological approach to the identification of severe mental illness involved identifying an arbitrary cut point on a carefully measured continuum of symptom severity—a dimensional approach. Psychiatrists, by contrast, relied on the *DSM-III* and its successors, with their underlying assumption of a clear status difference between a diseased and a healthy organism; the role of diagnosis was to make categorical distinctions between the "cases" that required treatment from those that didn't (APA, 1980).

Treatment preferences were the final and arguably most fundamental point of demarcation between the disciplines. While sociologists of mental health expected psychosocial treatments focused on the individual's environment to be efficacious, psychiatrists increasingly placed their faith in drugs that would correct neurochemical imbalances and thus alter the disease process (Kramer, 1993).

Within psychiatry, the new dominance of the psychopharmacological paradigm was reflected in soaring drug sales, rapid growth of membership in associations of biological psychiatry, and increasing rejection of Freudian and other psychodynamic perspectives. The NIMH turned away from sociologically oriented research in community settings to focus on drug trials for those diagnosed as severely mentally ill (Pearlin et al., 2007). By contrast, sociologists continued to seek in community surveys the external factors that increased the likelihood of depression and anxiety and the associated mental states whose amelioration could diminish the descent into more severe illness. Those with unremittingly severe depression were given the meaningless advice to "take arms against a sea of troubles" (Mirowsky & Ross, 2003, p. 277). Although some sociologists were less willing to eschew biological explanations for schizophrenia—our chapter author Alan Horwitz (2002) even distinguished schizophrenia as an illness with a biological cause—they still focused their attention on the effect of social stigma and other environmental factors on the course of the illness; understanding the role of any underlying neurobiological disruptions was not seen to be necessary (Mirowsky & Ross, 2003). Perhaps the zenith of this disciplinary divorce was reflected in the logo adopted for the American Sociological Association's (ASA) 2005 Annual Meeting in New York City, in which two teams on opposite sides of a mountain were engaged in a tug of war, with the taut rope pulled over the mountaintop indicating the intensity of the struggle—between biology and sociology.

Foundations for an Interdisciplinary Paradigm

But the fortifications of the unidimensional biological paradigm within psychiatry were already starting to crumble. First and foremost, the much heralded second-generation antipsychotic medications that had been developed on the basis of more specific neurobiological understandings of brain functioning were proving in repeated clinical trials to be no more effective than their first-generation precursors that had emerged from chance discoveries (Lieberman & Stroup, 2003). This was true for both general clinical efficacy and for "cognitive enhancement"; the first-generation drugs were in most cases as effective when they were used at doses low enough to avoid detrimental side effects. After a large NIMH-funded multisite test of the most promising second-generation antipsychotics (the CATIE trials) found only limited positive benefits and no sustained comparative advantage, drug companies began to withdraw from development of new psychotropic drugs and researchers began to question their assumptions about the role of the neurotransmitters that the second-generation drugs had targeted (Lieberman et al., 2005). A large multisite trial of treatments for depression (STAR-D) identified high rates of relapse despite treatment and failed to find advantages of particular pharmacological treatments over non-pharmacological treatments that were tested (Nelson, 2006; Rush, 2007).

Paradoxically, another key assumption of the biological paradigm was called into question by the increasingly sophisticated investigations made possible by the Human Genome Project. Despite concerted efforts by hundreds of research teams around the globe, attempts to find one or a handful of genetic variants that account for schizophrenia or other serious mental illnesses were failing. Even after what amounted to enormous fishing expeditions, genome-wide scans comparing persons suffering from schizophrenia to others in good health identified uncommon genetic variants that collectively could explain only a small fraction of cases; a large part of the heritability of schizophrenia remained unexplained or "missing" (van Dongen & Boomsma, 2013).[1] At the same time that these findings called into question the possibility of achieving the goal of simple genetic explanations, they also raised concerns about the biological reality underlying the clusters of symptoms that the *DSM-III* and its successors had so painstakingly used to demarcate diseases like schizophrenia. What psychiatrists had understood for a century to be one disease seemed instead to reflect symptoms, like a fever, of different disorders that could have various biological foundations (Keshavan et al., 2013).

The implications of genetic analysis for biologically based explanations of human behavior were also complicated by the rapid accumulation of evidence in the new field of epigenetics. Genes themselves cannot control bodily processes directly; they do so indirectly by causing the production of proteins that are carried throughout the body and stimulate other changes. What epigenetics revealed is that the environment to which genes are exposed influences whether they are activated to stimulate the production of specific proteins. Without the right trigger, a gene may not be expressed through protein production, and so its potential for shaping behavior may never be realized. Not only did this intermediary role of proteins complicate enormously the effort to identify the role of genes in behavior, it also revealed a mechanism for environmental action on genetic expression that made it impossible to maintain a clear distinction between biological and social factors (Keshavan, Chapter 2, this volume).

In turn, the polarization of biological and social explanations was crumbling in the face of advances in neurological research. Two discoveries were critical in the emergence of the unifying concept of a "social brain" (Burns, 2006). First, decades of neurobiological research identified specific neural structures and processes that had evolved to process social information and to respond to social stimulation (Kahneman, 2011). These structures and processes were connected closely to the centers for emotional processing that humans largely share with other animals, but they also engaged the areas of the brain that involve planning and reasoning and could not be separated from them. Reason could not be separated from emotion any more than behavior in pursuit of individual goals could be understood without regard to social context (Damasio, 1994).

The second neuroscientific advance that required bridging biology and sociology was the discovery of neuroplasticity (see Eack & Keshavan, Chapter 15, and Keshavan, Chapter 2, this volume). Rather than containing a neural endowment that was fixed by nature at birth, research revealed that the brain responded to social and other stimuli by growing new connections and, in the face of adversity, by allowing some connections to atrophy. A brain that is both social and plastic is one whose functioning can only be understood in a social context. The conception first proposed by Hubel and Wiesel in their Nobel prize–winning studies of visual system development now came to be seen as appropriate to the overall relation between the brain and the environment: living organisms adapt to their environment through changes in neural connections (Wiesel, 1981).

Advances in the understanding of human evolution created yet more pressure for convergence of biological and social explanation. Evolutionary biologists have long recognized that the evolution of the larger brain that made *Homo sapiens* a unique species—and the concomitant growth in human head size—required the birth of less mature human infants and therefore a longer period of dependence on maternal nurturance (Kaplan et al., 2009). This necessary dependence of human infants on their primary caretakers, usually their mothers, elicited other biological changes that encouraged infant-maternal attachment and therefore facilitated development of enduring family structures (Cassidy, Ehrlich, & Sherman, 2014; Zihlman & Bolter, 2004).

But early human sociality extended beyond the mother-child bond. There is evidence in the fossil record of the use of dwellings, and thus of ongoing intimate social ties, as far back as 1.9 million years ago (Roberts, 1993). Hunting big game required cooperation and thus encouraged development of social skills; the control of fire allowed longer and more intimate social contact; survival on the African savanna required cooperative identification of and reaction to threats (Turner, Chapter 3, this volume). Evidence from hunter-gatherer societies suggests that intense social cooperation within groups was the norm for ancestral humans (even while intergroup conflict was common) (Diamond, 2012; Thomas, 2006; Watanabe & Smuts, 2004). E. O. Wilson (2012) has suggested that selection in the process of evolution must not have been only for the fittest individuals but for more cooperative social groups. Recorded in the human genome and hence in human biology must be the consequences of pressures to engage effectively with others in your social group in order to maximize the chances of survival (Coan, Brown, & Beckes, 2014; De Dreu, 2014; Schutt, Chapter 10, this volume).

As sociologists became more skilled at identifying variation in the social environment, they also found increasing connections to human functioning at the biological level. Higher levels of social ties were associated with lower rates of chronic disease, longer lives, and less depression (Rutter, 2005). Sharp disruptions in the social environment increased the risk of maladies ranging from posttraumatic stress disorder (PTSD) to suicide, while active interventions to enhance social connectedness could delay the onset of dementia, lower the risk of PTSD, decrease the prevalence of violence, and prevent delays in child development (Hyman, 2000; Reiss, Plomin, & Hetherington, 1991; Sullivan, Neale, & Kendler, 2000).

Yet there could be no return to the period of unquestioned obeisance to environmental influence. The onset of schizophrenia among young adults in supportive and loving families (Takahashi, 2013), the imperviousness of autism to the most intense social manipulations (Hall & Kelley, 2013), and the difficulties of those with Asperger syndrome in relating to others (Griffith et al., 2012) each made it undeniable that the relationship between human biology and social functioning was reciprocal and ongoing. Accumulating evidence from genome-wide association studies with sample sizes exceeding 40,000 individuals suggested as many genetic variants associated with schizophrenia as have been identified in such other chronic medical diseases as diabetes and Crohn's disease (Ripke et al., 2013, 2014; Schizophrenia Working Group, 2014). Neither human thought nor human action could be understood without taking account of both nature and nurture (Panksepp et al., 2014). Neither biological nor social influence could themselves be understood apart from each other (Hyman, 2000; Kandel, 1998).

Enduring Questions

Different answers to two interrelated questions are at the core of the historical and interdisciplinary variation in identifying the appropriate relationship of biological and social factors in the explanation of serious mental illness. (1) *Is our sociality apart from or a part of our biological being?* If our bodies and brains evolved to maximize only our functioning as individuals, then we must understand our sociality as emerging from our interactions and not as inherent in our very being. But if the course of our evolution as a species and of our maturation as individuals is guided by the demands of our social environment, then any attempt to explain our sociality without taking account of our biology will be at best incomplete. (2) *Is the social world instantiated in our bodies?* Although it is undeniable that our social relations shape our personal accomplishments, the embodiment of social experience can easily be overlooked. From feelings of depression to symptoms of schizophrenia, our internal states are too easily interpreted as originating solely within us and belonging only to us.

The recent advances in neuroscience that we have described make it clear that earlier answers to these two questions have been reconsidered and that this reconsideration must be ongoing. The exciting new answers to these questions that have guided the research reported in this volume by neuroscientists, psychiatrists, psychologists, and sociologists also require attention to a third question: *What are the implications of the bidirectional influences between brain, mind, and society for our understanding of human orientations and behaviors?* Our answer to this question must integrate knowledge from each of our disciplines and findings from all levels of our world—from our genome to our globe. It is only when we have developed such an integrated understanding that the interdisciplinary foundation we seek will be completed.

Each of our chapters contributes to achievement of this goal; our tasks as editors are to make explicit connections, to develop general conclusions, and to suggest future directions. We begin with research on human evolution and on the neural architecture that evolution produced. The dense matrix of social ties that interpenetrates human functioning and underpins human society did not result from conscious human decisions or voluntary human actions but because social engagement was a defining feature of human evolution (Degler, 1991, p. 273). If we would not be human if our bodies were not attuned to social ties, then we cannot fully understand any aspect of human functioning without taking account of this essential biological substrate.

Social ties also shape the course of human development. Humans' lengthy period of postnatal dependence both requires close attachment between infant and mother and imbues social bonds with unique developmental significance. From family dynamics to peer influences to the social climate of organizations, the social context of neighborhoods, and the social supports available to the elderly, social ties continue to influence individual functioning throughout the life course. It is therefore no surprise that thinking about social ties is supported by unique cognitive processes and that the capacity for social cognition is essential for normal human functioning. Several chapters focus attention on the relationship between social ties, developmental processes, and the emergence of mental illness.

It is impossible to conceive of the larger social world without acknowledging the importance of social ties. Personal identities are defined largely through the nature of ties to others, and the manner in which social ties are structured both creates the distinctions between families, small groups, organizations, communities, and whole societies and determines how well they function. Neither human thought nor human action can be understood without taking account of the social context in which they occur; neither technological advances nor cultural achievements can be explained without consideration of the social processes through which they developed. Chapters in our final section focus on the macro social environment.

Our attention throughout the book on human mental health and illness keeps us focused on what is fundamental to the evolution of the human species, the development of human lives, and the functioning of human groups. When genetic anomalies or prenatal insults alter the neural connections required for social perception and emotion, conditions such as schizophrenia and autism spectrum disorders may result. When neural injury or disease damages the portions of the brain devoted to social relations, normal functioning becomes very difficult. Deficits in social engagement during human development are associated with infants' failure to thrive, children's social anxieties, adolescents' risk taking, and adults' risk of depression, among many other maladies. Extreme disturbances in the social environment have resulted in stunted growth among Romanian orphans, posttraumatic stress disorder among military veterans, ongoing violence in some inner-city neighborhoods, and increased suicide in the long-term unemployed.

We focus particular attention on schizophrenia, an illness that is characterized by marked social deficits and whose neurological basis is relatively well accepted. The research that several chapter authors review on schizophrenia serves as an exemplar of how the understanding of mental illness can be improved by taking into account social dimensions of neural, cognitive, and behavioral processes. At the same time, the research on schizophrenia raises provocative questions about the extent to which understanding of other illnesses may be improved by focusing more attention on social factors.

It is time for each of the medical and social science disciplines to recognize that understanding the link between biological and social processes is necessary for explaining human behavior. Our minds provide us with our feelings of individuality, but they can do so only because of our physical brains and they must do so not in isolation but in relation to the others with whom we interact. We possess a social brain because we must function in a social world, and that social world exists because of our social brains. In the words of evolutionary psychologists John Tooby and Leda Cosmides (1992), "The stuff of the mind is the stuff of the world" (pp. 72–73).

Note

1. Genome-wide scanning is becoming increasingly sophisticated, and the latest analyses suggest that genes that contribute to the risk of schizophrenia will continue to be identified (Schizophrenia Working Group, 2014).

References

American Psychiatric Association (APA). (1980). *Diagnostic and statistical manual for mental disorders* (3rd ed.). Washington, DC: American Psychiatric Association.

Banaji, Mahzarin R. (2006). Foreword. In J. T. Cacioppo, P. S. Visser, & C. L. Pickett (Eds.), *Social neuroscience: People thinking about thinking people* (pp. vii–x). Cambridge: MIT Press.

Bannister, Robert C. (1973). William Graham Sumner's Social Darwinism: A reconsideration. *History of Political Economy*, 5, 89–109.

Barkow, J. (Ed.). (2006). *Missing the revolution: Darwinism for social scientists.* New York: Oxford University Press.

Barkow, J., Cosmides, L., & Tooby, J. (Eds.). (1992). *The adapted mind: Evolutionary psychology and the generation of culture.* New York: Oxford University Press.

Black, E. (2003). *War against the weak: Eugenics and America's campaign to create a master race.* New York: Four Walls Eight Windows.

Bownds, M. D. (1999). *The biology of mind: Origins and structures of mind, brain, and consciousness.* Bethesda, MD: Fitzgerald Science Press. www.dericbownds .net/bom99/Ch01/Ch01.html

Burns, J. (2006). The social brain hypothesis of schizophrenia. *World Psychiatry*, 5, 77–81.

Bush, G. H. W. (1990). Presidential Proclamation 6158 by the President of the United States of America. July 17, 1990. www.loc.gov/loc/brain/proclaim.html. Accessed July 18, 2014.

Cacioppo, J. T., & Berntson, G. G. (1992). Social psychological contributions to the Decade of the Brain: Doctrine of multilevel analysis. *American Psychologist*, 47, 1019–1028.

Cacioppo, J. T., Visser, P. S., & Pickett, C. L. (Eds.). (2006). *Social neuroscience: People thinking about thinking people.* Cambridge: MIT Press.

Cassidy, J., Ehrlich, K. B., & Sherman, L. J. (2014). Child-parent attachment and response to threat: A move from the level of representation. In M. Mikulincer & P. R. Shaver (Eds.), *Mechanisms of social connection: From brain to group* (pp. 125–143). Washington, DC: American Psychological Association.

Coan, J. A., Brown, C. L., & Beckes, L. (2014). Our social baseline: The role of social proximity in economy of action. In M. Mikulincer & P. R. Shaver (Eds.), *Mechanisms of social connection: From brain to group* (pp. 89–104). Washington, DC: American Psychological Association.

Conti, G., & Heckman, J. J. (2012). *The economics of child well-being* (NBER Working Paper No. 18466). Cambridge, MA: National Bureau of Economic Research. www.nber.org/papers/w18466

Cooley, C. H. (1922). *Human nature and the social order.* New York: Scribner's.

Crews, Frederick. (1996). The verdict on Freud. *Psychological Science*, 7(2), 63–68.

Damasio, A. R. (1994). *Descartes' error: Emotion, reason, and the human brain.* New York: HarperCollins.

———. (2010). *Self comes to mind: Constructing the conscious brain.* New York: Pantheon.

Darwin, C. (1871). *The descent of man, and selection in relation to sex.* New York: Appleton.

———. (1872). *The expression of emotion in men and animals.* London: John Murray.

Decety, J., & Cacioppo, J. T. (Eds.). (2011). *The Oxford handbook of social neuroscience*. New York: Oxford University Press.

De Dreu, C. K. W. (2014). Oxytocinergic circuitry motivates group loyalty. In M. Mikulincer & P. R. Shaver (Eds.), *Mechanisms of social connection: From brain to group* (pp. 391–407). Washington, DC: American Psychological Association.

Degler, C. N. (1991). *In search of human nature: The decline and revival of Darwinism in American social thought*. New York: Oxford University Press.

Diamond, J. (2012). *The world until yesterday: What can we learn from traditional societies?* New York: Viking.

Durkheim, É. (1893 [1984]). *The division of labor in society*.With an introduction by Lewis A. Coser. Translated by W. D. Halls. New York: Free Press.

——. (1912 [1915]). *The elementary forms of the religious life: A study in religious sociology*. Translated by J. W. Swain. London: G. Allen & Unwin.

——. (1951 [1997]). *Suicide: A study in sociology*. New York: Free Press.

Engel, G. L. (1977). The need for a new medical model: A challenge for biomedicine. *Science, 196,* 129–136.

——. (1980). The clinical application of the biopsychosocial model. *American Journal of Psychiatry, 137,* 535–544.

Fiske, S., & Taylor, S. E. (1991). *Social cognition* (2nd ed.). Thousand Oaks, CA: Sage.

——. (2013). *Social cognition, from brains to culture* (2nd ed.). Thousand Oaks, CA: Sage.

Franks, D. D. (2010). *Neurosociology: The nexus between neuroscience and social psychology*. New York: Springer.

——. (2013). Why we need neurosociology as well as social neuroscience: Or—Why role-taking and theory of mind are different concepts. In D. D. Franks & J. H. Turner (Eds.), *Handbook of neurosociology* (pp. 27–32). New York: Springer.

Franks, D. D., & Smith, T. S. (Eds.). (1999 [2008]). *Mind, brain, and society: Toward a neurosociology of emotion*. Reprint of Volume 5, *Social perspectives on emotion*. Bingley, UK: JAI.

Franks, D. D., & Turner, J. H. (Eds.). (2013). *Handbook of neurosociology*. New York: Springer.

Freud, S. (1895 [1953]). Project for a scientific psychology. In S. Freud, J. Strachey, A. Freud, C. L. Rothgeb, A. Richards, Scientific Literature Corporation. *The standard edition of the complete psychological works of Sigmund Freud,* vol. 1 (pp. 283–397). London: Hogarth Press.

Galbis-Reig, D. (2004). Forgotten contributions to neurology, neuropathology, and anesthesia. *Internet Journal of Neurology, 3*(1), 8–21.

Garland, E. L., & Howard, M. O. (2009). Neuroplasticity, psychosocial genomics, and the biopsychosocial paradigm in the 21st century. *Health & Social Work, 34*(3), 191–200.

Goffman, E. (1961). *Asylums: Essays on the social situation of mental patients and other inmates*. Garden City, NY: Doubleday.

Gould, S. J. (1981). *The mismeasure of man*. New York: W. W. Norton.

Griffith, G. M., Totsika, V., Nash, S., & Hastings, R. P. (2012). 'I just don't fit any-where': Support experiences and future support needs of individuals with As-perger syndrome in middle adulthood. *Autism, 16*, 532–546.

Grob, G. N. (1994). *The mad among us: A history of the care of America's mentally ill.* New York: Free Press.

Hall, L., & Kelley, E. (2013). The contribution of epigenetics to understanding ge-netic factors in autism. *Autism,* October 14. [Epub ahead of print]

Hawkins, M. (1997). *Social darwinism in European and American thought, 1860–1945: Nature as model and nature as threat.* Cambridge: Cambridge University Press.

Healey, J. (2013a, April 5). Psychiatrist reported suspect in theater shooting as threat, *New York Times,* p. A12.

Healey, M. (2013b, October 10). Einstein's brain a wonder of connectedness. *Los Angeles Times.* articles.latimes.com. Accessed October 24, 2013.

Horwitz, A. V. (2002). *Creating mental illness.* Chicago: University of Chicago Press.

Hyman, S. E. (2000). The millennium of mind, brain, and behavior. *Archives of Gen-eral Psychiatry, 57,* 88–89.

Joyce, N., & Faye, C. (2010). Skinner air crib. *Observer, 23*(7). www.psychological science.org/index.php/publications/observer/2010/september-10/skinner-air -crib.html. Accessed August 28, 2013.

Kahneman, D. (2011). *Thinking, fast and slow.* New York: Farrar, Straus and Giroux.

Kandel, E. R. (1998). A new intellectual framework for psychiatry. *American Journal of Psychiatry, 155,* 457–469.

———. (1999). Biology and the future of psychoanalysis: A new intellectual framework for psychiatry revisited. *American Journal of Psychiatry, 156,* 505–524.

———. (2005). *Psychiatry, psychoanalysis, and the new biology of mind.* Washing-ton, DC: American Psychiatric Publishing.

———. (2006). *In search of memory: The emergence of a new science of mind.* New York: W. W. Norton.

Kaplan, H. S., Hooper, P. L., & Gurven, M. (2009). The evolutionary and ecological roots of human social organization. *Philosophical Transactions of the Royal Society B, 364,* 3289–3299.

Keller, A. G. (1910). William Graham Sumner. *American Journal of Sociology, 15,* 832–835.

Keshavan, M. S., Clementz, B. A., Pearlson, G. D., Sweeney, J. A., & Tamminga, C. A. (2013). Reimagining psychoses: An agnostic approach to diagnosis. *Schizo-phrenia Research, 146,* 10–16.

Kosik, K. S. (2003). Beyond phrenology, at last. *Nature Reviews Neuroscience, 4,* 234–239.

Kramer, P. D. (1993). *Listening to Prozac: The landmark book about antidepres-sants and the remaking of the self.* New York: Viking.

Lieberman, J. A., & Stroup, T. S. (2003). Guest editors' introduction: What can large pragmatic clinical trials do for public mental health care? *Schizophrenia Bul-letin, 29,* 1–6.

Lieberman, J. A., Stroup, T. S., McEvoy, J. P., Swartz, M. S., Rosenheck, R. A., Perkins, D. O., et al. (2005). Clinical Antipsychotic Trials of Intervention Effectiveness (CATIE): Effectiveness of antipsychotic drugs in patients with chronic
schizophrenia. *New England Journal of Medicine, 353,* 1209–1223.

Lieberman, M. D. (2013). *Social: Why our brains are wired to connect.* New York:
Crown.

Massey, D. S. (2002). A brief history of human society: The origin and role of
emotion in social life. 2001 Presidential Address, American Sociological Association. *American Sociological Review, 67,* 1–29.

———. (2005). *Strangers in a strange land: Humans in an urbanizing world.* New
York: Norton.

Mays, D. T., & Franks, C. M. (1980). Getting worse: Psychotherapy or no treatment—The jury should still be out. *Professional Psychology, 11,* 78–92.

McCulloch, A. (2001). Social environments and health: cross sectional natural
survey. *British Medical Journal, 323,* 208–209.

Mead, G. H. (1913). The social self. *Journal of Philosophy, Psychology, and Scientific Methods, 10,* 374–380.

Mikulincer, M., & Shaver, P. R. (Eds.). (2014). *Mechanisms of social connection:
From brain to group.* Washington, DC: American Psychological Association.

Mirowsky, J., & Ross, C. E. (2003). *Social causes of psychological distress* (2nd
ed.). Hawthorne, NY: Aldine de Gruyter.

National Institutes of Health (NIH). (2012). *An overview of The Human Genome
Project.* Washington, DC: National Human Genome Research Project, National
Institutes of Health. www.genome.gov/12011238

Nelson, C. A., Fox, N. A., & Zeanah, C. H. (2014). *Romania's abandoned children: Deprivation, brain development, and the struggle for recovery.* Cambridge, MA: Harvard University Press.

Nelson, C. J. (2006). The STAR*D study: A four-course meal that leaves us wanting
more. *American Journal of Psychiatry, 163,* 1864–1866.

Norman, G. J., Hawkley, L. C., Luhmann, M., Cacioppo, J. T., & Berntson, G. G.
(2013). In D. D. Franks & J. H. Turner (Eds.), *Handbook of neurosociology*
(pp. 67–81). New York: Springer.

Ochsner, K. N., & Lieberman, M. D. (2001). The emergence of social cognitive neuroscience. *American Psychologist, 56,* 717–734.

Panksepp, J., Solms, M., Schläpfer, T. E., & Coenen, V. A. (2014). Primary-process
separation-distress (PANIC/GRIEF) and reward eagerness (SEEKING) processes in the ancestral genesis of depressive affect and addictions. In M. Mikulincer & P. R. Shaver (Eds.), *Mechanisms of social connection: From brain to
group* (pp. 33–53). Washington, DC: American Psychological Association.

Parsons, Talcott. (1947). "Introduction." In T. Parsons (Ed.) & A. M. Henderson
& T. Parsons (Trans.), *Max Weber, The theory of social and economic organization* (pp. 3–86). New York: Free Press.

Pearlin, L. I., Avison, W. R., & Fazio, E. M. (2007). Sociology, psychiatry, and the
production of knowledge about mental illness and its treatment. In W. R.
Avison, J. D. McLeod, & B. A. Pescosolido (Eds.), *Mental health, social mirror*
(pp. 33–53). New York: Springer.

Perlez, J. (1996, March 25). Romanian 'orphans': Prisoners of their cribs. *New York Times,* pp. A1, A6.

Reiss, D., Plomin, R., & Hetherington, E. M. (1991). Genetics and psychiatry: An unheralded window on the environment. *American Journal of Psychiatry, 148,* 283–291.

Ripke, S., O'Dushlaine, Chambert, K., Moran, J. L., Kähler, A. K., Akterin, S., et al. (2013). Genome-wide association analysis identifies 13 new risk loci for schizophrenia. *Nature Genetics, 45,* 1150–1159.

Ripke, S., Neale, B. M., Corvin, A., Walters, J. T. R., Farh, K-H., Holmans, P. A., et al. (2014). Biological insights from 108 schizophrenia-associated genetic loci. *Nature, 511,* 7510, 421–427.

Ritter, M. (2007, October 19). DNA scientist is condemned for racial comments; Nobel laureate offers apology for remarks. *Boston Globe.*www.boston.com /news/world/europe/articles/2007/10/19/dna_scientist_is_condemned_for _racial_comments/

Roberts, J. M. (1993). *History of the world.* New York: Oxford University Press.

Rose, N., & Abi-Rached, J. M. (2013). *Neuro: The new brain sciences and the management of the mind.* Princeton, NJ: Princeton University Press.

Rothman, D. J. (1990). *The discovery of the asylum: Social order and disorder in the new republic* (Rev. 2nd ed.). Boston: Little, Brown.

Rush, A. J. (2007). STAR*D: What have we learned? *American Journal of Psychiatry, 164,* 201–204.

Rutter, M. (2005, October 25). *Why the different forms of gene-environment interplay matter.* Paper presented at the Judge Baker Children's Center Symposium, Children's Mental Health: Genes and Behavior, Boston, MA.

Ryan, W. (1971). *Blaming the victim.* New York: Random House.

Schizophrenia Working Group of the Psychiatric Genomics Consortium. (2014). Biological insights from 108 schizophrenia-associated genetic loci. *Nature, 511,* 421–427.

Schore, A. N. (1997). A century after Freud's Project: Is a rapprochement between psychoanalysis and neurobiology at hand? *Journal of the American Psychoanalytic Association, 45,* 804–840.

Segal, S. P., & Aviram, U. (1978). *The mentally ill in community-based sheltered care: A study of community care and social integration.* New York: John Wiley.

Skinner, B. F. (1987). Whatever happened to psychology as the science of behavior? *American Psychologist, 42,* 780–787.

Smith, T. S., & Franks, D. D. (1999). Introduction: Summaries and comments. In D. D. Franks (Ed.), *Mind, brain, and society: Toward a neurosociology of emotion in social perspectives on emotion* (Vol. 5, pp. 3–17). Stanford, CA: JAI Press.

Social Brain Conference. (2008). https://openlibrary.org/authors/OL7137473A /Barcelona_Social_Brain_Conference_(1st_2008_Barcelona_Spain)

Spencer, H. (1873). *The study of sociology.* London: Henry S. King. (Available at The Online Library of Liberty, A Project of Liberty Fund, Inc.)

Sullivan, P. F., Neale, M. C., & Kendler, K. S. (2000). Genetic epidemiology of major depression: Review and meta-analysis. *American Journal of Psychiatry, 157,* 1552–1562.

Sussman, R. W., & Chapman, A. R. (Eds.). (2004). *The origins and nature of sociality*. New York: Aldine de Gruyter.

Szasz, T. (1974). *The myth of mental illness: Foundations of a theory of personal conduct*. New York: Harper & Row.

Takahashi, S. (2013). Heterogeneity of schizophrenia: Genetic and symptomatic factors. *American Journal of Medical Genetics B: Neuropsychiatric Genetics, 162*, 648–652.

Tarnas, R. (1991). *The passion of the Western mind: Understanding the ideas that have shaped our world view*. New York: Ballantine.

Templeton, A. R. (1998). Human races: A genetic and evolutionary perspective. *American Anthropologist, 100*, 632–650.

TenHouten, W. D. (2013). *Emotion and reason: Mind, brain, and the social domains of work and love*. New York: Routledge.

Thomas, E. M. (2006). *The old way: A story of the First People*. New York: Farrar, Straus, Giroux.

Tooby, J., & Cosmides, L. (1992). The psychological foundations of culture. In J. H. Barkow, L. Cosmides, & J. Tooby (Eds.), *The adapted mind: Evolutionary psychology and the generation of culture* (pp. 19–136). New York: Oxford University Press.

Turner, J. H. (2007). *Human emotions: A sociological theory*. New York: Routledge.

Valenstein, E. S. (1986). *Great and desperate cures: The rise and decline of psychosurgery and other radical treatments for mental illness*. New York: Basic Books.

van Dongen, J., & Boomsma, D. I. (2013). The evolutionary paradox and the missing heritability of schizophrenia. *American Journal of Medical Genetics B: Neuropsychiatric Genetics, 162B*(2), 122–136.

Ward, J. W., & Warren, C. (Eds.). (2007). *Silent victories: The history and practice of public health in twentieth-century America*. New York: Oxford University Press.

Watanabe, J. M., & Smuts, B. B. (2004). Cooperation, commitment, and communication in the evolution of human sociality. In R. W. Sussman & A. R. Chapman (Eds.), *The origins and nature of sociality* (pp. 288–309). New York: Aldine de Gruyter.

Weatherall, D., Greenwood, B., Chee, H. L., Wasi, P. (2006). Science and technology for disease control: Past, present, and future. In D. T. Jamison, J. G. Breman, A. R. Measham, G. Alleyne, M. Claeson, D. B. Evans, et al. (Eds.), *Disease control priorities in developing countries* (2nd ed.). Washington, DC: World Bank. www.ncbi.nlm.nih.gov/books/NBK11740/

Weber, M. (1947). *The theory of social and economic organization* (A. M. Henderson, & T. Parsons, Trans.). New York: Free Press.

Wiesel, T. N. (1981). The postnatal development of the visual cortex and the influence of the environment. *Physiology or Medicine, 1981*, 61–83.

Wilson, E. O. (2012). *The social conquest of Earth*. New York: Liveright.

Zihlman, A., & Bolter, De. R. (2004). Mammalian and primate roots of human sociality. In R. W. Sussman & A. R. Chapman (Eds.), *The origins and nature of sociality* (pp. 23–52). New York: Aldine de Gruyter.

THE SOCIAL BRAIN

2.

The Evolution, Structure, and Functioning of the Social Brain

Matcheri S. Keshavan

As discussed in Chapter 1, the fields of neuroscience and social science were often in separate silos over much of the twentieth century. Fortunately, the advent of modern neuroscience techniques and conceptual advances has led to a considerable rapprochement between these disciplines, which has led to the emergence of the rapidly expanding interdisciplinary field of social neuroscience (Cacioppo & Berntson, 1992). Social processes interact with the brain continuously via genetic, endocrine, and metabolic factors, with a substantive and dynamic impact on health and disease risk. While the detailed exposition of the various aspects of social neuroscience (the "social brain") are beyond the scope of this chapter, a brief overview of the bidirectional effects of social and neural processes will be provided to the reader as a background to the subsequent chapters in this volume.

What Is the Social Brain?

The social brain is becoming increasingly better understood with the advent of lesion studies as well as neuroimaging technologies for probing social and emotional information processing. Based on her work in monkeys, Brothers (1990) originally proposed a circumscribed set of neural regions dedicated to social cognition, which included the amygdala, orbital frontal cortex, and temporal cortex as its major components. Subsequent work has expanded this circuitry to include other brain regions as well, such as the medial prefrontal and parietal cortices. Importantly, in recent years, there has been a shift away from considering these structures in isolation toward examining them as part of interconnected networks (Stanley & Adolphs, 2013).

As we navigate the social world, we need to understand others' emotions and intentions and relate them to our own mental states, so that we can make accurate predictions of our optimum behavior for day-to-day interactions. Broadly, cortical pathways connecting frontal executive circuits to phylogenetically older limbic regions of the brain are now known to support many of these social cognitive abilities (see Figure 1).

Some of the earliest and most well-studied aspects of social cognition as they relate to neurobiology concern social/emotional perception and regulation of emotion (Phillips, Drevets, Rauch, & Lane, 2003). Limbic structures of the brain have been consistently implicated in nearly every emotional task individuals have performed during functional brain imaging. The amygdala is perhaps the most studied brain region involved in emotion processing and has been shown to have a particularly critical role in the perception of emotion (Adolphs, 2001) and regulation of emotion (Banks, Eddy, Angstadt, Nathan, & Phan, 2007). Beyond the limbic system, other medial temporal structures have also been implicated in emotion processing, particularly emotion perception. For example, the fusiform gyrus, an elongated structure within the medial temporal cortex, is commonly activated when processing facial emotions (Kanwisher, McDermott, & Chun, 1997). Current models suggest that the sensory systems direct emotional data to both limbic and prefrontal circuits, and as the amygdala and other limbic structures become active, prefrontal areas of the brain (e.g., dorsolateral and orbitofrontal prefrontal cortices) work to regulate the activity of these limbic regions to reduce arousal and lend assignment of importance (sometimes considered salience) to emotional experience (Perlman & Pelphrey, 2011).

The ability to understand others is a key aspect of social cognition. With regard to the input and processing of social information, such as in social cue perception, medial prefrontal structures have been commonly implicated. Studies of theory of mind (Völlm et al., 2006), social perception (Pelphrey & Carter, 2008), and emotion recognition (Harris, McClure, van den Bos, Cohen, & Fiske, 2007) have helped define a unique medial prefrontal social processing network that is active above and beyond the primary visual system. This network includes such areas as the medial pre-

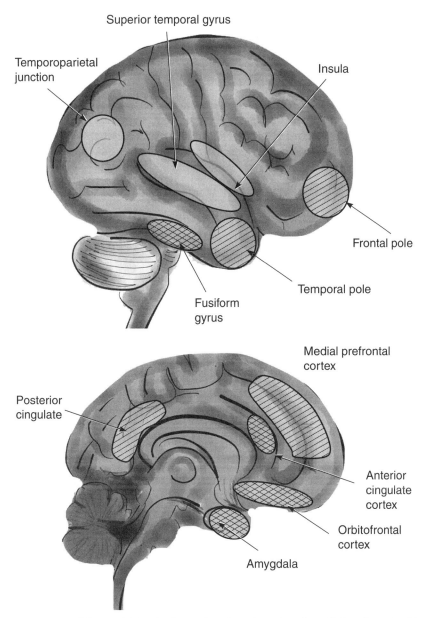

FIGURE 2.1. The social brain. Lateral regions (2.1a) and medial regions (2.1b) represented here include the structures that comprised the original list proposed by Adolphs (2001), but the increasing understanding of these structures functioning as networks is represented in the figure (social/emotional perception: cross-hatch; self-perception/mentalizing: hatch; mirror/action-perception: blank). It is to be noted that these brain regions may have highly overlapping functions.

frontal cortex, orbitofrontal cortex, cingulate, and ventral lateral prefrontal cortex, all of which have been shown to be involved in the processing of social information. This frontal and medial prefrontal cluster of regions appears to be uniquely tuned to social stimuli. Lateral temporal areas have also been shown to have a role in particular aspects of social information processing. For example, superior temporal and the temporoparietal junction regions are two of the most common temporal structures activated when individuals are asked to identify the mental states and intentions of others (Saxe, 2006). In recent years, neuroscientists (Rizzolatti & Criaghero, 2004) have identified neurons in the monkey brain (and later, albeit controversial, in the human brain) that may mediate empathy and our ability to understand the actions and intentions of other people. These "mirror" neurons are, for example, activated when an individual either engages in or observes another person in an action such as picking up a cup of tea with intent to drink from it or to take it off the table. The regions of the brain thought to contain these neurons include the inferior frontal and premotor regions. Understanding these circuitries can provide important clues to identify what causes disorders such as schizophrenia and autism.

Another important aspect of social cognition is the ability to reflect upon the self. Functional magnetic resonance imaging (fMRI) studies in healthy subjects have shown that self-reflective processing involves the activation of midline cortical structures (e.g., medial prefrontal cortex [MPFC] and posterior cingulate cortex [PCC]) as well as parts of the lateral temporal cortex (e.g., superior temporal sulcus [STS]) (Frith & Frith, 2003). These areas during self-reflection show increased activation during the retrieval of self-specific information, in contrast to tasks that involve focusing on physical or semantic aspects of stimuli. These same brain areas are considered "nodes" of the brain's resting state, or "default mode network" (DMN). Activity of the DMN during rest is thought to reflect "internal mentation" (Buckner, Andrews-Hanna, & Schacter, 2008).

Taken together, the social cognitive neural networks are becoming increasingly defined as a set of interconnected brain regions that require a considerable amount of communication and connectivity to process and interpret a fast-paced and dynamic social world.

How Does the Social Brain Develop?

Humans, like their closest primate relatives, the great apes, are not programmed to be highly social and do not naturally organize themselves into permanent groups. In a highly innovative conceptualization of the evolution of the social brain and its vicissitudes, Jonathan Turner (Chapter 3, this volume) argues that natural selection led to enhanced use of subcortical regions of the hominin (human ancestor) brain mediating emotions, making humans more social and group oriented. This was paralleled by the vastly expanded connectivity and functionality of association networks, such as the frontal, temporal, and parietal cortices, in the service of increasing cognitive control of an increasing range of emotions. Turner points out that this has its costs—that of increase in stress and the consequent risk for psychopathology.

Development of the human brain and of cognitive and emotional processes follows a somewhat similar process, bringing into mind the old notion of "ontogeny recapitulates phylogeny." While not everyone agrees with this view, some analogy may be drawn between phylogenic processes and the development of the human brain. Childhood is characterized by a reliance on concrete thinking processes and parental input for formal and informal rules to navigate the social world (the so-called primary socialization). Adolescence brings with it the requirement for novel, largely unscripted social situations (like the hominins faced) and therefore a need to develop novel, appropriate responses to unrehearsed situations, a process termed *secondary socialization* (Selman & Schultz, 1990). These situations induce a range of emotional responses, which the adolescent brain is initially less able to address effectively. During adolescence, brain networks subserving emotional processes mature earlier than those involved in cognitive control and reasoning (i.e., higher-order association networks). Components of the social brain such as the prefrontal and lateral temporal cortex, discussed earlier, develop and establish mature connectivity relatively late (Klapwijk et al., 2013). Adolescence and early adulthood are therefore a period of a maturational imbalance, with the emotional response systems already in place and the top-down social cognitive control systems still developing (Keshavan et al., 2014a). Not surprisingly, this brings with it the increased likelihood of stress and risk for psychopathology, as will be addressed in several chapters of this book.

How Does Brain Chemistry Determine Social Behavior and Social Cognition?

The ongoing interaction between the organism and its environment leads to a state of dynamic equilibrium, termed *homeostasis*. When the organism's ability to adapt to environmental demands is exceeded, it leads to stress. Such interaction is mediated by a major part of the endocrine system, the hypothalamic-pituitary-adrenal (HPA) axis. This system involves the hypothalamus, which activates the pituitary via a peptide, corticotrophin-releasing factor, and in turn the adrenal, which releases cortisol. The response of the HPA axis, which regulates many bodily processes such as the immune system, digestion, mood, and energy storage, can be adaptive in the short term; however, if excessive and prolonged, the HPA response, involving the release of cortisol, could serve as a double-edged sword, disrupt homeostasis, and increase the risk of disease. Work by Bruce McEwen (2012) has shown that chronic exposure to stress-related cortisol release can lead to shrinkage of neuronal dendrites, predisposing psychiatric disorders such as depression.

Over the past two decades, two other neuropeptides, oxytocin and vasopressin, have been increasingly studied underlying social behaviors. Oxytocin, which has been previously known to play an important role in childrearing in mammals, is now known to underlie attachment and social bonding behaviors (Insel & Young, 2001; McCall & Singer, 2012). Vasopressin, which has been known to underlie kidney function, has in recent years been associated with long-term pair bonding and male aggression. Genetic variations in the receptors of these peptides have been found to be related to species differences and social behavior. In recent years, these observations have led to efforts to develop oxytocin and vasopressin as potential therapeutic agents in addressing social impairments in disorders such as autism and schizophrenia. Studies of socially active neuropeptides may therefore offer new directions in understanding relationships between the brain and social behavior (Yamasue et al., 2012).

How Do Socioenvironmental Factors Shape the Brain?

The enormous impact of environmental factors on the brain is enabled by a unique property of the brain, neuroplasticity. In recent years, experimental neuroscience has revealed that the brain changes with the introduction of new experiences and with the training of new perceptual, cognitive, or motor skills. There are at least two ways in which neuroplasticity occurs in developmental contexts. Very early in development, experience and its resulting neuronal activity can shape neuronal response properties irrespective of an organism's attention to a stimulus. This process of *experience-expectant neuroplasticity* leads to lasting alterations in brain structure and function and is often conceptualized to occur within a finite window, a so-called critical period. Maladaptive experiences or insults to the developing nervous system during these critical periods, as described in Behen and Chugani's work (Chapter 12, this volume), can have lasting behavioral consequences.

A qualitatively different process, *experience-dependent neuroplasticity,* occurs *throughout* development. This process involves changes in neuronal activity that represents meaningful stimuli and behaviors, particularly those associated with learning and reward; such activity in turn effects lasting cortical representations (Greenough, Black, & Wallace, 1987). Maladaptive learning (particularly during the extended critical period for development), followed by enduring alterations in neuronal networks, can help us understand how psychiatric symptoms develop, then stabilize and become chronic.

Neuroplastic processes related to learning can be harnessed for therapeutic purposes across a wide range of disorders (Keshavan et al., 2014b). Cognitive enhancement approaches, elaborated by Eack in Chapter 15 of this volume, focus on identifying the impaired representational systems that are relevant to a given illness and then training such processes via implicit learning mechanisms in order to improve the speed and accuracy of task-relevant information processing, as well as strengthen the fidelity and reliability of distributed neural responses underlying critical cognitive and socioaffective operations. Growing knowledge of the specific processing anomalies, developmental features, and distributed neural circuits that characterize various psychiatric illnesses will inform the next generation of cognitive training approaches, *including their content and timing*. This requires a constant iterative process, bridging cognitive, affective, and developmental neuroscience with clinical treatment development.

How Do Psychosocial Experiences Affect the Genetic Blueprint and Expression?

It is clear from Paul Nestor's review (Chapter 4 of this volume) that variations in structural integrity of social brain circuits can explain diverse psychopathological symptoms, including social, language, and emotional behaviors in serious mental illnesses such as schizophrenia. What causes these brain changes in the first place? It is nowadays widely agreed that most major mental illnesses such as schizophrenia have a substantive basis in heredity (Schizophrenia Working Group, 2014). A term that is frequently used to represent the contribution of heredity is *heritability* (which is the proportion of the disease variation that can be explained by genetic factors). On a 0 to 1 scale, the higher the number, the more heritable the disease. Given the high heritability of major mental illnesses (e.g., approximately .7, or 70 percent in schizophrenia), it is likely that alterations in brain structure and function stem from genetic risk factors. Indeed, brain structural alterations and impairments in social and neurocognitive functions such as those described in patients with schizophrenia are also observed, albeit to a smaller extent, in nonpsychotic adolescents at familial risk for this illness (Keshavan et al., 2005; Thermenos et al., 2013). Clearly, variations in DNA sequence account for a substantive proportion of variations in psychosocial deficits in psychiatric disorders. However, since few disorders have a heritability approaching 1, environmental factors are clearly important (see, for example, Walder et al., 2014). While our DNA sequence determines individual variations in expression and transmission of phenotypic characteristics across generations, it is important not to ignore the environmental contributions to these processes.

The dynamic interplay between the genome and our environmental experiences is embodied in the concept of epigenetics—the study of factors that alter the activity of genes without altering the underlying DNA sequence. Advances in molecular biology have increasingly illuminated the mechanisms by which environment shapes biological processes. Examples of such mechanisms are DNA methylation (addition of a methyl group to a nucleotide, which forms the backbone of the DNA) and modification of histones (proteins around which DNA is wrapped), all of which serve to modify gene function without altering the underlying sequence of DNA. Further, noncoding RNA molecules (called microRNAs) can also alter gene expression. These fascinating molecules can "silence" the function of a gene by acting on messenger RNAs (molecules that carry information from genes to places in the cell where proteins are synthesized).

Social experiences across the life span in a variety of species have been shown to have broad effects on behavior, including stress responsivity, learning/memory, and reproductive behavior via epigenetic pathways as described above. Such influences on the genetic blueprint and biology may eventually persist across generations (Champagne, 2008).

Of relevance to Behen and Chugani's work in Chapter 12 (this volume), there is postmortem evidence for childhood adversity to affect gene expression. Thus, individuals with a history of childhood abuse have decreased hippocampal gene expression associated with increased DNA methylation compared to nonabused subjects (McGowan et al., 2009). Orphans raised in institutions show overall higher levels of DNA methylation compared to children raised by their biological parents (Naumova et al., 2011). Epigenetics may therefore shed light on critical questions on the timing, specificity, and stability of the effects of social environments on human development.

Conclusions

The nature of being human is to live in continuous interaction with each other and the social world. We construct our social world by engaging our complex apparatus of the social brain, and in turn, the mind and the brain are constructed dynamically by interactions with the social world. As Dunbar (2009) has suggested, the demands of living in large, complex societies may have led to selection for large brains, especially those involved in social abilities, in primates. However, the more complex systems also have their costs, accounting for uniquely human psychopathological disorders such as schizophrenia and autism. Understanding the bidirectional relationships between social influences and changes in the nervous system in a non-reductionistic framework is therefore likely to advance understanding of both the social brain and the social world.

Over the past two decades, social neuroscience has greatly expanded at least in part due to the advent of novel neuroimaging techniques. While a lot has been learned about the distributed neural and hormonal systems that may underlie social processes, many complex challenges continue (Stanley & Adolphs, 2013). First, fMRI studies are not always easy to interpret and often provide correlative data, making causal inferences difficult to establish. Any single discipline such as cognitive neuroscience or lesion studies may fall short of efforts to understand complex social constructs that operate at a macro level. Thankfully, exciting new technologies are now available at the single cell level, such as optogenetics (Deisseroth, 2011). While these techniques are too invasive for human studies at this time, they are likely to be applied to human neuroscience in the not too distant future. The relationship between neural networks and social behaviors is likely to be better elucidated by mining large data sets that will be available across species and across research domains such as the Allen Brain Atlas for the mouse (www.brain-map.org/), the Human Connectome Project (www.humanconnectome.org/), and the Brain Research through Advancing Innovative Neurotechnologies (Brain) project just recently announced by President Obama (www.nih.gov/science/brain/). Increasingly, social scientists and neuroscientists are beginning to utilize a common language and moving toward collaboration. One may therefore expect that in the next two decades, several large questions facing the interface between the social brain and the social world will be effectively and collaboratively addressed.

We have referred to several chapters in this section and elsewhere in the volume that address the key questions central to the interface between the social brain, social world, and psychopathology. First, Jonathan Turner (Chapter 3) provides an account of how the brain has evolved to adapt to the social, interpersonal nature of human mental processes. Second, Paul Nestor and colleagues (Chapter 4) and Christine Hooker (Chapter 5) review their and others' work elucidating the neural structural under-pinnings of disrupted social cognitive functions in schizophrenia, a dis-order that is highly heritable. Third, Michael Behen and Harry Chugani (Chapter 12) review their and others' work on Romanian orphans, illus-trating how development of the social brain may be affected by early envi-ronmental factors such as psychosocial deprivation that disrupt attach-ment. Fourth, Shaun Eack and Matcheri Keshavan's chapter (Chapter 15) provides insights into how psychosocial treatments designed to improve social cognitive processes might reverse some of the abnormalities seen in a serious disorder like schizophrenia. Together, these chapters highlight the importance of understanding how the social brain is put together, how genetic risk might interact with adverse psychosocial and biological environmental influences to lead to psychopathology, and how psycho-social interventions, acting on the "plastic" brain, can potentially reverse such impairments and the underlying neural deficits. The key neurosci-ence concepts summarized in this introduction will place these chapters in perspective.

References

Adolphs R. (2001). The neurobiology of social cognition. *Current Opinion in Neuro-biology*, 11, 231–239.

Banks, S. J., Eddy, K. T., Angstadt, M., Nathan, P. J., & Phan, K. L. (2007). Amygdala-frontal connectivity during emotion regulation. *Social Cognitive and Affective Neuroscience*, 2, 303–312.

Brothers, L. (1990). The social brain: A project for integrating primate behavior and neurophysiology in a new domain. *Concepts in Neuroscience*, 1, 27–51.

Buckner, R. L., Andrews-Hanna, J. R., & Schacter, D. L. (2008). The brain's de-fault network: Anatomy, function, and relevance to disease. *Annals of the New York Academy of Sciences*, 1124, 1–38.

Cacioppo, J. T., & Berntson, G. G. (1992). Social psychological contributions to the decade of the brain: Doctrine of multilevel analysis. *American Psycholo-gist*, 47, 1019–1028.

Champagne, F. A. (2008). Epigenetic mechanisms and the transgenerational effects of maternal care. *Frontiers in Neuroendocrinology, 29*, 386–397.

Deisseroth, K. (2011). Optogenetics. *Nature Methods, 8*, 26–29.

Dunbar, R. I. (2009). The social brain hypothesis and its implications for social evolution. *Annals of Human Biology, 36*, 562–572.

Frith, U., & Frith, C. D. (2003). Development and neurophysiology of mentalizing. *Philosophical Transactions of the Royal Society of London, 358*, 459–473.

Greenough, W. T., Black, J. E., & Wallace, C. S. (1987). Experience and brain development. *Child Development, 58*, 539–559.

Harris, L. T., McClure, S. M., van den Bos, W., Cohen, J. D., & Fiske, S. T. (2007). Regions of the MPFC differentially tuned to social and nonsocial affective evaluation. *Cognitive and Affective Behavioral Neuroscience, 7*(4), 309–316.

Insel, T. R., & Young, L. J. (2001). The neurobiology of attachment. *Nature Reviews Neuroscience, 2*, 129–136.

Kanwisher, N., McDermott, J., & Chun, M. M. (1997). The fusiform face area: A module in human extrastriate cortex specialized for face perception. *Journal of Neuroscience, 17*, 4302–4311.

Keshavan, M. S., Diwadkar, V. A., Montrose, D. M., Rajarethinam, R., & Sweeney, J. A. (2005). Premorbid indicators and risk for schizophrenia: A selective review and update. *Schizophrenia Research, 79*, 45–57.

Keshavan, M. S., Giedd, J., Lau, J., Lewis, D. A., & Paus, T. (2014a). Changing adolescent brain and the pathophysiology of psychotic disorders. *Lancet Psychiatry, 1*, 549–558.

Keshavan M. S., Vinogradov, S., Rumsey, J., Sherrill, J., & Wagner, A. (2014b). Cognitive training in mental disorders: Update and future directions. *American Journal of Psychiatry, 171*, 510–522.

Klapwijk, E. T., Goddings, A. L., Burnett Heyes S., Bird, G., Viner, R. M., & Blakemore, S. J. (2013). Increased functional connectivity with puberty in the mentalising network involved in social emotion processing. *Hormones and Behavior, 64*(2), 314–322.

McCall, C., & Singer, T. (2012). The animal and human neuroendocrinology of social cognition, motivation and behavior. *Nature Neuroscience, 15*, 681–688.

McEwen, B. S. (2012). Brain on stress: How the social environment gets under the skin. *Proceedings of the National Academy of Sciences of the United States of America, 109*(Suppl. 2), 17180–17185.

McGowan, P. O., Sasaki, A., D'Alessio, A. C., Dymov, S., Labonte, B., Szyf, M., Turecki, G., & Meaney, M. J. (2009). Epigenetic regulation of the glucocorticoid receptor in human brain associated with childhood abuse. *Nature Neuroscience, 12*, 342–348.

Naumova, O. Y., Lee, M., Koposov, R., Szyf, M., Dozier, M., & Grigorenko, E. L. (2012). Differential patterns of whole-genome DNA methylation in institutionalized children and children raised by their biological parents. *Developmental Psychopathology, 24*, 143–155.

Pelphrey, K. A., & Carter, E. J. (2008). Brain mechanisms for social perception: Lessons from autism and typical development. *Annals of the New York Academy of Sciences, 1145*, 283–299.

Perlman, S. B., & Pelphrey, K. A. (2011). Developing connections for affective regulation: Age-related changes in emotional brain connectivity. *Journal of Experimental Child Psychology*, 108, 607–620.

Phillips, M. L., Drevets, W. C., Rauch, S. L., & Lane, R. (2003). Neurobiology of emotion perception I: The neural basis of normal emotion perception. *Biological Psychiatry*, 54(5), 504–514.

Rizzolatti, G., & Craighero, L. (2004). The mirror-neuron system. *Annual Review of Neuroscience*, 27, 169–192.

Saxe, R. (2006). Why and how to study theory of mind with fMRI. *Brain Research*, 24, 57–65.

Schizophrenia Working Group of the Psychiatric Genomics Consortium. (2014). Biological insights from 108 schizophrenia-associated genetic loci. *Nature*, 511, 421–427.

Selman, R. L., & Schultz, L. H. (1990). *Making a friend in youth*. Chicago: University of Chicago Press.

Stanley, D. A., & Adolphs, R. (2013). Toward a neural basis for social behavior. *Neuron*, 80, 816–826.

Thermenos, H. W., Keshavan, M. S., Juelich, R. J, Molokotos, E., Whitfield-Gabrieli, S., Brent, B. K., & Seidman L. J. (2013). A review of neuroimaging studies of young relatives of persons with schizophrenia: A developmental perspective from schizotaxia to schizophrenia. *American Journal of Medical Genetics, B: Neuropsychiatric Genetics*, 162, 604–635.

Völlm, B. A., Taylor, A. N., Richardson, P., Corcoran, R., Stirling, J., McKie, S., Deakin, J. F., & Elliott, R. (2006). Neuronal correlates of theory of mind and empathy: A functional magnetic resonance imaging study in a nonverbal task. *Neuroimage*, 29, 90–98.

Walder, D. J., Faraone, S. V., Glatt, S. J., Tsuang, M. T., & Seidman, L. J. (2014). Genetic liability, prenatal, stress and family environmental risk factors in the Harvard Adolescent Family High Risk for Schizophrenia study. *Schizophrenia Research*, 157, 142–148.

Yamasue, H., Yee, J. R., Hurlemann, R., Rilling, J. K., Chen, F. S., Meyer-Lindenberg, A., & Tost, H. (2012). Integrative approaches utilizing oxytocin to enhance prosocial behavior: From animal and human social behavior to autistic social dysfunction. *Journal of Neuroscience*, 32, 14109–14117.

3.

The Neurology of Human Nature

Implications for the Sociological Analysis
of Health and Well-Being

Jonathan H. Turner

T HERE ARE NOW very large literatures on the psychology of health, happiness, and well-being as well as a rapidly developing sociological literature on the relationship between emotions and health. In this chapter, my goal is to bring what can be termed *evolutionary sociology* (as distinct from the arguments of *evolutionary psychology*) into the more applied study of health questions (Maryanski & Turner, 1992; Turner & Maryanski, 2005, 2008, 2015). Humans are like any other animal and have evolved under pressures from natural selection and, at times, the other three forces of evolution (mutation, genetic drift, and gene flow). Understanding these selection pressures and how they rewired the primate and, more generally, the mammalian brain can perhaps offer some insight into the dynamics of human behavior; these dynamics affect human health, happiness, and well-being. In pursuing evolutionary sociology, several important findings about hominin (those primates on the evolutionary line to humans) and human evolution emerge. First, humans are evolved apes and, like all of the great apes, do not possess bioprogrammers, or genetically driven behavioral propensities hardwired in the neurology of the brain, for group affiliation. Most mammals have these bioprogrammers to form and remain in troops, pods, herds, and other group-like social formations. Second, hominins or those ape-like species on the human line of evolution and then humans became more social and capable of forming groups and other sociocultural formations over eight million years of evolution, but these formations were, and still are, *indirectly* created and sustained initially by heightened emotions and other neurologically driven behavioral propensities. Third, heightened emotional capacities, coupled with the fragility of group formations among humans, inevitably lead to high levels of emotional stress when the interpersonal processes sustaining group affiliations become problematic.

Thus, by understanding (a) the rewiring of the ape brain during hominin evolution, (b) the selection forces that took away bioprogrammers for group behaviors among apes during primate evolution, and (c) the interpersonal processes by which humans form and sustain groups, we gain more empirical and conceptual purchase in explaining the relationship among group affiliations, social support, and well-being. This relationship is, however, always problematic for a species that evolved from low-sociality apes, and as a consequence, we should expect high levels of distress, anxiety, unhappiness, and lowered well-being and health among animals who are so precariously social and who must use emotions rather than genetically controlled bioprogrammers to create and sustain social relations and group affiliations (Turner, 2007).

These assertions may, at first, seem rather extreme, and so, let me qualify them at the outset. The emphasis on the rewiring of the human brain does not mean that hominin and human brains are radically different from primate brains or mammalian brains more generally. The neocortex gets most of the attention in neurological analysis as applied to social science because the human neocortex is so large, relative to body size. Still, the structures evident in chimpanzee brains are still present in humans; the most significant differences are the overall size of the neocortex, the more pronounced asymmetry of the left temporal lobe (which is also asymmetrical in apes) for language production, the additional association cortices around the inferior parietal lobe (where the temporal, parietal, and occipital lobes meet) that, as we will see, provide the basic wiring for language production (which great apes also reveal since this new wiring occurred during primate rather than human evolution), and the more extensive neuronets connecting the neocortex to the subcortical portions of the brain. The same is true in the subcortical portions of the brain where, as I will emphasize, emotions are generated; the subcortical structures involved in emotional arousal and storage of emotion-tagged memories (before being eventually transferred to the frontal lobe) are, on average, twice as large as those in our closest primate relatives (the common chimpanzee) and evidence more connectivity. Still, despite scale differences, relative to body size, and connectivity, these structures in humans are roughly the same as those in primates and mammals more generally. Thus, as rewiring occurred over seven million years, natural selection did not change the basic structure of the primate brain; indeed, evolution is a conservative process that retains structures and, in the case of the brain, altered them to make hominins and then humans more emotional and intelligent than other mammals, although the intelligence of dolphins, whales, and elephants relative to humans is still ambiguous. Indeed, as MacLean's (1990, 1993) famous portrayal of the triune brain emphasizes, this progression from the ancient brain of reptiles remains basically the same, even as neocortical areas evolved over and around this "reptilian brain." Indeed, radical discontinuities are unlikely because mutations on the brain will almost always be maladaptive, and so, as I will emphasize, most changes in the primate, hominin, and human brains were caused by directional selection on existing structures, modifying them over time in terms of their size and connectivity.

Evolutionary Sociology

The New Science of Evolutionary Sociology

For most of its history, evolutionary analysis in sociology involved (1) the portrayal of stages in societal evolution from simple to more complex societies (e.g., Hebert Spencer, 1874–1896; Durkheim, 1893/1947; Gerhard Lenski, 1964, 2005; Talcott Parsons, 1966, 1971; Turner, 2003) and (2) rather speculative portrayals, often implicit, of human nature. The challenge posted by the emergence of sociobiology (e.g., Wilson, 1975, 1978) and, later, evolutionary psychology (e.g., Cosmides & Tooby, 1992) generated a defensive reaction among most sociologists because it was perceived that these approaches were highly reductionist and not capable of explaining the emergent properties of culture and social structure of most interest to sociologists. This defensiveness led to a general suspicion about any analysis that adopted Darwinian ideas incorporated into the Modern Synthesis of evolutionary theory. These suspicions were not wrong, but they did make it difficult for sociologists to use the tools of biology to address the second form of evolutionary analysis that has always existed in sociology: the analysis of human nature or, put differently, the search for the hardwire behavioral capacities and propensities of humans. Some sociologists adopted sociobiological models (e.g., van den Berghe, 1974, 1975; Lopreato & Crippen, 1999), while others adopted those from evolutionary psychology (e.g., Kanazawa & Still, 2000; Hopcroft, 2010), and these are, along with stage models of societal evolution, a part of the new evolutionary sociology. But there is a newer form of evolutionary sociology that addresses many of the same issues as sociobiology and evolutionary psychology (that is, what is the biological basis of behavior of humans and, by extension, their creations: social structures and culture?). This newer approach—adopted here in this chapter—does not make many of what are considered extreme assertions (e.g., maximization of fitness, modular structures of the brain). Rather, this brand of evolutionary sociology borrows key ideas from biology, such as a concern with the fitness consequences of evolved traits, the use of cladistic analysis to trace behavioral propensities of ancestors to present-day great apes and humans, the ecological shifts in habitats and niches of human primate ancestors, and the (directional) selection pressures that drove anatomical and neuroanatomical evolution of primates, hominins, and humans. The result is a Darwinian approach that seeks to overcome what sociologists perceive as the weaknesses of sociobiology and evolutionary psychology. My goal in this chapter is to demonstrate the utility of this form of evolutionary sociology for understanding the behavioral propensities of humans as an evolved ape and the implications of these propensities for human happiness and health.

A Brief History of Primate Evolution

The starting point of this new form of evolutionary sociology draws upon the large literature on the behaviors and relational patterns among various species of primates. These hard data are then used to make inferences on the selection pressures on primates caused by these organization patterns to evolve in the ancestors of present-day primates, including the last common ancestor of present-day great apes and hominins who eventually evolved into humans. In this way, we are to gain purchase on the innate behavioral propensities of humans (e.g., Turner, 2007; Turner & Maryanski, 2005; Maryanski & Turner, 1992) and on the implications of these behaviors for human health.

The reason for this emphasis on primate evolution is that humans are evolved apes, and the evolution of our neuroanatomy as it affects stress, distress, well-being, and health can only be understood by understanding how the brains of primates in general and the great apes in particular were wired and rewired during the course of hominin evolution. Primate evolution began sixty-five million years ago when small rodent-like mammals climbed or clawed their way into the arboreal habitats of Africa. Humans are, first of all, the product of the selection pressures imposed by the arboreal habitat on the basic mammalian anatomy and neuroanatomy and, later, the result of the selection pressures imposed by the African savanna on species of apes that were forced back down to the ground as the forest of Africa began to recede some ten to fourteen millions years ago.

The early selection pressures arising from adapting the basic mammalian anatomy to a three-dimensional arboreal habitat led to key anatomical changes in primates. Perhaps the most important of these pressures was for movement away from olfactory dominance of senses to visual dominance, where auditory and haptic sense modalities become subordinated to vision and where visual acuity increases with both color and stereographic vision. Most important, the rewiring of the brain to achieve this visual dominance created a by-product: the development of the association cortices around the inferior parietal lobe that became an important preadaptation or what Steven Jay Gould termed *spandrels*. This by-product is the neurological capacity for language in more intelligent primates like present-day great apes (Geschwind, 1965a, 1965b, 1965c, 1985; Geschwind & Damasio, 1984)—a point to be taken up later.

For much evolution from thirty million to around twenty-three million years ago, there was not much difference between apes and monkeys. Then, around twenty-three million years ago, monkeys got the upper hand in the arboreal habitat and began to dominate the core and more verdant areas of the trees, thereby pushing apes to the terminal feeding areas high in the forest. It is not clear why monkeys became more dominant, especially since apes are on average bigger and stronger than monkeys, but the key adaptation may have been the capacity of monkeys to eat unripe fruit (something apes still cannot do) and thereby secure a critical food resource earlier than apes. In any event, the niches of the core of trees and the terminal feeding areas of the arboreal habitat are vastly different. Monkeys could sustain larger and more permanent groups in the core areas of the arboreal habitat because there is more room, stronger structural support from thick branches, and significantly more food. In contrast, larger animals like early apes trying to survive in the terminal feeding areas could not support permanent groups because there was not enough food, structural support in ends of branches, or physical room. The result was that natural selection *took away* from apes, if they had existed in the first place, bioprogrammers for group formation. Apes would need to reveal the fission-fusing pattern evident among contemporary great apes—breaking groups apart so that their members can find food resources and, perhaps, occasionally coming together in temporary gatherings when food resources were more plentiful. Thus, the social structures of apes and monkeys began to diverge, with monkey societies being built around groups held together by matrilines of related females and patterns of male dominance and with apes evidencing no propensities for tight-knit groups and only a general sense of who belongs in the larger community (Maryanski, 1986, 1987, 1992, 1993, 1995, 1996).

The niches of apes at the tops of trees, feeding on the scarce food resources on the undersides of branches, also led to additional anatomical changes. At the level of neuroanatomy, apes became more intelligent than monkeys because the terminal feeding areas of the arboreal habitat are more dangerous, where one false step means death by gravity. Along with these neuroanatomical changes, apes developed (a) greater dexterity and strength in hands and fingers; (b) stronger wrists, arms, and shoulders; and (c) the capacity to brachiate or rotate the arm in the shoulder joint 360 degrees and thereby swing from branch to branch.

Thus, over twenty million years of divergent evolution, apes became smarter than monkeys. Because of increased intelligence, the great apes were able to possess the potential capacity for language (generated, as noted above, by the transformation to visual dominance). Monkeys do not possess this capacity because they do not have the requisite level of intelligence that, apparently, must accompany changes in the association cortices around the inferior parietal lobe where the parietal (haptic/touch), temporal (auditory), and occipital (vision) lobes meet in the neocortex. This preadaptation for language was thus available twenty million years ago among larger, more intelligent apes, *if* its enhancement by natural selection would promote increased fitness. In the upper reaches of the arboreal habitat, the breakdown of bioprogrammers for group formation was highly adaptive, but it altered the basic mammalian tendency to form groups, troops, pods, packs, herds, and other group-like formations, and, more significantly, it would dramatically decrease fitness of apes if forced to live on the two-dimensional African savanna filled with predators. As I will emphasize further, this lack of stable group formation is very important in understanding "human nature" as it evolved along the hominin line because this nature has the consequences for human health and well-being.

Another important mode of analysis is comparative sociology among apes and monkeys where their respective social structures are examined. Alexandra Maryanski (1987, 1988, 1992, 1993, 1995, 1996), my frequent coauthor (e.g., Maryanski & Turner, 1992; Turner & Maryanski, 2005; Turner & Maryanski, 2008), did such an analysis by reviewing all extant field studies on apes in order to compare the structures evident among apes and representative samples of monkeys. The results—as briefly mentioned above—were startling. Monkeys evidence stable group structures, built around female matrilines created and sustained by the fact that females never leave their natal group. Male monkeys, in contrast, leave their natal group and are replaced by immigrating males from other groups that then compete for dominance. Thus, the transfer patterns of adolescents reaching puberty became critical to understanding the social structures of monkeys and apes as well. Unlike females in monkey societies, female apes *all* leave their natal community at puberty and migrate to another community, *never to return;* they are replaced by females migrating from other communities. Note that I did not mention natal group because these are not stable or permanent among the great apes; the only stable social structure among the great apes is the larger, regional community, with groups forming and disbanding within this community. For orangutans and gorillas, males also leave their natal community, but for common chimpanzees, who are the most closely related to humans, males remain in their natal community, moving about it in temporary groups or often alone and, when necessary, gathering to defend the home range with true violence from incursion by males from other communities (females, of course, are welcome because they are needed to replace the emigrating females that were born in the community). Thus, the only really strong ties in great ape communities are between females and their prepuberty offspring (a virtual universal among all mammals); paternity is not known among apes because great apes are highly promiscuous and, hence, there are no strong father-offspring ties. There are, however, some stronger ties that can form within gorilla and chimpanzee communities. Among chimpanzees, brothers can often form strong bonds and help each other out in the somewhat low-key competition for dominance in a community; chimpanzees males can also form lifelong bonds with their mothers, often visiting them, but not forming a stable "family group" or ever having sexual relations with them, even though the mother and all other males in the community are potential sexual partners. Among gorillas, a lead silverback male may try to dominate a group in which other males and females with offspring may cluster for a time, but females tend to use the lead male as a babysitter so that she can sneak off and have sexual relations with other males. This "harem group," however, breaks apart once the female's children leave their natal community and the female no longer needs the babysitting services of the lead silverback. In contrast to gorillas and chimpanzees, orangutans form virtually no strong ties; only the mother-offspring ties last, at least until puberty, when males and female offspring leave their natal community. Otherwise, males wander alone, and females move about with their prepubescent offspring in the forests of Asia. Males will hang around females for a relatively short time when mating, but within a couple of weeks, they will have left their temporary mates. Thus, orangutans are highly solitary, evidencing no strong ties among adults. And, among other species of great apes, where some temporary groupings occur, females are still strangers to each other because they have immigrated from other communities, and while they may hang out to allow their offspring to play, they do not form strong or permanent bonds.

With data like those arrayed by Maryanski, she was also able to perform cladistic analysis, which seeks to discover the social structures of the common ancestor to humans and the great apes. In simplified form, the logic of cladistic analysis is this: those traits that all members of related species possess are likely to have been traits of their last common ancestor. Thus, female transfer at puberty, the lack of local and stable group structures, and promiscuity among adults were likely traits of the behavior and social structures of the last common ancestor to humans and present-day great apes. To assume differently would require the assumption that such novel behaviors for mammals evolved separately among closely related species. For gorillas and orangutans, males also leave their natal community, and so, it is likely that this too was a trait of the last common ancestor to humans and the great apes, with the chimpanzee pattern of the male staying in his natal community evolving since the split with the last common ancestor.

The bottom line of Maryanski's analysis is that the social relations and networks of the last common ancestor were probably very much like contemporary orangutans who are virtually solitary except for the hardwire mammalian bioprogrammer for females to attend to their young until they are able to care for themselves. All other ties are nonexistent or weak and temporary. Cladistic analysis thus allows us to see in the distant past and observe what might seem like counterintuitive behavioral patterns of low sociality, individualism, weak ties, mobility, separation, and lack of permanent groups among the last common ancestors of present-day great apes and humans. This finding is only counterintuitive because notions of humans as "naturally" social, family-oriented, and group-organizing animals are so ingrained in Western philosophy and social science that they are rarely questioned, even when the data are staring them in the face. I emphasize this point because it runs against so much thinking in the social sciences and humanities: humans are naturally social and naturally group living animals. To be sure, humans have become dramatically more social than their great ape cousins over the last seven to eight million years of hominin evolution, but again, natural selection is generally conservative and retains and then supplements these features, although it is clear that natural selection eliminated most if not all of the typical bioprogrammers of apes for group formation, typical of monkeys. There must have been intense selection pressures for such a radical change, but it is one that eventually led to the extinction of most apes over the last 10,000 years and of all savanna-dwelling apes except one, humans. Maryanski's cladistic analysis documents this dramatic change, and to this day, great apes do not form permanent or stable social groupings, but they do recon a home range or larger community within which members move about forming and disbanding temporary groups. Coupled with the fact that great apes do not have families, because paternity is never known, only community as a more meso- or macro-level social formation was available for selection on hominins.

Thus far, I have emphasized that ecological analysis of selection pressures generated by habitats and niches, analysis of behavior and social structural formations among species closely related to humans, and then cladistic analysis yielding insight into the behavioral and organizational propensities of the last common ancestor to apes and hominins/humans are critical to evolutionary sociology and the search for "human nature." The final mode of analysis in the new evolutionary sociology is *comparative neuroanatomy*. By comparing the brains of humans and great apes, we can see where natural selection was working as it rewired the brain of the last common ancestor to humans/hominins and the great apes. Unlike many claims by evolutionary psychology (e.g., Cosmides & Tooby, 1992), the basic modules directing behaviors and propensities to form particular forms of social relations/structures evolved long before the Pleistocene, which only covers the last few million years of hominin evolution. The basic structure of the mammalian brain goes back past sixty-five million years when the first mammals began to ascend into arboreal habitat, and the basic structure and function of the higher primate brain has existed for at least twenty million years—long before the Pleistocene. Thus, we should not be looking for new modular structures driving human nature but, rather, *alterations of very old structures*. In general, as I emphasized at the outset, what is evident in comparing the brains of humans and the great apes is that, compared to apes and controlling for body size, key structures among humans are much larger and evidence more connectivity with larger bundles of neurons connecting all regions of the brain. Thus, evolutionary sociology must also depend on another new field in sociology, *neurosociology* (Franks, 2010; Franks & Turner, 2013). And, to put perhaps a too polemic point on it, neurosociology emphasizes continuity of the brain because it does not posit any new modules for specific behaviors; indeed, the modules of the brain are ancient, going back to the reptiles and early mammals. The rewiring of the mammalian brain, then, involved generating new subassemblies of existing brain modules inherited from reptiles and early mammals. These subassemblies are not modular but, instead, are rather diffuse with increased size to particular structures and alternation or intensification of the functions in some of these structures, coupled with dramatically increased connectivity within and between the structures of the neocortex and subcortex. If anything, the brain is probably somewhat less modular in that the changes during hominin evolution involved increased connectivity across both neocortical and subcortical brain structures. For example, the subcortical structure known as the amygdala is the ancient reptilian center for both fear and anger as an emotional response to danger, and it is still discrete in mammals but, in humans, it is twice as large as in great apes (see Table 3.1), with most of this increase in the size of the amygdala due to additional layers of neuronets generating happiness and pleasure in this ancient area dedicated to fear and anger responses; see Eccles, 1989). Moreover, it is clear that the amygdala was also usurped by natural selection as a pivotal node for bundling neurons between the prefrontal cortex (where decision making occurs) and subcortical emotion centers. Let me offer another example. The septum in mammals is the center where the pleasure associated with sex is generated, but in humans, it is twice as large as it is in chimpanzees. Since chimpanzees are highly promiscuous and enjoy sex immensely, we need to wonder why natural selection would enlarge a structure that was already adequate for ensuring reproduction. What new emotional effects does this enlarged structure have for humans? One possible answer, highly speculative, is that the emotions associated with "love" and more permanent male-female bonding (something that does not occur among the great apes) might be one explanation for why the septum was under such heavy selection. That is, new emotions were created to form a very important type of group, the nuclear family, which was the structural foundation of the first human societies.

The arguments of evolutionary psychology on special-function modules evolving to solve adaptive problems during the Pleistocene have elements of teleology, reminiscent of the old sociological functionalism. We do not need this kind of illegitimate teleology but, instead, the simple understanding that directional selection can alter or add functions to existing modules like the amygdala or septum. In so doing, the discreteness of the older modules decreases as these modules become part of more inclusive subassemblages across cortical and subcortical areas of the brain. Moreover, these subassemblages involve connections among modules of the brain that evolved with reptiles and later with early mammals. They did not emerge in the Pleistocene. For example, even somewhat discrete areas of the brain for language production (Broca's area) and for uploading language into the brain's mode of thinking (Wernicke's area) are, as it turns out, not so discrete; they run across the entire left frontal and temporal lobes into the association cortices around the inferior parietal lobe (which became preadaptations for language use, as is evident in great ape capacities for language). But more fundamentally, the asymmetries that these areas reveal on the left temporal lobe *already existed* because they are evident in the great apes and, hence, are likely to be millions of years old, emerging long before the Pleistocene. Once again, then, selection was working on already *existing modules*, not creating new ones.

Also, evolutionary psychology ignores some very basic evolutionary dynamics. One is that large mutations are generally harmful, and the larger the mutation, the greater is the likelihood that it will diminish rather than increase fitness (Fisher, 1930). Furthermore, mutations of any magnitude in such a complex system as the brain, where structures are highly interdependent, are likely to be harmful. Rather, it is more likely that directional selection on existing brain structures of hominins is the key to understanding the transformations evident in the human brain. Directional selection can work very rapidly, as can be seen by the following thought experiment. The size of existing modules, inherited from reptiles and early mammals, may affect fitness, and since the size of any brain system probably distributes itself as a normal curve, the favored size (typically a tail of the curve where the size of the brain system is larger) will become the new bell curve for the next generation of phenotypes, with each successive generation moving the brain structure to ever-larger size as the smaller sized phenotypes and underlying genotype are selected out. The same is true to connectivity among structures, which probably varies on a normal curve and might also be affected by very small mutations that did not disrupt brain functioning. In either case, directional selection on the tail of the distribution describing higher connectivity will, over a number of generations, rewire the brain toward increased connectivity, mostly by directional selection on *existing* brain structures rather than new modules created by mutations.

This line of argument makes the comparative analysis of the brain somewhat easier. We do not have to postulate the existence of new modules, which are rarely specified in evolutionary psychology, but rather, we look for alterations in existing brain systems, especially with respect to changes in size and connectivity. In my view, this shift in methodology emphasizes the continuity of the mammalian brain, which, while rewired here and there, was not dramatically changed in its basic structure and function. And since we have animals such as the common chimpanzee that share 99 percent of our genetic material, a comparative analysis of their brains with the human brain can tell us a great deal about what natural selection was doing to the hominin brain when the ancestors of today's chimps split away from the hominin ancestors of humans. We do not have to posit a new structure for every fitness-enhancing behavioral capacity; instead, we redouble efforts to understand how various brain systems affect behavioral propensities in chimpanzees and humans.

If this kind of comparative neuroanatomy is pursued, we will be able to determine behaviors that are hardwired and those that are not, and we will be able to see how selection worked on the brain of hominins (when compared to chimpanzee brains) to wire up the human brain. This job is actually made much easier than might otherwise be the case because many of the behaviors that are often seen as unique to humans *are also evident in the great apes* and, hence, are very old adaptive behaviors in primates and mammals more generally. Selection just worked to enhance them among hominins and then humans, and so by comparing size and connectivity among brain systems between the great apes and humans, we can learn how natural selection went about enhancing those hardwired behaviors that enhanced fitness of hominins. We do not need to speculate about the existence of new modules because we can see changes in structures and their connections by simply noting the obvious differences between the great ape and human brains. These differences are the "smoking guns" of what natural selection was doing over the last seven million years. So, as will be evident very shortly, much of what is often considered to be unique to humans is not. Moreover, because of the existence of spandrels and preadaptations in the brain, such as those association cortices responsible for language abilities in great apes, many of the key modules, if we still want to call them that, already existed and were, in essence, just waiting there for selection to grab onto them and enhance their powers. They did not need to be created; they already existed.

Another virtue of this kind of comparative neuroanatomy is that we can work both ways in discovering the brain systems responsible for various behaviors. We can look at brain assemblages and stimulate them to see the behavioral outcomes, or we can observe behaviors in great apes, monkeys, and even mammals in general and see what areas of the brain "light up" on functional magnetic resonance imaging and other imaging technologies when these behaviors are emitted. Moreover, by examining diseased or damaged areas of the brain, we can often learn about the behaviors that are driven by particular regions if they had not been damaged or diseased.

Thus, once we abandon the unfounded speculation of evolutionary psychology about the emergence of new modules and just focus on behaviors evident in all humans and often in other primates and mammals as well, we can conduct searches for the systems that generate these behaviors. And, as will become evident, these systems have been around *long before* the Pleistocene—often by tens of millions of years.

Another fact simplifying our search is that the neocortex of the hominin brain did not grow dramatically in size until rather late in hominin evolution. With *Homo habilis* at around three million years ago, the first significant increase in the modal size of the hominin brain from 375 cc of chimpanzees (and Australopithecines on the hominin line) to around 500 cc occurred. Then, not until *Homo erectus* at around two million years ago does the brain jump some more to a modal size of around 750 to 850 cc, although some *Homo erectus* brains were in the 900 cc range. Then, with *Homo sapiens,* the brain jumps again to the 1,250 to 1,350 cc range. Most of this growth over the last three million years was to the neocortex, but I believe that subcortical areas were growing much earlier, but this growth would be less evident in endocasts than would neocortical growth. The fact that so many subcortical brain structures are twice the size of those in the great apes, controlling for body size (Stephan, 1983; Stephan & Andy, 1969, 1977; Stephan, Baron, & Frahm, 1988; Eccles, 1989), means that many of the unique capacities of humans are driven by enhancements of subcortical areas of the brain generating emotions, allowing for the storage of unconscious memories, and facilitating repression of unpleasant emotions. Since health and well-being are related to emotions, many of the problems of humans today arise from the subcortex filled with modules inherited from reptiles and early mammals millions of years before the Pleistocene. And, I would argue that selection first began working here in the subcortex, thereby making many of the questions of well-being related to the operation of truly ancient brain systems rather than to the more recent enlargements of the hominin and human neocortex (Turner, 2000).

How, then, do we get analytical purchase on the neurology of human natures that employs all of the elements of evolutionary sociology that, by necessity, I have briefly outlined above? My answer is to look at the literature summarizing those behavioral capacities that are evident in nonhuman primates and mammals. This literature can give us a baseline of what natural selection was enhancing during hominin evolution as it was generating the neurology behind human nature.

I approach the problem by emphasizing, once again, the unique problems that hominins faced as evolved apes. The basic problem is that, as the forest in Africa began to recede and the great savannas expanded, many arboreal primates were forced to begin living a more terrestrial lifestyle. The savanna was filled with many more predators than exist today, and so animals that could not form herds, packs, prides, and troops were at a great disadvantage in securing food and protecting themselves. Monkeys would be far more fit than apes on the savanna because they have strong group structures, and the fitness of savanna-dwelling monkeys can be seen today when, for example, baboons march across the savanna in almost military style, with smaller females and offspring surrounded by bigger males in front, on the flanks, and the rear of a troop that marches across the open country. Few predators would attack such a well-oiled phalanx. In contrast, apes have many liabilities in the open country, including the following: they are slow and cannot outrun predators, they get highly emotional when anxious (screaming and shouting) and thereby attract more predators, they do not have a highly sensitive sense of smell (the dominant sense for most mammals) and thus cannot sense predators in hiding, their vision is often obscured by high grasses and bushes so that they cannot take advantage of their high visual acuity, and, most important, they do not have strong bioprogrammers for cohesive and stable groups, an absolute must for an animal with all of the other liabilities it possessed when living on the savanna. Monkeys have many of the same liabilities as apes, but not the critical one—lack of group organization. This one large difference led to a very different evolutionary history between monkeys and apes trying to adapt to the open country savanna. Thus, it should not be surprising that over the last ten million years, a great extinction among species of apes has occurred, while monkeys have been able to flourish in a wide variety of habitats because of their cohesive troops. Indeed, no ape except humans can survive on the open-country savanna today.

So, the most important question is, how did hominins become more social and group oriented than contemporary apes, particularly if Maryanski's cladistic analysis is correct that humans' last common ancestor with the great ape line was virtually solitary like the present-day orangutan? How did natural selection overcome this liability of all apes that sought to survive on the African savanna? Most could not, and they went extinct, but somehow selection hit upon a solution for rewiring the great ape brain to be more social. Surprisingly, as will become very evident below, there were many behavioral propensities evident in primates and mammals that could, with enhancement by natural selection, lead to increased sociality and social bonding among an evolving terrestrial ape, and yet, these apparently were not enough. Something more was needed, and this something was a dramatic increase in the size and connectivity of those subcortical areas of the brain that generate emotions. So, despite some promising capacities for sociality that were already hardwired in the primate brain, they were not sufficient to forge more stable groupings, with the consequence that most species of apes went extinct over the last ten million years. Today, what is left from the carnage imposed by natural selection is a few subspecies of gibbons/siamangs, two subspecies of chimpanzees (common and bonobo), two subspecies of gorillas (lowland and highland), one species of orangutan, and one species of humans. There are, then, less than two handfuls of apes left on the planet from what once were hundreds, if not thousands, of species of apes.

Enhancing Emotional Capacities

As Table 3.1 emphasizes, the neocortex is three times larger among humans compared to great apes, controlling for body size, but what is equally interesting is that, on average, key subcortical areas of the brain where emotions are generated are twice as large. Why should this be so? It is not a matter of speculation since these differences can be measured and have been (notes at bottom of Table 3.1), and the differences tell us what natural selection was doing: increasing emotionality of hominins compared to the last common ancestor that they shared with present-day great apes. It appears, then, that emotions were one of the keys to strengthening group ties among weak-tie apes and hominins. Otherwise, there would be no need for selection to have increased their relative size and, moreover, their connectivity, which is not measured by the data in Table 3.1.

How were emotions enhanced? Robert Plutchik (1980, 2002) was the first to posit an evolutionary analysis of how the brain can produce a greater variety of emotions beyond those that are considered primary and hard-

TABLE 3.1. Relative Size of Ape and Human Brains Compared to *Tenrecidae**

	Apes (*Pongids*)	Humans (*Homo*)
Subcortex		
Diencephalon	8.57	14.76
Thalamus		
Hypothalamus		
Amygdala	1.85	4.38
Centromedial	1.06	2.52
Basolateral	2.45	6.02
Septum	2.16	5.48
Hippocampus	2.99	4.87
Transition cortices	2.38	4.43
Neocortex	61.88	196.41

*Numbers in columns denote how many times larger than *Tenrecidae* components of the human and ape brain are, controlling for body size. Thus, *Tenrecidae* represents a value of 1, and the numbers listed are how many times greater than 1 (for *Tenrecidae*) a particular suborcortical or neocortical brain component is. By doing the measurements in this way, comparisons between the relative size of humans and apes brains are made easier.

Data sources: Stephan (1983), Stephan and Andy (1969, 1977), and Eccles (1989).

wired into mammalian neuroanatomy. Plutchik was not alone in developing this explanation, but his analysis was the most influential. The analysis must start with some determination of which emotions are primary—something over which there is not complete consensus. Plutchik posited eight primary emotions: fear, anger, sorrow, disgust, expectancy, joy, surprise, and acceptance. Then he argued that these emotions are very much like a color wheel, with "mixes" among these emotions generating a larger palate of secondary and tertiary emotions. Just how this occurs neurologically, he could not explain, nor can anyone do so today. The basic idea is, I think, correct but his analysis of how mixing occurs is not quite correct. I do not think that the brain is as precise as Plutchik implies, nor can we be confident that his portrayal of what emotions are primary is accurate. In Table 3.2, I have arrayed the postulated primary emotions of prominent thinkers in a variety of fields. As is evident, Plutchik's count of primary emotions—eight—is about modal among this group, but as is evident, some schemes have more and some less primary emotions.

I would argue that the actual number is much smaller because all of the secondary and tertiary emotions in Plutchik's and others' scheme can be generated by combining just four primary emotions: fear, anger, sadness, and happiness (Turner 1987, 1996a, 1996b, 1996c, 1997, 1998, 1999, 2002). Moreover, if we examine the range of emotions among most mammals, it appears to array itself around just a few primary emotions, although even here there are no definitive answers. At one time, I had "surprise" as a primary emotion, and thus my scheme is not too far from Plutchik's and others' in the table. I am limiting the number because, among the great apes, researchers indicate that complex emotions like shame and guilt are not evident (Boehm, 2012). There are variants of these four primary emotions, to be sure, and the more intelligent the mammal, the greater are the variants of the four primary emotions that I emphasize. But, for an animal like humans whose ancestors had to overcome the lack of strong bioprogrammers for kinship and, more generally, for stable groups, expanding the emotional repertoire could be critical to increasing the strength of social bonds and group cohesion.

I speculate that natural selection first worked on hominins to gain control of emotions because apes do not have high levels of cognitive control of their emotions, and it is likely that such was the case for our last common ancestor with present-day great apes. With this control, the palate of emotions from the four primary emotions could be expanded dramatically and used to forge more nuanced social bonds. Table 3.3 offers some examples of this variation from low to higher-intensity primary emotions.

Then, if selection favored a more complex palate of emotions, and it must have, since apes do not reveal this enlarged palate, two primary emotions

TABLE 3.2. Varying Numbers of Hypothesized Primary Emotions

Fewer Primary Emotions (3–6)

Sroufe (1979): pleasure, fear, anger
Kemper (1987): satisfaction, fear, anger, depression
Arnold (1960): flight, fight, defensive, aggression
Johnson-Laird and Oatley (1992): fear, anger, sadness, disgust
Gray (1982): hope, anxiety, anger, sadness
Fehr and Russell (1984): happiness, fear, anger, sadness
Trevarthen (1984): happiness, fear, anger, sadness
Turner (1996): happiness, fear, anger, sadness, surprise
Scott (1980): pleasure, love, fear, anxiety, anger, loneliness
Arnold (1960): flight, fight, defensive, aggression
Epstein (1984): joy, love, fear, anger, sadness
Arieti (1970): satisfaction, fear, tension, rage, unpleasure, appetite
Ekman (1984): happiness, fear, anger sadness, surprise, disgust

Moderate Number of Primary Emotions (7–8)

Darwin (1872): pleasure, joy, affection, terror, anger, astonishment, pain
Plutchik (1980): joy, fear, anger, sadness, surprise, disgust, anticipation, acceptance
Fromme and O'Brien (1982): joy, elation, satisfaction, fear, anger, grief, resignation, shock
Panksepp (1982): fear, panic, rage, sorrow, loneliness, grief, expectancy
Malatesta and Haviland (1982): joy, fear, anger, interest, pain, brownflash, knitbrow

Higher Number of Primary Emotions (11–12)

Emde (1980): joy, fear, anger, sadness, surprise, disgust, shame, shyness, distress, guilt, interest
Izard (1977/1992): enjoyment, fear, anger, contempt, surprise, disgust, shame, shyness, distress, guilt, interest
Osgood (1966): joy, quiet, pleasure, fear, anxiety, anger, sorrow, amazement, disgust, interests, expectancy, boredom

Note: Virtually all scholars posit variants of *happiness, sadness, anger,* and *fear* as primary emotions. Moreover, a majority keep the count low to less than six primary emotions.
Data sources: Turner (2000, pp. 68–69) and Turner and Stets (2005, pp. 14–15).

can be combined to produce additional variants of emotions, as illustrated in Table 3.4, where a greater amount of primary emotions, combined in some unknown neurological way, generates an additional palate of emotions. And finally, as illustrated in Table 3.5, I think that the final step in this process of directional selection was to produce emotions that may be unique to humans: shame and guilt. These are the emotions of social control because shame is an intense feeling of inadequacy in one's inability to

TABLE 3.3. Range of Variation of Primary Emotions

Emotions	Intensity of Emotions		
	Low	Medium	High
Variants of satisfaction-happiness	content sanguine serenity gratified	cheerful buoyant friendly amiable enjoyment	joy bliss rapture jubilant gaiety elation delight thrilled exhilarated
Variants of aversion-fear	concern hesitant reluctance shyness	misgivings trepidation anxiety scared alarmed unnerved panic	terror horror high anxiety
Variants of assertion-anger	annoyed agitated irritated vexed perturbed nettled rankled piqued	displeased frustrated belligerent contentious hostility ire animosity offended consternation	dislike loathing disgust hate despise detest hatred seething wrath furious inflamed incensed outrage
Variants of disappointment-status	discouraged downcast dispirited	dismayed disheartened glum resigned gloomy woeful pained dejected	sorrow heartsick despondent anguished crestfallen

Data source: Turner (1999a, 1999b).

TABLE 3.4. First-Order Elaborations of Primary Emotions

Primary Emotions		First-Order Elaborations
Satisfaction-happiness		
Satisfaction-happiness + *aversion-fear*	*can generate*	wonder, hopeful, relief, gratitude, pride, reverence
Satisfaction-happiness + *assertion-anger*	*can generate*	vengeance, appeased, calmed, soothed, relish, triumphant, bemused
Satisfaction-happiness + *disappointment-sadness*	*can generate*	nostalgia, yearning, hope
Aversion-fear		
Aversion-fear + *satisfaction-happiness*	*can generate*	awe, reverence, veneration
Aversion-fear + *assertion-anger*	*can generate*	revulsion, repulsion, antagonism, dislike, envy
Aversion-fear + *disappointment-sadness*	*can generate*	dread, wariness
Assertion-anger		
Assertion-anger + *satisfaction-happiness*	*can generate*	condescension, mollification, rudeness, placation, righteousness
Assertion-anger + *aversion-fear*	*can generate*	abhorrence, jealousy, suspiciousness
Assertion-anger + *disappointment-sadness*	*can generate*	bitterness, depression, betrayed
Disappointment-sadness		
Disappointment-sadness + *satisfaction-happiness*	*can generate*	acceptance, moroseness, solace, melancholy
Disappointment-sadness + *aversion-fear*	*can generate*	regret, forlornness, remorseful, misery
Disappointment-sadness + *assertion-anger*	*can generate*	aggrievement, discontent, dissatisfaction, unfulfillment, boredom, grief, envy, sullenness

meet expectations of others, whereas guilt involves feelings that one has violated moral codes. Emotions like these control individuals, and they are essential to permanent group arrangements.

In reading across these tables, beginning with the variants of primary emotions, it is evident that, for purposes of forging permanent bonds, three of the four primary emotions are negative in that they do not promote solidarity, as many sociological studies document. Let me emphasize that negative emotions, particularly fear and anger, can be highly adaptive because they push animals to avoid danger and, if trapped, to engage in aggressive defense against predators. This is why, no doubt, they are so ancient and

TABLE 3.5. The Structure of Second-Order Emotions: Shame, Guilt, and Alienation

Constituent Primary Emotions	Shame	Guilt	Alienation
1	Disappointment-sadness (at self)	Disappointment-sadness (at self)	Disappointment-sadness (for self)
2	Assertion-anger (at self)	Aversion-fear (for self)	Assertion-anger (at situation)
3	Aversion-fear (for self)	Assertion-anger (at self)	Aversion-fear (for self)

Note: Numbers in left column denote the rank-ordering of relative valences of the constituent primary emotions making up second-order emotions.

why a structure like the amygdala evolved among reptiles. Negative emotions emitted in groups where individuals are held together by hardwired bioprogrammers do not represent the same problem as would be the case for animals like hominins using emotions to overcome their lack of bioprogrammers. To some extent, first-order elaborations (combinations of two primary emotions) and second-order elaborations (combining the three negative emotions to produce shame and guilt) increase the number and variety of emotions that can be used to forge more nuanced social bonds, although some very intense negative emotions, such as emotions for vengeance, can emerge from combinations of anger and happiness. Thus, the negativity of emotions—from the perspective of needs to achieve higher levels of social solidarity—can create problems for human happiness and adjustment. To experience negative emotions, especially powerful ones like shame and guilt, is painful, often leading to repression of emotions and their transmutation into one of the negative components of shame and guilt—most typically, *diffuse anger* from shame and *diffuse anxiety* from guilt. The expression of these emotions is highly disruptive to social relations among humans and, thereby, poses dangers of breaking social bonds and lowering group solidarity.

Moreover, as I explore below, when reviewing the behavioral capacities and propensities of great apes (and, to varying degrees, mammals more generally), it would seem that there already existed a large array of propensities that could have been selected upon and enhanced to the point of creating strong bonds and group solidarities. And yet, this apparently was not the case because humans also reveal a large palate of emotions, many of which are essential to social control and group solidarity but many of which work against solidarity in groups. So, why was enhancing emotions essential when negative emotions can work against group solidarity? Despite these liabilities, enhancing emotions must have been essential because, otherwise, we cannot explain how the subcortical areas of the human brain became so much larger, more connected, and enhanced in their power during hominin evolution. To understand why enhancement of emotions occurred, we first need to summarize what the data show on the hardwired behavioral propensities among great apes (and other primates and mammals) to see if they were sufficient for group formation without higher levels of emotionality.

Hardwired Behavioral Capacities and Propensities

In reviewing literatures on neurology and primates, it is clear that there are a number of hardwired behavioral capacities and propensities that the last common ancestor to present-day great apes and the ancestors of humans possessed. These are all available for natural selection to work on, and enhancement of each would increase hominin and eventually human sociality, bonding, and group formation. And, as I will argue, these expanded neurological capacities, coupled with emotions that can be aroused can help explain the nature, direction, and intensity of stress as it affects human psychological well-being and health. Let me begin with the first set of neurological features of primates that were subject to selection during hominin and human evolution.

Early Selection on Primate Neuroanatomy for an Emotion-Based Language

Visual Dominance. One of the earliest changes in the basic mammalian anatomy during primate evolution was selection for visual dominance over haptic and auditory sense modalities, thereby subordinating other sense modalities to vision (Maryanski & Turner, 1992; Passingham, 1982, pp. 51– 55). This shift to visual dominance would make interaction among conspecifics primarily a visual rather than an olfactory or auditory process, even with the eventual development of the capacity for speech. Moreover, as emphasized earlier, this large shift in sense modalities created a spandrel or preadaptation for language, which initially would be visually based rather than auditory based.

Language Capacity. The great apes—that is, chimpanzees, gorillas, and orangutans—are all able to learn and use language at the level of a three-year-old human child (Geschwind, 1965a, 1965b, 1965c, 1970; Geschwind & Damasio, 1984; Rumbaugh & Savage-Rumbaugh, 1990; Savage-Rumbaugh & Lewin, 1994; Savage-Rumbaugh et al., 1988, 1993; Bickerton, 2003). This ability indicates that the preadaptation created by the shift to visual dominance can be used, if needed, and if needed, it could be selected upon and enhanced. Yet, because apes do not the possess the anatomical equipment to make fine-tuned speech possible, it is not likely that the first languages among humans' hominin ancestors were auditory, or based upon spoken phonemes and morphemes organized by a syntax. Rather, natural selection would take the easiest route to increasing language abilities, if these would enhance hominin fitness. This route would be to use the dominant visual sense modality. And so, a visually based language could, therefore, have emerged during hominin evolution *long before* auditory, or speech-based language, could evolve. As a consequence, selection for the neurology necessary for language production built around visual cues and use would not have to "wait" for the more difficult anatomical changes needed for spoken language—that is, complex changes in the frontal and parietal lobes controlling facial and lip movements necessary for speech, opening up the focal tract to free up room for a larynx capable of fine-grained vocalizations, gaining control of tongue and lips for articulated auditory-based language, and other key anatomical changes Duchin (1990).

Attention to Eyes and Gaze. Great apes, just like humans, have the behavioral propensity to follow the gaze and eye movements of others (Hare et al., 2001, 2006; Povinelli, 2000; Povinelli and Eddy 1997; Itakura, 1996; Baizer et al., 2007; Tomasello et al, 2001; Tomasello and Call 1997; Ikamoto et al., 2002). This capacity argues that apes and, hence, all hominins and humans are wired to look at eyes, to follow gazes, and to interpret their meanings—thus making interaction in groups a process of watching face and, particularly, eye movements. This conclusion is supported by the propensity for face monitoring for signs of action of conspecifics, particularly for emotional content (Leslie, et al., 2004; Gazzaniga & Symlie, 1990). And so, if selection were going to increase fitness, it would install the propensity that we see today among humans: reading of emotions by paying attention to facial expressions more generally but eyes and eye movements more specifically. It may not have been necessary for selection to enhance this propensity, per se, but it is very likely that selection focused the emerging language of emotions on face and eyes as primary sources of information about the emotional states of others and secondarily on more general body countenance.

Infant Abilities to Read Emotions. Within the first weeks of life, human infants can imitate the facial expressions of their caretakers (Emde, 1962; Ekman, 1984; Sherwood et al., 2004), especially those associated with emotions such as smiles and frowns. This ability and, indeed, propensity precedes the capacity to babble sounds producing speech phonemes by well over a year. Developmental stages are sometimes indicative of evolutionary stages in the distant past, and the fact that facial movements and expressions of adult caretakers can be imitated almost immediately after birth by infants, whereas auditory sounds signaling language often take two years to develop, suggests that reliance on facial cues, particularly those indicating emotional states, are hardwired into ape and thus hominin and human neuroanatomy and were more critical than auditory sounds in emerging groupings among hominins. From birth, then, humans are wired for reading and reproducing signs of emotions, thus ensuring that the first images of self were be tagged with high levels of emotional content.

Face and the Production of Meanings. Apes have the capacity to communicate very subtle meanings and to coordinate instrumental actions through nonverbal signals, especially by eyes and face (Menzel, 1971; Mitani, Watts, & Muller 2002; Turner & Maryanski, 2008). Chimpanzees can, for example, coordinate hunts and killings of baboons through the visual channel without any auditory output, indicating that there already existed in the last common ancestry a proto-language for concerted, collective action in groupings—albeit in the case of chimpanzees temporary and fluid groups—by relying of facial and eye gestures, and if these episodes of temporary coordination could be extended to form more permanent groupings, natural selection had an existing capacity and propensity on which to select, long before hominins developed anything close to human speech communication.

Learning Body Language. Human children, as well as infant apes, have the propensity to imitate appropriate facial and body signals and behaviors, eventually adding them to their own behavioral repertoire in order to communicate to others (Tomonaga, 1999; Subiaul, 2007; Horowitz, 2003; Gergely & Csibra, 2006). Again, the wiring for imitating and learning nonverbal signals indicates that there was a hardwired behavioral propensity to rely on nonverbal "body language" in group contexts, which would produce a visually based language system without much auditory content.

Cortical Control of Subcortical Emotional States. For a visually based language of emotions to evolve on the behavioral capacities and propensities of the great apes, and hence the last common ancestor of apes and humans, control of emotional outburst would be critical. The fact that humans have such dramatically increased cortical control of emotions compared to the great apes indicates that selection had probably started increasing neocortical control of emotions long before the neocortex began to grow during late hominin evolution. This control in humans occurs through projections of axons (Raghante et al., 2008; Sherwood, 2007; Sherwood et al., 2004). This difference between apes and humans argues for the conclusion that controlling emotions had fitness-enhancing value for hominins on the savanna, primarily by inhibiting emotional outbreaks that would attract predators and, as I argue, for the instrumental control of emotional expressions as the first language among hominins. This control was perhaps necessary since the subcortical areas of the human brain are twice as large as those among the great apes, controlling for body size (Stephan, 1983; Stephan & Andy, 1969, 1977; Eccles, 1989). Thus, there was selection on subcortical areas of the brain that dramatically increased hominin emotionality long *before selection* began to increase the size of the hominin neocortex and, at the same time, selection began to work on the neocortex to gain control of these emotions if they were to be used as the basic mode of solidarity-generating communication among hominins.

The Prefrontal Cortex and Emotional Control. The larger decision-making prefrontal cortex among humans compared to apes indicates how natural selection increased control of humans over emotions (Semendeferi et al., 2002). The enlarged prefrontal cortex of humans compared to that of apes indicates that selection favored not only control of emotions but also use of emotions to provide the markers of utility or reward-value in making decisions (Damasio, 1994), and if this capacity enhanced fitness, it could also be used for additional control on emotions and for their use for more instrumental purposes in an emotion-based language system. This process probably began slowly, but one hypothesis would be that even before the overall neocortex began to grow, the prefrontal cortex was already developing new capacities to control emotions and, also, to use emotions in communication and in making judgments about fairness and reciprocity in exchange relations. All of these changes in the neuroanatomy of the evolving hominin brain would significantly increase cooperation and group organization and, hence, fitness among hominins.

The Late Arrival of Speech. As noted above, fine-tuned speech is not possible among great apes and, hence, humans' early hominin ancestors because they would not have had key anatomical structures for finely articulated speech.

This led to reliance on vision, which, among all primates, is highly developed and would not require any new structures. The recent discovery that the mutations on genes involved in the development of the anatomical alterations for fine-grained speech have been under selection for *only* about 200,000 years—about the time that *Homo sapiens* have existed—adds further evidence that communication among hominins was not auditory but, rather, visually based. This startling discovery (Enard et al., 2002a, 2002b) suggests, then, that speech was a late arrival in the evolution of hominins and, indeed, may only have emerged with the evolution of *Homo sapiens*. If such is the case, then interpersonal processes and patterns of group formation among hominins were not based upon speech but a language of a different kind, most likely a system of phonemes and syntax revolving around emotions signaled and read through facial and body gestures. This was not a quasi-language but *the first and most primal language of hominins and, hence, humans.* Auditory language was piggy-backed onto body language during the early evolution of humans or, at best, the late evolution of *Homo erectus,* and hence was a supplement to hominins' and humans' primal language based on visual communication of emotional states. Indeed, when people seek to form bonds of solidarity, they use visually based emotional states to do so more than speech.

In sum, then, it is evident that natural selection had a great many neurological capacities on which to select for language, but a visually based language probably built from emotions that reveal phonemes and a syntax— just as emotions when strung out in a series of gestural displays—"speaks" to people (Turner, 2000). If one doubts the capacity of such body language to communicate meanings, turn off the sound on a foreign language film and observe how easy it is to "follow the storylines," especially the emotional dispositions of the actors. Thus, the neurological capacity to use emotions as a language existed with the last common ancestor of humans and the great apes, and as a result, it was available for further selection if developing an emotion-based language would enhance fitness. And, for species of ape-like primates without powerful bioprogrammers for group formation (in contrast to monkeys), selection may well have hit upon these already-in-place neurological capacities to increase social bonding through emotions and social solidarity among weak-tie apes. Moreover, I would argue that this language of emotions enhancing sociality and solidarity could be used to develop proto moral codes because linguistic moral codes depend upon emotions to exert their power over humans.

Yet, social bonding and solidarity would not have to depend solely on neurological capacities for a visually based language. Primates today and, hence, those hominin primates on the human clade reveal(ed) other hardwired behavioral propensities that increase sociality. If subject to further enhancement by selection on tail ends of the bell curves, these additional nonlinguistic propensities for sociality could also serve as mechanisms for enhancing social ties among weak-tie primates. Once again, these mechanisms existed long before culture emerged in the hominin line, and so, we can gain more confidence that many of the processes that create and sustain groups are *not* constructed solely by culture but, instead, by behavioral propensities that have been part of primates for millions of years. Let me list the most important of these.

Selection on Nonlinguistic Behavioral Capacities

Empathy. Great apes have the capacity to read the facial and body gestures of conspecifics and develop a sense of empathy with other apes (deWaal, 1996, 2009). It is clear that the great apes, particularly chimpanzees—humans' closest primate relative—can empathize with conspecifics by reading gestures, especially those revealing emotional states but also instrumental states as well. And then, on the basis of this reading develop such complex emotional states as *sympathy* and engage in efforts to help those fellow chimpanzees experiencing *distress* and other negative emotions. Thus, what George Herbert Mead (1932) termed *role-taking* is possible, and moreover, even more in-depth role-taking of emotional states, or what we could term *emotion-taking* (Turner, 2013a, 2013b), is built into the neurology of humans' closest relatives, which means that it was part of the hominin neuroanatomy and, thus, could be subject to further selection if empathy would have fitness-enhancing consequences. The fundamental capacity for interaction outlined by Mead—interaction with gestures carrying common meanings and, I would add, emotional states—was already in place; it did not have to arise from mutations or, perhaps, even much selection on tail ends of the bell curve describing its distribution in the hominin genome.

Rhythmic Synchronization. Primates rather easily fall into rhythmic synchronization of bodies, especially involving emotions, via mirror neurons (Schutz-Bosbach & Pinz, 2007; Rizzolatti et al., 2002). Mirror neurons were first discovered in monkeys, and it is now clear that they are also part of ape and human neurology. The neurons generating responses of others are activated, at least to a degree, in the same areas of the brain as those observing these responses. Thus, the capacity for role-taking and empathy is hardwired into higher-primate mirror neurons, and if role-taking and empathy would have fitness-enhancing value by creating bonds of solidarity, they were available for further selection—although perhaps such selection was not needed. The capacity to fall into rhythmic synchronization, as emphasized by Collins (2004), is a neurological process as much as a culturally constructed pattern of behavior. It has been part of the higher-primate genome for millions of years and, thus, was part of the hominin and human genome.

Carnival. The propensity of chimpanzees to engage in a practice described by researchers as "carnival" is very similar to what humans do in various festivals seen around the world (e.g., New Orleans, Rio). Émile Durkheim (1912/1965) described these as "effervescence" among periodic gatherings of Arunta aboriginals around Alice Springs, Australia. What they signal is that hominins probably possessed the neurological propensity at gatherings of conspecifics to ramp up collective emotional states in a festival-like way and, in so doing, display heighten emotions and group solidarity with others. Thus, even moderately weak-tie animals like chimpanzees and, perhaps, humans' last common ancestor have the tendency to overcome their weak-tie pattern of relations for solidarity-generating emotions to be aroused in periodic gatherings of conspecifics. Such a capacity was probably only periodic, but as Goffman (1958, 1967) and Collins (2004) have emphasized in their respective extensions of Durkheim's basic insight, humans do this on a more frequent but less intense way during virtually all interpersonal encounters and interaction rituals. Thus, the propensity for carnival, if selected on, could be extended to almost all interaction rituals on a dramatically less intense scale but with the same solidarity-generating consequences, if such selection enhanced fitness by building solidarities that could be carried across encounters over time.

New Variants of Primary Emotions. As I emphasized in Tables 3.3, 3.4, and 3.5, humans reveal the capacity to experience variants among primary emotions, particularly among *happiness, fear, anger,* and *sadness* (Darwin, 1872; Turner, 2000; Parr, 2001). This capacity needs to be analyzed in relation to the capacity for carnival-like exuberance evident among humans' closest relative, the common chimpanzee. This exuberance is built around *collective happiness,* and if natural selection worked to lower the intensity but still retain the solidarity-generating effects of carnival-like behaviors, the capacity for carnival can be considered a preadaptation for more normal interaction rituals evident in all encounters of face-to-face human interaction (Goffman, 1967; Collins, 2004). To lower the level of exuberance but retain what Émile Durkheim (1912/1965) saw as "effervescence" in human interaction, it would be important to create more lower-key variants of *happiness* in the emotional repertoire of hominins forging new kinds of social bonds. Lower-key interaction rituals generate solidarity, but without exhausting individuals—as often happens during human carnivals and parties. The great apes have a comparatively large repertoire of emotional variants of primary emotions, but not to the extent of humans. And thus, as the last common ancestors of humans and chimpanzees were under selection pressures to develop more enduring and stable solidarities, the necessary diversity of emotional states, particularly those around variants of *happiness,* were available for selection to work on as carnival was downsized to interaction rituals revolving around rhythmic synchronization and positive emotional arousal leading to solidarity at the group level.

Note, however, such solidarity does not rely on culture, beliefs, or norms; solidarity can exist and, indeed, does occur in more intense forms among chimpanzees, *without* cultural props. Indeed, like language more generally, the cultural embellishment and perhaps normative regulation of carnival and its lower-key variants in interaction rituals are simply add-ons to *already extant neurological* capacities that humans share with common chimpanzees and, of course, their hominin ancestors. The dramatic increase in the relative size of subcortical areas of the brain where emotions are generated signals that selection was enhancing emotionality among hominins, perhaps not the more intense emotions (although these could have been a by-product of larger subcortical neurosystems) but the quieter emotions that sustain interactions and work to forge more enduring social bonds.

Reciprocity. The propensity for reciprocity in the give-and-take of resources is evident in apes and, indeed, in many higher animals (Cosmides, 1989; deWaal, 1989, 1991, 1996; deWaal & Brosnan, 2006). And, it is particularly developed in apes and humans, and as the vast sociological literature on exchange processes among humans so clearly documents, it is one of the central dynamics of human interaction and group formation (e.g., Lawler et al., 2009; Hechter, 1987; Molm, 1997). With expanded emotional repertoires, coupled with the capacities listed above, it is not difficult to see how natural selection enhanced this sense of reciprocity, creating a need for reciprocity and arousing negative emotions and negative sanctions when reciprocity is not honored. Thus, to the degree that reciprocity is involved in exchanges of resources, including solidarity-generating emotional resources, it was available for selection to work on and, once again, does not require culture. Reciprocity can, of course, be normatively regulated by culture, but its power comes from nonsymbolic neurology and the power of emotions.

Judgments of Fairness and Justice. Primates reveal the behavioral propensity to compare shares of resources with others in making judgments of fairness in the distribution of resources (Bronson & de Waal, 2003; Bronson et al., 2005). Monkeys and apes both evidence this behavioral propensity, especially when interacting with humans in the laboratory. A capuchin monkey, for example, will stop exchanging with a trainer (exchange behaviors for food) if this monkey can see another monkey getting more food for the same behaviors. In chimpanzees, the emotions can be even more dramatic, as was the tragic case of individuals who brought a birthday cake to their ape who had lived with them before being retired to a home for aging primates; the two other apes in the compound viciously attacked the persons distributing this valued resource (a cake) because they had been excluded. Thus, rather complicated calculations of justice and fairness involving shares of resources, behaviors produced to receive these resources, and comparisons of one's resources with those received by others can, again, occur without culture. What is necessary is the capacity to arouse emotions over these calculations, with fairness and unfairness generating *automatic* emotional arousal without invoking a moral yardstick calibrated in terms of cultural symbols. Again, judgments are not the force driving fairness; rather, the subcortically generated emotions attached to these cognitive deliberations in the prefrontal cortex are what put the teeth and power into morality, not statements of rights and wrongs (the latter only generate morality *if* tagged with emotions). So noncultural morality exists neurologically in chimpanzees, being built from more general mammalian and primate propensities of expectations for reciprocity in resource exchanges.

While the notion of noncultural morality may seem an oxymoron, this reaction is an artifact of bias in sociology toward social constructivist arguments. But, it can be argued on the evidence from primate studies that morality is deeply sedimented in human neuroanatomy and evident very early in primate evolution, as is revealed in monkeys and apes today. Again, culture can give more power, focus, and complexity to morality, but it is *not morality's driving force.* Thus, to the extent that morality enhances solidarity and binds individuals to groups, it was available for selection to work on long before the neurological capacity for symbolization with arbitrary signs and the consequent development of beliefs and ideologies evolved in hominins, although the in-place neurological potential for language was available for selection to work on. But, for a noncultural morality, it is selection on emotion centers in the subcortex and perhaps the neocortical control of emotions (in the prefrontal cortex) that had to evolve *before* morality could become cultural and be enshrined in speech texts and beliefs.

Self. The ability to recognize an image in a mirror as a reflection of self as an object in the environment exists among all of the great apes (Gallup, 1970, 1979, 1982) and among a few other higher mammals (elephants, dolphins, and probably whales). All of the capacities listed above are dramatically enhanced if this rudimentary sense of self-recognition is enhanced. When animals can see themselves as objects vis-à-vis others in encounters and groupings, they are more likely to evaluate themselves in reference to what they perceive to be the expectations of others, the expectations for reciprocity, the expectations for fairness and justice in distributions of resources, and the expectations that come with empathy and role-taking. By simply enhancing sense of self as "an object in the environment" (as G. H. Mead, 1934, phrased the matter), self-directed and controlled behavior involving expectations, emotions, and noncultural morality can evolve.

Thus, to the degree that seeing oneself as an object in social environments increases the power of groups to control an organism and, in fact, increases self-control through self-evaluation vis-à-vis others and groupings, it could have fitness-enhancing consequences for weak-tie animals that do not also have strong bioprogrammers for pod, troop, or herd behaviors. Selection could have hit upon enhancing the capacity to see oneself as an object in relation to others, and it is a short step to seeing oneself as an object in the eyes of others to experiencing the evaluations of others. And so, in conjunction with increasing the complexity and nuance of emotions, new kinds of self-emotions such as feelings of *pride* and *shame* (as emphasized by Charles Horton Cooley, 1902/1964) could emerge. As a result, self-control through the language of emotions could be achieved millions of years before cultural forms of morality evolved. Culture would, of course, grant greater power to efforts to verify identities in the eyes of others and groups, just as it would for enhancing all of the processes described above, but culture alone could not have these effects unless capacities for identity formation *had already evolved* beyond what we see in apes, who do not evaluate self in terms of complex emotions like *shame* and *guilt* (Boehm, 2012).

Thus, culture alone is almost powerless in promoting group solidarity and group bonds *without* extant bioprogrammers for group cohesion, which for apes were lost twenty million years ago. And so, *without* the enhancement of all the behavioral capacities that I have listed above, the underlying neurosystems producing them had to evolve *beyond the rudimentary base we see in the great apes* before culture could "super-charge" all of them in making humans an even more social and group-oriented animal.

And, this may be the reason that the neocortex did not grow much beyond that evident in contemporary chimpanzees for millions of years of hominin evolution. It could not have fitness-enhancing effects *until* all of the neurologically based behavioral capacities listed above had been enhanced to varying degrees by natural selection working on the tail end of distributions of neurological structures. Each enhancement would increase sociality and group solidarity to some extent, allowing low-sociality hominins to become more group oriented and, hence, more able to survive in the open-country, savanna habitat. At some point, these enhancements could be dramatically extended by growing the neocortex and building an auditory language employing arbitrary signs and symbols on top of the emotion-based primal language of hominins. And, as this language evolved and as cultural codes emerged, the behavioral propensities that apes and hominins always possessed would become conflated with culture and constitute the basic core of all those group processes described by social psychologists and sociologists more generally.

From all of the neurological capacities briefly reviewed in the last two sections, we can draw some conclusions about the biases of the interpersonal mechanisms that emerged as selection began to work on these extant neurological capacities. Most fundamentally, interaction would have a visual bias since primates are visually dominant (very rare among mammals). The most important interpersonal mechanisms for increasing bonding and group solidarity are likely to be based upon visual readings of face and body, especially with respect to emotions. Along with this visual bias came the rudimentary capacity for language, and so it is likely that visually based mechanisms of interpersonal behavior were dramatically enhanced by natural selection to produce a language system based upon (a) visual phonemes and morphemes produced by face and body and (b) syntactical conventions for ordering emotional phonemes and morphemes to produce more complex meanings (just as present-day great apes do today when they learn human language). The great apes are programmed to use imitation of face and body signals, and thus there would be a built-in propensity to learn those that carried meanings and allowed for increased attachments to conspecifics. Moreover, since chimpanzees already possess the capacity for empathy, a bias toward reading emotional gestures signaling affective states in others already existed in the common ancestor of chimpanzees and humans.

The emotionality of apes would bias the reading of face and body gestures toward expressions of emotions, but the lack of control of emotions by apes and, no doubt, the last common ancestor of apes and hominins would be problematic for the survival of early hominins on the savanna. Survival on the savanna, then, probably had to begin with natural selection rewiring connections between the neocortex, especially the prefrontal cortex, to give hominins neocortical control over emotional outbursts. Once this control existed, it could be selected upon to expand the repertoire of emotions among hominins and eventually the capacity to use implicit syntax to string together emotional phonemes in a proto-language of emotions. And given the propensity to read gestures for empathy, this capacity would bias directional selection toward exchanges of emotional states to produce intersubjectivity on an emotional level and, thereby, increase bonding and group-level solidarity.

The fact that apes already reveal the capacity for rhythmic synchronization would further bias the formation of an emotionally based language for establishing rhythms in communication among conspecifics as a solidarity-generating mechanism. And, when we add to this conclusion the recent data indicating that the mutations responsible for fine-tuned and articulated speech in the human measure are very recent, we have further evidence that the language of emotions was likely to be the primal and primary language for communicating emotional states, just as this language is today when humans rely on visual cues about emotions to signal and interpret others' emotional responses. Furthermore, chimpanzees and hence the common ancestor of chimpanzees and humans engage in "carnival" or what Durkheim (1912/1965) termed "collective effervescence" in festivals of solidarity-generating group-level emotional displays. Auditory-based (spoken) language would have come after the language of emotions and thereby have been secondary to communicating emotions, just as they are today in humans. Adding to this conclusion is the ability of human infants to imitate primary emotions of caretakers within two weeks of birth, long before speech centers are activated. Since developmental sequences are often reflective of evolutionary sequences, this would suggest that the language of emotions came millions of years before capacities for articulated speech and is still the primal and primary language of humans.

Stress is itself an emotional state, but equally important, it generates additional negative emotional states. Since emotions were the basis of hominin survival on the savanna, human well-being and health revolve around the emotions aroused during stressful interactions and the capacities of individuals to manage these emotions. Indeed, as much as we tend to see speech and culture as the hallmarks of what it means to be human, far more primal and primary is the emotionality of humans. When emotions turn negative, they pose an ancient problem for not only individuals but the social order. One set of mechanisms for controlling the problem of negative emotional arousal under conditions of stress is to activate repression and other defense mechanisms. In expanding neocortical control over emotions with growth in the prefrontal cortex and thereby increasing their diversity and use as intentional signals of meaning, natural selection may have produced yet another preadaptation: the ability to repress or reconceptualize negative emotions, which dramatically increases the complexity of the relationship among stress, emotional arousal, health, and psychological well-being. The capacity of great apes to recognize themselves in a mirror was clearly enhanced during hominin evolution since much human behavior is motivated and constrained by images of self that are seen in what Charles Horton Cooley (1902/1964) termed "the looking glass self" composed of the gestures of others. An enhanced sense of self as an object in all environments would further bias individuals to read the emotional responses of others toward self and, when necessary, to repress those responses that reflect negatively on self.

This self-referential bias of perceptions would be enhanced further by existing hardwired behavioral propensities for reciprocity and calculations of justice. Monkeys and apes already reveal neurologically driven propensities for reciprocity and implicit calculations of fairness and justice in exchanges of resources. The presence of these behavioral propensities in hominins would further the biases discussed above, with the result that interactions would be dramatically charged up with emotions and feelings about self and others when reciprocity and justice were not evident in exchanges of resources among hominins. And later, these behavioral propensities would bias and, indeed, provide the neurological impetus for the formation of culture and language toward articulation of moral codes, charged by the power of emotions from the primal language of emotions. Such codes would have "teeth" and power when complex moral emotions like shame and guilt became part of the emotional repertoire of hominins or, perhaps, only humans. Without these emotional underpinnings, morality has no power; only when individuals can evaluate self in relation to moral codes and experience *shame* or *pride* when moral imperatives of cultural codes are realized or violated can culturally imposed proscriptions and prescriptions have power. And this is a very special kind of power because these emotions lead individuals to impose self-control on their behaviors, thereby reducing the monitoring and sanctioning costs of others. Thus, building on the neurology of reciprocity and justice already wired into hominins, coupled with the expansion of emotionality and especially emotions directed at a more salient sense of self, culturally based morality could gain even more traction. Thus, culture as we know could not have evolved without the neurological substrate for increasing social bonds, but once it evolved, it could double the pain and well-being of individuals because with morality comes the truly powerful and stressful emotions of *guilt* and *shame*. And these emotions, because they are so painful, increase the likelihood that they will be repressed, thereby compounding and convoluting the emotions driving stress and undermining health and well-being.

The Fragility of Human Interaction

In reviewing the behavioral capacities and propensities of primates and apes, and presumably, the last common ancestor of apes and humans, it becomes clear why human interaction is biased toward the reading of emotions, especially those about self, as well as reciprocity and justice—all of which add intensity to emotional responses like stress. What is surprising to me is that if we look down the list of behaviors subject to selection in the last section, it is difficult to see why enhancing these alone would not have been sufficient to increase group bonds among hominins. Yet, it is clear that this was probably not the case because most apes went extinct over the last ten million years, and as the comparative measurements of subcortical areas of the brain responsible for emotions make clear, selection also pushed hominins and then humans to become highly emotional by enlarging centers of emotions and the connectivity among these centers as well as between these subcortical subassemblages and the neocortex, especially the prefrontal cortex. Without emotional overlays, enhancement of the behavioral propensities examined above was apparently not sufficient to increase bonding and group solidarity to a level promoting fitness, whereas expanded emotional capacities, coupled with these other neurologically based capacities, were enough to allow hominins to survive the open-country savanna. But, while increased emotionality makes high levels of solidarity possible, it also makes human social relations rather fragile, especially in the absence of hardwired propensities for group formation, per se.

The lists of neurologically based behavioral capacities and propensities outlined above constrained the evolution of the interpersonal mechanisms by which hominins and then humans could forge social bonds. Without underlying bioprogrammers for group formation, building social relations of solidarity in groups was much more costly than it would be in organisms with strong bioprogrammers for group, pod, pack, troop, or herd behaviors. For humans today must *actively work* at interpersonal relations because they must, at a minimum, (a) visually monitor others and the reactions of others to self-presentations; (b) invoke relevant aspects of culture and display prescribed emotional states, even if they are not actually felt; (c) determine the status and roles of others in social contexts, while playing appropriate roles and behavior in accordance with status designations for self; (d) monitor the motive states of others, while presenting to others the motives and needs driving self; (e) constantly make attributions for any interpersonal action of self or others; and (f) in general, emit very complex and subtle behavioral outputs toward others, while interpreting a complex array of visual, auditory, and, at times, haptic (touch) responses of others.

Thus, even without further elaboration, the complexity of the list in the last sentence documents that interpersonal behavior occurs along many dimensions and operates at many levels. A great deal can easily go wrong because of this complexity of the interaction process, per se, especially without the stabilizing force of function-specific neurologically based bio-programmers for affiliation and group behaviors, as is the case with most mammals.

Breaches to interactions immediately arouse negative emotions in self and others, causing considerable stress even in relatively mundane interactions (if one doubts this, consider how you feel when a sales clerk seems rude; the negative emotional arousal is instantaneous, often intense, and sometimes even long-lasting). Thus, as natural selection enhanced hominins' and then humans' emotional capacities as the basis for forming social bonds, it set up the potential for negative emotions when interactions are breached. Another reason for the fragility of interaction is that with increases in the size of the prefrontal cortex, (a) the expansion of the neurons connecting the prefrontal cortex to subcortical emotions centers and (b) modification in the size of the hippocampus allows for use of defense mechanisms, including repression (Schmeing et al., 2013). With repression, negative feelings about self are pushed below the neocortex and not fully experienced in their original form. Moreover, emotions will tend to transmute into new negative forms, thus breaking the connection between the original causes of negative emotions that have been repressed (Turner, 2007). Thus, emotional responses can become highly convoluted once repressed; they can be lost to full self-awareness, while still evident visually to others; they can become transmuted to new negative emotions (e.g., shame can be transmuted to anger, guilt to anxiety, both shame and guilt to depression); and attributions about the causes of emotions will often be wildly inaccurate, thereby making dealing with negative feelings that much more difficult. The result is that interaction is made that much more complex because the real emotions driving interpersonal relations can become difficult for self and others to determine, thereby making the interaction that much more fragile.

Stress, Well-Being, and Health

Neurology and Social Structure

Given the neurology of apes, especially a neurology charged up by dramatically increased emotionality, we should expect that humans as evolved apes would experience stress and that persons' well-being and health would be affected by this neurology, which was jury-rigged together by natural selection to increase, at some potential costs, sociality and group solidarities. Large-brained animals with a jury-rigged set of neurologically based propensities supercharged by emotions and a dramatically expanded neocortex would naturally experience stress, remember the emotions accompanying this stress, repress some of these memories, and worry about those experiences and the emotions attached to them. And the effects of stress would be doubly enhanced because the viability of group affiliations and verification of self would always be on the line when interpersonal processes failed and caused breaches to interaction.

While members of hunting and gathering bands experienced stress and conflict (see Boehm, 2012), the low level of complexity of bands and the nuclear kinship units from which they were built may have reduced the rates of stressful and conflictual interactions, while making it easier to restore order. Yet, as the complexity of human societies increased, this complexity itself would add one more source of stress to interpersonal relations, for several reasons: (a) complexity always increases uncertainty and risk, which, in turn, increases stress; (b) large, complex sociocultural formations can take much of the capacity to manage interpersonal relations out of the hands of individuals and, instead, impose these relations on individuals in groups, thereby often making them more stressful; (c) constraints of structures and their cultures in complex systems can also make stress chronic because it may not be possible to exit these structures and their cultures, with chronic stress systematically generating a range of negative emotions over time, perhaps a lifetime; (d) stress, when supercharged by the failure to meet basic needs for identity-verification, reciprocity, and fairness, which are built into humans' enhanced neurology, will not only be chronic but more intense; and (e) stress and the complicated emotions that it can generate, such as shame and guilt, will often be repressed and transmuted into emotions like defuse anger, anxiety, and sadness, which not only compounds the original repressed stress but also makes present and future interpersonal relations more difficult and stressful.

Ironically, it is humans' lack of bioprogrammers for groups that makes the macro-societies generating these additional sources of stress possible. Few organisms on earth form macro-societies and, with the exception of humans, none are very large. Indeed, most are tiny (insects), and their members are genetically programmed to play roles vis-à-vis others playing the same or different roles. Since most mammals are group oriented, they cannot forge a macro-society because their group bonds are too strong; they cannot easily interact with strangers or large numbers of members playing differentiated roles, as can insects and humans. Indeed, humans are huge animals compared to insects, and yet, we can construct societies that number into the hundreds of millions and even billions, probably because we are at our core a low-sociality ape whose natural social unit is the larger community rather than local groups. Thus, with culture and language, humans have been able to forge macro-societies and survive, but at a certain cost: the increased likelihood that some of the many and complex relations that humans have in diverse network structures can be breached, arousing stressful emotions that affect well-being and long-term health.

As a relevant side note, the popularity of social media and texting comes, I would hypothesize, from the fact that texting enables people to cut down on face-to-face interactions, which are often emotionally taxing and fraught with the potential for emotionally charged breaches. People may gravitate to social media to sustain a sense of group inclusion, low-key implicit verification of self and identities, and low-cost psychic profits in exchanges of resources without much interpersonal work. Indeed, as some literature on stress indicates, the very existence of social relations, per se, increases people's sense of well-being, even if these relations are never drawn upon. The feeling that one is included in networks and groups and that one could draw upon them for help is enough to enhance well-being, whereas when people actually seek help from these relations, they experience stress for lots of neurologically based reasons, such as the need to reciprocate, the sense that justice and fairness demands this reciprocation, the sense of self-degradation that comes with having to seek assistance from others, the work involved in sympathy dynamics involved in seeking help from group members (Clark, 1997), and the need to open and sustain for a time more intense interpersonal relations. All of these are stressful to an evolved ape, and some data on health and well-being document that such is the case, as is summarized below.

Social Support and Stress

It is, then, one of the ironies of hominin evolution that the very mechanisms that allow humans to create groups and emotionally gratifying social bonds can also be stressful because the very process of interaction is so fragile and conditional, becoming more complicated with increases in the complexity of social structures and the dynamics of repression. Yet, despite many needed qualifications, there are several generalizations that emerge from the psychological literature on health and well-being. First, stress, particularly chronic stress, reduces happiness, well-being, and long-term health, and thus those social structures that systematically generate such stress can have negative consequences on well-being and health. However, looking at the psychological studies through the eyes of a sociologist, I would offer the following hypothesis specifying forces that might mitigate the stress: if persons are of higher status in social structures, giving more orders than receiving them, and if they are able to develop supportive social networks, regardless of status, the effects of inequality on stress levels of individuals will decline, as will the harmful effects of stress on well-being and health. Yet, because human social relationships are so fragile, tenuous, and loaded with potential negative emotions, it is not easy under any circumstances to develop longer-term supportive networks under any conditions, especially those revolving around inequalities. Such systems of inequality tend to be shame-generating machines because they are built on authority and the constant threat of negative sanctions and often the need for subordinates to repress their shame and even the anger that often arises from shame when it is repressed and transmuted to an emotion that does not so directly attach self.

Second, social support reduces psychological distress and the accompanying negative emotions, such as variants of fear and sadness (Sarason, Sarason, & Gurung, 1997; Fleming Baum, Gisriel, & Catchel, 1982; Lin, Ye, & Ensel, 1999). Moreover, having social support has positive effects on health (Berkman 1995), which are probably partly mediated through the stress-reducing effects of social networks and other forms of social capital, especially those that verify identities, while allowing individuals to successfully navigate through interaction rituals. And since lack of physical health is highly stressful, the relationships between high levels of stress and health are reciprocal.

The relationship between distress/health and social support is complicated by the nature of social support. If social support is intrusive (Shumaker & Hill, 1991) and/or does not meet up with a person's needs (Thoits, 1995), then it forces individuals to engage in interactions that, themselves, are stress generating. Thus, once again, social support that a person feels is present, without having to be drawn upon, is often more comforting than actual support, and even if social support is not particularly intrusive, the very process of having to acknowledge it has effects on meeting needs revolving around self-verification and fair exchanges of resources. The more social support forces individuals to manage identities or recalculate costs/investment/rewards vis-à-vis others, the more this social support will generate stress.

Individuals who are good at falling into rhythmic synchronization in interaction rituals will generally gain social support from others because positive emotions have been aroused in such encounters (Collins, 2004). Indeed, a lifetime of encounters generating positive emotions and social support lowers the accumulated stress that individuals will have experienced and, thereby, has positive effects on health because individuals will have accumulated a large reservoir of positive emotional energy to ride out temporary episodes of stress. Data clearly indicate that consistent social support generates greater interpersonal fluency, and vice versa (Kessler et al., 1992; Taylor, 2011). Moreover, individuals who have interpersonal skills are typically able to manage stress when it does arise, and from success in managing stress, they experience positive emotions toward self and a sense of efficacy, thereby further increasing their sense of well-being and healthy consequences of such well-being.

There is a very large literature in psychology on personality, health, disease, and healing (Friedman, 2011). Much of the psychological literature has searched for "personality types" and "syndromes of conditions" affecting disease, health, and self-healing, with what appear to be inconsistent results (see Kern & Friedman, 2011; Friedman & Martin, 2011). It may be that a more sociological approach can inform this literature, in several respects.

First, the interpersonal processes in encounters are critical to understanding the activation of stress. Human interaction is directed by enhanced neurological capacities that evolved from the neurology of the last common ancestor to humans and contemporary great apes. The more people can consistently fall into rhythmic synchronization, meet needs for self-verification, arouse positive emotions toward self and others, and avoid activating defense mechanisms that repress negative emotions like shame and guilt, the more likely they are to avoid stress, effectively manage it when it occurs, and thereby enjoy the sense of well-being and health effects of lives lived without great distress and the negative emotions that chronic distress inevitably arouses.

Second, from a sociological perspective, we should seek out the basic types of situations that increase the likelihood that people will be able to fall into rhythmic synchronization, arouse positive emotions, meet needs to verify self, and avoid activation of defense mechanisms. Any social structure that does not allow individuals to meet basic needs for self-verification, that causes breaches in the interpersonal flow, or that forces people to experience high levels of shame (that must be repressed) will be a tension-generating machine that causes distress and, over time, poor health. Certain types of structures are more likely to have these negative effects—those with linear systems of authority, those whose incumbents reveal cultural differences that must constantly be negotiated, and those that are subject to constant change might be one list of candidates for sociocultural stress machines. Whether these structures be families, workplaces, schools, churches, and so on, it is their underlying structure and culture that matters because these affect the underlying (and evolved) neurology of humans as they seek to meet needs for self-verification, to achieve a sense of justice and fairness in exchanges of resources, to carry off smooth interactions with others by falling into rhythmic synchronization and by arousing positive emotions, and to avoid the negative emotional effects of repression of powerful emotions like shame. Thus, rather than look for personality types, it might be better to look at a person's biography of encounters and the extent to which these encounters have facilitated activation of the evolved mechanisms in human neurology for forming positive social bonds and group solidarity.

Conclusions

I have, it appears, run out of space, but I have also extended my analysis beyond my knowledge as well. I am not an expert on health and well-being or in any significant way part of the emerging research tradition on human happiness. What I have tried to bring to the table here is some idea of what evolutionary sociology, coupled with some ideas from micro-sociology, might add to what are now vast literatures in psychology and, to a lesser extent, sociology. Stress and distress are inevitable for an animal wired to be more emotional and having to rely upon activation of complex interpersonal mechanisms to create and sustain groups. Interaction, per se, involves a certain level of low-level stress, sometimes positive stress but stress that can escalate rather dramatically when needs for self-verification, rhythmic synchronization, reciprocity, and fairness are not met and when interpersonal behaviors become breached. Each and every interaction runs these risks, and the potential for breaches from these risks is why people must work rather hard to open, sustain, and close episodes of interaction against the backdrop of few, if any, direct bioprogrammers for group formation and against powerful palates of emotions, the majority of which are biased by the preponderance of negative over positive emotions. Social bonds and solidarities are formed with positive emotions aroused when people's transaction needs are met, when their interpersonal actions enable them to avoid breaches, and when their emotional experiences do not involve shame and guilt that may have to be repressed.

The relatively small bands that were forged during hominin and human evolution allowed persons to sustain viable encounters, to meet needs, and to avoid the pitfalls of repression. Surely, such was not always the case, because conflict, murder, and executions were part of hunter-gatherer societies, but for the most part, when conflicts could not be resolved, individuals and families simply went their own way because densities of population were so low. At the peak of hunting and gathering, there were probably no more than 6.5 million people on earth compared to the 6.7 billion today. The hunting and gathering band, which organized humans for 95 percent of their time as a distinct species of ape, was not a cage; it was easy to fly the coup. As societies became more macro and complex, however, individuals became increasingly "caged" in structures from which they could not so easily escape and, moreover, to put people in structures where their needs could not always be met, where power often made interaction problematic, and where repression became more common (Maryanski & Turner, 1992). Human neurology and the emotional basis of all human interactions evolved in small and flexible groups, and perhaps it is a tribute to human adaptability that we can now organize ourselves into macro, mass societies, but it should not be surprising that problems of health and well-being accompany the new social cages in which we must live. In many ways, it is remarkable that such an emotionally charged animal, capable of self-defeating repression of powerful negative emotions and having to work hard at sustaining even basic social relations, can survive, can even prosper in large-scale societies. However, given our neurology and the history of its evolution, there would inevitably be emotional costs and consequences for well-being and health.

References

Baizer, J. S., Baker, J. F., Haas, K., & Lima, R. (2007). Neurochemical organization of the nucleus *paramedinaus dorsalis* in the human. *Brain Research*, 1176, 45–52.

Berkman, L. F. (1995). The role of social relations in health promotion. *Psychosomatic medicine*, 57, 245–254.

Bickerton, D. (2003). Symbol and structure: A comprehensive framework for language evolution. In M. S. Christianisen & S. Kirby (Eds.), *Language evolution: The states of the art.* Oxford, UK: Oxford University Press.

Bronson, S. F., & de Waal, F. B. M. (2003). Fair refusal by Capuchin monkeys. *Nature*, 511, 128–140.

Brosnan, S. F., Schiff, E. C., & de Waal, F. B. M. (2005). Tolerance for inequity may increase with social closeness in chimpanzees. *Proceedings of the Royal Society of London*, 272, 253–258.

Clark, C. (1997). *Misery loves company: Sympathy and everyday life.* Chicago: University of Chicago Press.

Collins, R. (2004). *Interaction ritual chains.* Princeton, NJ: Princeton University Press.

Cooley, C. H. (1902 [1964]). *Human nature and the social order.* New York: Schocken.

Cosmides, L. (1989). The logic of social exchange: Has natural selection shaped how humans reason? *Cognition, 31*, 187–276.

Cosmides, L., & Tooby, J. (1992). Cognitive adaptations for social exchange. In J. H. Barkow, L. Cosmides, & J. Tooby (Eds.), *The adapted mind: Evolutionary psychology and the generation of culture.* New York: Oxford University Press.

Damasio, A. R. (1994). *Descartes' error: Emotion, reason, and the human brain.* New York: G. P. Putnum.

Darwin, C. (1872). *The expression of the emotions in man and animals.* London, UK: John Murray.

deWaal, F. B. M. (1989). Food sharing and reciprocal obligations among chimpanzees. *Journal of Human Evolution, 18*, 433–459.

———. (1991). The chimpanzee's sense of social regularity and its relation to the human sense of justice. *American Behavioral Scientist, 34*, 335–349.

———. (1996). *Good natured: The origins of right and wrong in humans and other animals.* Cambridge, MA: Harvard University Press.

———. (2009). *The age of empathy: Nature's lesions for a kinder society.* New York: Three Rivers Press.

de Waal, F. B. M., & Brosnan, S. F. (2006). Simple and complex reciprocity in primates. In P. Kappeler & C. P. van Schaik (Eds.), *Cooperation in primates and humans: Mechanisms and evolution* (pp. 85–106). Berlin: Springer-Verlag.

Duchin, L. (1990). The evolution of articulate speech: Comparative anatomy of the oral cavity in Pan and Homo. *Journal of Human Evolution, 19*, 687–697.

Durkheim, É. (1893 [1947]). *The division of labor in society.* New York: Free Press.

———. (1912 [1965]). *The elementary forms of the religious life.* New York: Free Press.

Eccles, J. C. (1989). *Evolution of the brain: Creation of self.* London: Routledge.

Ekman, P. (1984). Expression and the nature of emotion. In K. Scherer & P. Edman (Eds.), *Approaches to emotion* (pp. 319–343). Hillsdale, NJ: Lawrence Erlbaum.

Emde, R. N. (1962). Level of meaning for infant emotions: a biosocial view. In W. A. Collins (Ed.), *Development of cognition, affect and social relations* (pp. 1–37). Hillsdale, NJ: Lawrence Erlbaum.

Enard, W. M., Przeworski, M., Fisher, S. E., Lai, C. S., Wiebe, V., Kitano, T., Monaco, A. P., & Pääbo, S. (2002a). Molecular evolution of FOXP2, a gene involved in speech and language. *Nature, 418*, 869–872.

Enard, W., Khaitovich, P., Klose, J., Zöllner, S., Heissig, F., Giavalisco, P., Nieselt-Struwe, K., Muchmore, E., Varki, A., Ravid, R., Doxiadis, G. M., Bontrop, R. E., & Pääbo, S. (2002b). Intra-and interspecific variation in primate gene expression patterns. *Science, 296*, 340–343.

Fisher, R. A. 1930. *The genetical theory of natural selection.* Oxford, UK: Oxford University Press.

Fleming, R., Baum, A., Gisriel, M. M., & Catchel, R. J. (1982). Mediating influences of social support on stress at Three Mile Island. *Journal of Human Stress, 8*, 14–22.

Franks, D. S. (2010). *Neurosociology.* New York: Springer.

Franks, D. S., & Turner, J. H., (Eds.). (2013). *Handbook of neurosociology.* New York: Springer.

Friedman, H. S. (2011). Personality, disease, and self-healing. In H. S. Friedman (Ed.), *The Oxford handbook of health psychology* (pp. 215–240). New York: Oxford University Press.

Friedman, H. S., & Martin, L. R. (2011). *The longevity project: Surprising discoveries for health and long life from the landmark eight-decade study.* New York: Hudson Street Press.

Gallup, G. G., Jr. (1970). Chimpanzees: Self-recognition. *Science, 167,* 88–89.

———. (1979). *Self-recognition in chimpanzees and man: A developmental and comparative perspective.* New York: Plenum.

———. (1982). Self-awareness and the emergence of mind in primates. *American Journal of Primatology, 2,* 237–248.

Gazzaniga, M. S., & Smylie, C. S. (1990). Hemisphere mechanisms controlling voluntary and spontaneous mechanisms. *Annual Review of Neurology, 13,* 536–540.

Gergely, G., & Csibra, G. (2006). Sylvia's recipe: The role of imitation and pedagogy. In N. J. Enfield & S. C. Levinson (Eds.), *The transmission of cultural knowledge.* Oxford, UK: Oxford University Press.

Geschwind, N. (1965a). Disconnection syndromes in animals and man, Part I. *Brain, 88,* 237–294.

———. (1965b). Disconnection syndromes in animals and man, Part II. *Brain, 88,* 585–644.

———. (1965c). Disconnection syndromes in animals and man. *Brain, 88,* 237–285.

———. (1970). *The Organization of language and the brain.* In Y. Grodzinsky & K. Amunts (Eds.), *Broca's Region.* Oxford, UK: Oxford University Press.

———. (1985). Implications for evolution, genetics, and clinical syndromes. In S. Glick (Ed.), *Cerebral lateralization in non-human species.* New York: Academic Press.

Geschwind, N., & Damasio, A. R. (1984). The neural basis of language. *Annual Review of Neuroscience, 7,* 127–147.

Goffman, E. (1958). *The presentation of self in everyday life.* New York: Penguin.

———. (1967). *Interaction ritual.* Garden City, NY: Anchor Books.

Hare, B., Call, J., & Tomasello, M. (2001). Do chimpanzees know what conspecifics know? *Animal Behavior, 61,* 139–59.

———. (2006). Chimpanzees deceive a human competitor by hiding. *Cognition, 101,* 495–514.

Hechter, M. (1987). *Principles of group solidarity.* Berkeley: University of California Press.

Hopcroft, R. L. (2010). *Sociology: A biosocial introduction.* Boulder, CO: Paradigm.

Horowtiz, A. C. (2003). Do chimps ape? Or apes human? Imitation and intention in humans (homo sapiens) and other animals. *Journal of Comparative Psychology, 1117,* 325–336.

Ikamoto, S., Tomonaga, M., Ishii, K., Kawai, N., Tanaka, M., & Matsuzawa T. (2002). An infant chimpanzee (pan troglodytes) follows human gaze. *Animal Cognition*, 5, 107–114.

Itakura, S. (1996). An exploratory study of gaze-monitoring in non-human primates. *Japanese Psychological Research*, 38, 174–180.

Izard, C. E. (1977 [1992]). *Human emotions*. New York: Plenum.

Kanazawa, S., & Still, M. C. (2000). Why men commit crimes. *Sociological Perspectives*, 18, 434–437.

Kern, M. L., & Friedman, H. S. (2011). Personality and differences in health and longevity. In T. Chamorro-Premuzic, A. Furnham, & S. von Stumm (Eds.), *The Wiley-Blackwell handbook of individual differences* (pp. 469–497). New York: Wiley-Blackwell.

Kessler, R. C., Kendler, K. S., Heath, A., et al. (1992). Social support, depressed mood, and adjustment to stress: A genetic epidemiologic investigation. *Journal of Personality and Social Psychology*, 62, 257–272.

Lawler, E. J., Thye, S., & Yoon, J. (2009). *Commitment in a depersonalized world*. New York: Russell-Sage.

Lenski, G. (1964). *Power and privilege: A theory of social stratification*. New York: McGraw-Hill.

———. (2005). *Ecological-evolutionary theory: Principles and applications*. Boulder, CO: Paradigm.

Leslie, K. R., Johnson-Frey, S. H., & Grafton, S. T. (2004). Functional imaging of face and hand imitation: Towards a motor theory of empathy. *Neuroimage*, 21, 601–607.

Lin, N., Ye, X., & Ensel, W. M. (1999). Social support and depressed mood: A structural analysis. *Journal of Health and Social Behavior*, 40, 344–359.

Lopreato, J., & T. Crippen. (1999). *Crisis in sociology: The need for Darwin*. New Brunswick, NJ: Transaction Press.

MacLean, P. D. (1990.) *The triune brain in evolution: Role in paleocerebral functions*. New York: Plenum Press.

———. (1993). Cerebral evolution of emotion. In M. Lewis, J. M. Haviland (Eds), *Handbook of emotions*. New York: Guilford Press.

Maryanski, A. (1986). African ape social structure: A comparative analysis. Ph.D. diss., University of California.

———. (1987). African ape social structure: Is there strength in weak ties? *Social Networks*, 9, 191–215.

———. (1992). The last ancestor: An ecological-network model on the origins of human sociality. *Advances in Human Ecology*, 2, 1–32.

———. (1993). The elementary forms of the first proto-human society: An ecological social network approach. *Advances in Human Evolution*, 2, 215–241.

———. (1995). African ape social networks: A blueprint for reconstructing early hominid social structure. In J. Steele & S. Shennan (Eds.), *Archaeology of human ancestry* (pp. 67–90). London: Routledge.

———. (1996). Was speech an evolutionary afterthought? In B. Velichikovsky & D. Rumbaugh (Eds.), *Communicating meaning: The evolution and development of language*. Mahwah, NJ: Erlbaum.

Maryanski, A., & Turner, J. H. (1992). *The social cage: Human nature and the evolution of society.* Stanford, CA: Stanford University Press.

Mead, G. H. (1934). *Mind, self, and society.* Chicago: University of Chicago Press.

Menzel, E. W. (1971). Communication about the environment in a group of young chimpanzees. *Folia Primatologica, 15,* 220–232.

Mitani, J., Watts, D., & Muller, M. N. (2002). Recent developments in the study of wild chimpanzee behavior. *Evolutionary Anthropology, 11,* 9–25.

Molm, L. D. (1997). *Coercive power in exchange.* Cambridge, UK: Cambridge University Press.

Osgood, C. E. (1966). Dimensionality of the semantic space for communication via facial expressions. *Scandinavian Journal of Psychology, 7,* 1–30.

Panksepp, J. (1982). Toward a general psychobiological theory of emotions. *Behavioral and Brain Sciences, 5,* 407–467.

Parr, L. A. (2001). Cognitive and physiological markers of emotional awareness in chimpanzees. *Animal Cognition, 4,* 223–229.

Parsons, T. (1966). *Societies: Evolutionary and comparative perspectives.* Englewood Cliffs, NJ: Prentice-Hall.

———. (1971). *The system of modern societies.* Englewood Cliffs, NJ: Prentice-Hall.

Passingham, R. E., (1982). *The human primate.* Oxford, UK: Freeman.

Plutchik, R. (1980). *Emotion: A psychoevolutionary synthesis.* New York: Harper & Row.

———. (2002). *Emotions and life: Perspectives from psychology, biology, and evolution.* Washington, DC: American Psychological Association.

Povinelli, D. J. (2000). *Folk physics for apes: The chimpanzees' theory of how the world works.* Oxford, UK: Oxford University Press.

Povinelli, D. J., & Eddy, T. J. (1997). Specificity of gaze-following in young chimpanzees. *British Journal of Developmental Psychology, 15,* 213–222.

Raghanti, M. A., Stimpson, C. D., Marcinkiewicz, J. L., Erwin, J. M., Hof, P. R., & Sherwood, C. C. (2008). Differences in cortical serotonergic innervation among humans, chimpanzees, and macaque monkeys: A comparative study. *Cerebral Cortex, 18,* 584–597.

Rilling, J. K., & Insel, T. R. (1999). The primate neocortex in comparative perspective using magnetic resonance imaging. *Journal of Human Evolution, 37,* 191–223.

Rizzolatti, G. L., Fadiga, L., Fogassi, L., & Gallese, V. (2002). From mirror neurons to imitation; Facts and speculations. In W. Pinz & A. N. Melzoff (Eds.), *The imitative mind: Development, evolution, and brain bases.* Cambridge, UK: Cambridge University Press.

Rumbaugh, D., & Savage-Rumbaugh, E. S. (1990). Chimpanzees: competencies for language and numbers. In W. Stebbins & M. Berkley (Eds.), *Comparative Perception* (Vol. 2). New York: John Wiley.

Sarason, B. R., Sarason, I. G., & Gurung, R. A. R. (1997). Close personal relationships and health outcomes: A key to the role of social support. In S. Duck (Ed.), *Handbook of personal relationships.* New York: John Wiley.

Savage-Rumbaugh, E. S., Seveik, R., & Hopkins, W. (1988). Symbolic cross-model transfer in two species. *Child Development, 59,* 617–625.

Savage-Rumbaugh, E. S., Murphy, J., Seveik, J., Brakke, K., Williams, S. L., & Rum-baugh, D. (1993). *Language comprehension in the ape and child* (Mono-graphs of the Society for Research in Child Development No. 58). Chicago: University of Chicago Press.

Savage-Rumbaugh, E. S., & Lewin, R. (1994). *Kanzi: The ape at the brink of the human mind.* New York: John Wiley.

Schmeing, J. B., Kehyayan, A., Kessler, H., Do Lam, A. T., Fell, J., Schmidt, A. C., & Axmacher, N. (2013). Can the neural basis of repression be studied in the MRI scanner? New insights from two free association paradigms. *PLoS One,* 8(4), e62358. doi: 10.1371/journal.pone.0062358.

Schütz-Bosbach, S., & Prinz, W. (2007). Prospective coding in event representation. *Cognitive Processing,* 8, 93–102.

Semendeferi, K., Lu, A., Schenker, N., & Damasio, H. (2002). Human and great apes share a large frontal cortex. *Nature Neuroscience,* 5, 272–276.

Sherwood, C. C. (2007). The evolution of neuron types and cortical histology in apes and humans. In T. M. Preuss & J. H. Kaas (Eds.), *Evolution of nervous systems 4: The evolution of primate nervous systems.* Oxford, UK: Academic Press.

Sherwood, C. C., Holloway, R. L., Erwin, J. M., Schleicher, A., Zilles, K., & Hoff, P. R. (2004). Cortical orofacial motor representation in Old World mon-keys, great apes, and humans. *Brain behavior and evolution,* 63, 82–106.

Shumaker, S. A., & Hill, D. R. (1991). Gender differences in social support and physical health. *Health Psychology,* 10, 102–111.

Spencer, H. (1874–1896 [1898]). *The principles of sociology* (3 vols.). New York: Appleton Century.

Stephan, H. (1983). Evolutionary trends in limbic structures. *Neuroscience and Biobehavioral Review,* 7, 367–374.

Stephan, H., & Andy, O. J. (1969). Quantitative comparative neuroanatomy of primates: An attempt at phylogenetic interpretation. *Annals of the New York Academy of Science,* 167, 370–387.

———. (1977). Quantitative comparison of the amygdala in insectivores and pri-mates. *Acta Antomica,* 98, 130–153.

Stephan, H., Baron, G., & Frahm, H. (1988). Comparative size of brains and brain components. In H. Steklis & J. Erwin (Eds.), *Neurosciences* (vol. 4). New York: Alan Liss.

Subiaul, F. (2007). The imitation faculty in monkeys: Evaluating its features, distri-bution, and evolution. *Journal of Anthropological Science,* 85, 35–62.

Taylor, S. E. (2011). Social support. In H. S. Friedman (Ed.), *Oxford handbook of health psychology.* Oxford, UK: Oxford University Press.

Thoits, P. A. (1995). Identity-relevant events and psychological symptoms: A cau-tionary tale. *Journal of Health and Social Behavior,* 36, 72–82.

Tomasello, M., & Call, J. (1997). *Primate cognition.* Oxford, UK: Oxford Univer-sity Press.

Tomasello, M., Hare, B., & Fogleman, T. (2001). The ontogeny of gaze following in chimpanzees, *Pan troglodytes,* and rhesus macaques, *Macaca mulatta. An-imal Behavior,* 61, 335–343.

Tomonaga, M. (1999). Attending to the others' attention in macaques' joint attention or not? *Primate Research*, 15, 425.

Turner, J. H. (1987). Toward a sociological theory of motivation. *American Sociological Review*, 52, 15–27.

———. (1996a). The evolution of emotions in humans: A Darwinian-Durkheimian analysis. *Journal for the Theory of Social Behaviour*, 26, 1–34.

———. (1996b). Cognition, emotion, and interaction in the big-brained primate. In K. M. Kwan (Ed.), *Social processes and interpersonal relations*. Greenwich, CN: JAI Press.

———. (1996c). Toward a general sociological theory of emotions. *Journal for the Theory of Social Behavior*, 29, 132–162.

———. (1997). The evolution of emotions: The nonverbal basis of human social organization. In U. Segerstrale & P. Molnar (Eds.), *Nonverbal communication: Where nature meets culture*. Hillsdale, NJ: Erlbaum.

———. (1998). The evolution of moral systems. *Critical Review*, 11, 211–232.

———. (1999). The neurology of emotions: Implications for sociological theories of interpersonal behavior. In D. Franks (Ed.), *The sociology of emotions*. Greenwich, CT: JAI Press.

———. (2000). *On the origins of human emotions: A sociological inquiry into the evolution of human affect*. Stanford, CA: Stanford University Press.

———. (2003). *Human institutions: A new theory of societal evolution*. Boulder, CO: Rowan and Littlefield.

———. (2007). *Human emotions: A sociological theory*. Oxford, UK: Routledge.

———. (2013a). The neurological basis of the evolution of human sociality. In D. Franks & J. H. Turner (Eds.), *Handbook of neurosociology*. New York: Springer.

_____. (2013b). Neurology and interpersonal behavior: The basic challenge for neurosociology. In D. Franks and J. H. Turner (Eds.), *Handbook of neurosociology*. New York: Springer.

Turner, J. H., & Maryanski, A. (1975). *Man in society: A biosocial view*. New York: Elsevier.

———. (2005). *Incest: Origins of the taboo*. Boulder, CO: Paradigm.

———. (2008). *On the origins of societies by natural selection*. Boulder, CO: Paradigm.

_____. (2015). The prospects and limitations of evolutionary theorizing in the social sciences. In J. H. Turner, R. Machalek, & A. Maryanski (Eds.), *Handbook on evolution and society: Toward a more explanatory social science*. Boulder, CO: Paradigm Press.

Wilson, E. O. (1975). *Sociobiology: The new synthesis*. Cambridge, MA: Harvard University Press.

———. (1978). *On human nature*. Cambridge, MA: Harvard University Press.

4

In Search of the Functional Neuroanatomy of Social Disturbance in Schizophrenia

Paul G. Nestor, Victoria Choate, and Ashley Shirai

DISTURBANCES IN BOTH sociality and cognition have long been considered central to the psychopathology of schizophrenia. Indeed, Kraepelin (1919), Bleuler (1924), and Kretschmer (1934) all emphasized disease-related changes in not only cognition but also in sociality, with the latter expressed primarily in a signature constellation of affective, attitudinal, and behavioral predispositions referred to as schizoid personality. Some forty years later, P. E. Meehl (1962) introduced as a latent genetic liability for schizophrenia the construct of schizotypy, a personality syndrome defined by a particular set of cognitive and social traits that was hypothesized to represent the behavioral expression of disease vulnerability. In the Meehl model, schizotypy, which reflected the configuration of cognitive slippage, interpersonal aversiveness, ambivalence, and anhedonia, originated from an inherited central nervous system integrative defect identified as "schizotaxia" (Meehl, 1962, 1975, 1989, 1990). From Meehl's influential work spawned a body of research that cast schizotypy as fundamental to understanding disease risk. Subsequent longitudinal studies used psychometric scales of psychotic proneness developed to measure various aspects of schizotypy (e.g., Chapman, Edell, & Chapman, 1980). Perhaps most striking of these studies was that of Kwapil (1998), which showed that scores on the schizotypy scale of social anhedonia specifically predicted a diagnosis of schizophrenia spectrum disorder at a ten-year follow-up evaluation.

More recently, researchers have begun to examine these disease-related changes in sociality and cognition through the lens of evolutionary neuroscience (Burns, 2004, 2006; Crespi & Badcock, 2008). From this perspective, the organizing theoretical principle is that the selective pressures driving the evolution and development of the primate brain are social rather than ecological (see Emery, 2000). The principal hypothesis undergirding these theoretical works is that schizophrenia reflects a disturbance in the development and function of the so-called social brain (Burns, 2004, 2006; Crespi & Badcock, 2008). The social brain, a term originating from comparative studies (Brothers, 1990), is hypothesized as a dominant model for understanding the evolution of cognition in primates and the attendant massive expansion in their neocortex volume. It has gained wide empirical support ranging from neuroimaging studies that have correlated increased gray matter volume with larger social networks in macaques (Sallet et al., 2011) as well experimental evidence showing that tasks of social (e.g., observational learning) but not physical (e.g., spatial memory) cognition distinguish 2.5-year old human children from their nearest primate relatives, chimpanzees and orangutans (Herrmann et al., 2007; Herrmann et al., 2010; van Schaik et al., 2012). Thus, there is growing converging evidence favoring the social brain hypothesis. That is, neither demands for "more" general intelligence, nor specific ecological and environmental challenges of greater adaptive intelligence, can fully account for why primates have such unusually large brains (Hermann et al., 2007). Rather, the answer to this evolution puzzle is that the selective pressures of social behavior drove the phylogenetic expansion of the neocortex (Humphrey, 1976; Dunbar & Schultz, 2007).

The chapter investigates the role of the social brain in schizophrenia using multiple modalities: neuropsychological, structural neuroimaging, self-report inventories, and symptom rating scales. We examine in schizophrenia the relationship of the social brain and social cognition, that is, how disease-related changes in specific brain structures may be linked to the neuropsychology and symptom expression of the illness. We focus on specific aspects of social cognition: social attention, motivational decision making, and particular positive and negative symptoms. With structural brain imaging, we explore functional neuroanatomy of social cognition in schizophrenia, focusing on magnetic resonance imaging (MRI)–generated gray matter volumes of the orbital frontal cortex, superior temporal gyrus, and fusiform gyrus, as well as the white matter fiber tract of the cingulum bundle, as assessed by diffusion tensor imaging (DTI). We begin by first briefly examining the functional neuroanatomy of the human social brain and then examine the relationship of specific brain regions with particular aspects of social cognition in schizophrenia.

Social Brain

Brothers (1990) was one of the first scientists to propose that there is a specific set of brain regions dedicated to social cognition. She identified as principal regions the amygdala, orbital frontal cortex, and temporal cortex, which together formed what she referred to as the social brain. In support of her proposal, she drew on experimental evidence pointing to social isolation in monkeys after lesions to the amygdala (Kling & Brothers, 1992) and disrupted affiliation behaviors following lesions to the orbital frontal cortex (Raleigh & Steklis, 1981). Additional support came from studies that demonstrated that recordings of neurons in the superior temporal sulcus responded to particular feature of faces, such as gaze direction and expression (Perrett et al., 1992). Subsequent functional brain imaging studies would provide new evidence for the neural basis of social cognition (e.g., Adolphs, 2003). And as Frith (2007) outlined, two additional social brain regions were identified: the medial prefrontal cortex and the adjacent anterior cingulate cortex.

In support for these areas as key social brain regions, Frith (2007) emphasized that neural imaging studies have consistently demonstrated that both medial prefrontal and paracingulate areas play a prominent role in "reading" the mental state of others. These abilities, called mentalizing, form the basis of "having a theory of mind" (Premack & Woodruff, 1978), which in turn allows for the human capacity to apprehend that behavior is caused by mental states (Frith, 2007). And as Frith also stressed, there is now strong empirical support for a "mirror system" in both monkeys and humans that serves the vital function of allowing us to grasp the intentions of others and to empathize with their emotions (see also Frith & Frith, 2010). The mirror system is hypothesized to operate via mirror neurons, which were first discovered in the inferior frontal cortex and inferior parietal cortex in macaque monkeys (Rizzolatti et al., 1996). In humans, direct evidence of mirror neurons per se has recently been provided by single-cell recordings in medial temporal and frontal cortices while subjects observed the execution of actions (Mukamel et al., 2010).

Over the past two decades, the neurochemistry of social behavior has also emerged as a rich topic of investigation. Indeed, neuropeptides of oxytocin and vasopressin have been identified as key neuromodulators of social cognition and behavior related to pair bonding, attachment, peer recognition, and social memory (Donaldson & Young, 2008; Lee et al., 2009). Ancient neuropeptides homologous to oxytocin and vasopressin date back to 700 million years ago and have been found across diverse organisms, including hydra, worms, insects, and vertebrates (Donaldson & Young, 2008). In mammals, the hypothalamus produces oxytocin and vasopressin, which are then transported to the pituitary and released into the bloodstream or projected to various brain sites (Donaldson & Young, 2008).

Converging evidence for the role of these neuropeptides in social behavior is evident in studies ranging from knockout mice to human genetics to functional neural imaging. For example, as Krueger et al. (2012) noted, mice bred without the oxytocin receptor show disrupted social behaviors in the form of aggression and mother-offspring interactions (Nishimori et al., 2008). This effect, however, can be reversed with the injection of oxytocin (Ferguson et al., 2001). In addition, the vasopressin receptor V1a subtype gene, AVPR1A, is highly polymorphic (Donaldson & Young, 2008), and one particular APVRIA variant (RS3) has been shown to be directly linked to the quality of bonding in a large sample ($n = 522$) of Swedish men, with these same results also pointing to an association of the RS3 genotype of these males to the quality of their marriages as perceived by their spouses (Walum et al., 2008). Another line of support comes from behavioral studies demonstrating that participants, after administration of intranasal oxytocin, increased their trust, as measured by money shared with another in economic exchange games (Kosfeld et al., 2005). And complementing these findings are functional neural imaging studies that have consistently shown that across different experimental paradigms, oxytocin decreases activity in the amygdala, which is known to be highly responsive to threatening or fearful stimuli (Baumgartner et al., 2008; Petrovic et al., 2008; Kirsch et al., 2005). As Donaldson and Young (2008) noted, the dampening effect of oxytocin on amygdala responsiveness to threat may aid social interaction by lowering potentially negative, anxiety-related associations.

These neuropeptides are polymorphic in their function, acting as extrinsic neurotransmitter modulators within synapses or as neurohormones altering receptors far from the point of their release (Donaldson & Young, 2008). While markedly diverse in their brain expression patterns, both oxytocin and vasopressin receptors are tightly coupled with dopaminergic receptors in the reward centers of the brain. These centers code and coordinate appetitive responses to pleasurable emotions linked to reinforcing stimuli. Pair-bonding, for example, engages the neural reward circuitry of reinforcement learning modulated by concomitant dopaminergic and neuropeptide (vasopressin and oxytocin) receptors (Donaldson & Young, 2008). As Frith and Frith (2010) pointed out, reinforcement learning via prediction error represents an all-purpose mechanism that is engaged in the processing of both social and nonsocial salient information (see also Behrens et al., 2009). These same widely distributed reward circuits begin in midbrain dopamine neurons, extending to the ventral striatum and spanning throughout the brain with key sites of amygdala, orbital frontal cortex, and anterior cingulate cortex (Behrens et al., 2009). Thus, this all-purpose mechanism of prediction error learning via reward is not specifically social but rather is critical for the development of cognition in general. It is thought to be the crucial learning mechanism for highly evolved traits of human expertise related to both sociality and abstract reasoning.

Simply put, we generate and maintain expectancies about real-world contingencies based on past experiences. And it is when our expectancies are unmet, called "prediction errors," that we learn to adjust our action and thoughts accordingly. In a recent functional MRI (fMRI) study, Behrens et al. (2008) compared fMRI activation of learning via prediction error across social and nonsocial tasks. For the social task, an informant told the subjects what their responses should be before each trial of the experiment. Thus, a subject presumably came to expect certain outcomes, based on the message received from the informant. Prediction errors occurred when the message turned out to be unexpectedly wrong (or unexpectedly right). The results indicated that prediction errors for the social task corresponded with heightened activity in the posterior temporal sulcus. By contrast, prediction errors for trials on the nonsocial task elicited greater activity in the striatum. This finding for nonsocial tasks follows a long line of research linking reward prediction to dopaminergic activity in the ventral striatum, which is thought to be significantly compromised in schizophrenia (Koch et al., 2008; Murray et al., 2008; Walter et al., 2009).

For example, in people with schizophrenia, including first-episode psychosis patients, some of whom had not been exposed to antipsychotic medication, there is strong neuroimaging evidence of reduced neural response in the ventral striatum to reward-related prediction errors (Koch et al., 2008; Murray et al., 2008; Walter et al., 2009). In addition, recent fMRI studies have pointed to an aberrant pattern of neural activity in schizophrenia marked by exaggerated responses in the right ventral striatum to expected rewards and blunted responses in the left ventral striatum to unexpected rewards (Morris et al., 2006. Moreover, increased negative symptom severity correlated with exaggerated neural activity in the ventral striatum in schizophrenia, suggesting that the disease may compromise brain responses in reward pathways (Morris et al., 2006).

This all-purpose prediction mechanism is thus central to the instrumental reward learning system of the brain. Among its most vital functions are the neural computations mediating social preference and valuation (Behrens et al., 2009). As a key system of the social brain, reward learning via prediction serves as an important neural mechanism underlying the theory of mind processes that are engaged when considering the intentions of others. As Frith and Frith (2010) emphasized, "Perhaps the most important attribute of the social brain is that it allows us to make predictions about people's actions on the basis of their mental states" (p. 671).

Research Design

In the following section, we examine recent studies from our laboratory that aimed to examine the relationship of the anatomy of the social brain in healthy controls and in persons with schizophrenia. We employed a research design in which the same subjects are assessed in two or more functional or behavioral domains thought to reflect social cognition as well as imaged in two or more anatomical regions of interest. There are two principal advantages to this research design. First, by comparing two or more measures of both function and brain regions of interest, single and double dissociations in function and anatomy can be empirically tested. Second, in this research design, each subject in effect serves as his or her own comparison for both behavioral and brain structural imaging results. The critical within-group comparisons are thus less influenced by between-group differences in factors that are known to influence neuropsychological performance in patients as well as in control subjects. As such, the likelihood is increased that observed cognitive deficits reflect, in part, underlying disease-related brain disturbance.

Our research and theoretical approach can therefore be cast within the new and burgeoning social brain sciences. To wit, neural computations of social behavior are conceptualized as carried out across networks of widely distributed brain areas (e.g., Behrens et al., 2009). Here neuroimaging techniques are directed toward elucidating functionally and anatomically connected networks of brain regions that may be involved in the myriad aspects of human sociality. The emphasis is on identifying coordinated networks of brain areas in relation to sociality; the idea of networks is important both conceptually and heuristically as it debunks the pernicious phrenology that had in the distant past haunted the search for anatomizing cognition and sociality (see, e.g., Knight, 2007). Equally important is the concept of sociality and the difficulty differentiating and quantifying its many facets. The concept is now commonly framed in reference to social cognition, which in turn is defined as a complex set of representations of internal bodily states, knowledge of self, perceptions of others, and inter-personal motivations that is supported by a widely distributed network of diverse brain regions, including the temporoparietal junction, the temporal sulcus, and the temporal poles, as well as the paracingulate cortex and the adjacent medial prefrontal cortex, extending to orbital frontal sectors (Adolphs, 2003; Amodio & Frith, 2006).

To summarize, the research design of many of our studies involves mul-timodal brain imaging. These techniques provide complementary yet dis-tinct imaging of brain anatomy, as for example, MRI gray matter volume and DTI-fractional anisotropy of white matter. The former may be viewed as an index of local neuronal assemblies and the latter as a measure of the structural highways of the brain. However, in some studies, we had avail-able only one of these measures (e.g., studies examining MRI gray matter of particular regions of the orbital frontal cortex) (Nestor et al., 2013). Yet even our research designs with only one brain imaging modality (e.g., MRI) always allowed for the comparison of the anatomy of at least two specific brain regions with neuropsychological performance on at least two distinct tasks. In other words, we specifically design our studies to test for a double dissociation between two distinct brain areas and two distinct functions. A *double dissociation,* a term dating back to the studies of Teuber (1955), is important because it provides arguably the strongest neuropsychological evidence for linking specific cognitive functions to discrete brain regions (e.g., Plaut, 1995). And thus, for the aim of this current chapter, a double dissociation framework can be used to address whether different aspects of social cognition are mediated by separable neural systems and whether these functional-anatomical relationships hold for both healthy adults and persons with schizophrenia.

Orbital Frontal Cortex, Cingulum Bundle, and Sociality

Since the iconic case of Phineas Gage (see, e.g., Damasio et al., 1994), the orbital frontal cortex (OFC) has long been thought to play an important role in social cognition. More recent neuroimaging studies have suggested that the anterior cingulate cortex (ACC) represents another key site in the social brain network (see, e.g., Eisenberger et al., 2003). For example, a prominent neuropsychological theory posits a dorsal-cognitive/ventral-emotional functional dissociation within the ACC (Bush et al., 2000). In support for this division of labor, fMRI studies have demonstrated differ-ential brain activity in dorsal but not ventral ACC for cognitive conflict, measured by tasks such as the Stroop (Botvinick et al., 2004; Carter et al.,

1998). By contrast, tasks involving social evaluation and feedback, along with related emotional processes, have revealed an opposite pattern of differential brain activity in the ventral but not dorsal ACC sector (Somerville et al., 2006; Whalen et al., 1998). For this chapter, an important question is the anatomical connectivity of the ACC to other putative social brain areas. In this regard, it is important to emphasize that the ACC projects to multiple cortical and subcortical sites, including the OFC through its major pathway, the cingulum bundle (CB), considered the most prominent white matter tract in the limbic system. Indeed, the CB furnishes both input and output to the dopamine-rich ACC and lateral and ventral medial prefrontal sites, including the OFC, as well as to the amygdala, nucleus accumbens, and medial dorsal thalamus (Goldman-Rakic, Selemon, & Schwartz, 1984; Pandya & Seltzer, 1982; Vogt, Rosene, & Pandya, 1979). The ACC thus has extensive connections, traversing through the CB, transmitting signals to multiple sites, including key multiple social brain regions, such as the OFC and the amygdala. DTI allows us to examine the microstructural white matter integrity of the CB pathway that we hypothesize plays a central role in social cognition.

Whereas the CB may represent a key structural highway connecting the social brain, the OFC is considered a central hub in this expansive neural circuitry. The OFC is among the most polymodal regions of the brain receiving multisensory inputs of taste, smell, auditory, visual, and somatosensory as well as visceral signals, due to its wide and deep connections to functionally diverse cortical and subcortical regions, including the amygdala, cingulate cortex, insula, hypothalamus, hippocampus, striatum, and its neighboring dorsolateral prefrontal cortex (Kringelbach, 2005). The OFC is located between the frontopolar gyri rostrally, the anterior perforated substance caudally, the inferior frontal gyrus laterally, and the ventromedial margin of the cerebral hemisphere medially (Duvernoy, 1999; Chiavaras & Petrides, 2000). Its anatomically heterogeneous sulcogyral morphology (Ono et al., 1990; Chiavaras & Petrides, 2000; Nakamura et al., 2007) is thought to be reflective of the rich molecular processes underlying neuronal migration, local neuronal connection, synaptic development, and lamination and formation of cytoarchitecture (Rakic, 1988; Armstrong, Myers, & Smith, 1995).

In light of such structural and functional diversity, researchers have focused on dividing the OFC into distinct subregions. Duvernoy (1999), for example, used the major orbital sulci to divide the OFC into five subregions of gyrus rectus and medial, anterior, posterior, and lateral orbital gyri. More recently, Nakamura et al. (2008), in an effort to mitigate differences arising from variability of OFC sulcogyral morphology, particularly the H-shaped sulcus (Chiavaras & Petrides, 2000), used a three-dimensional (3D) MRI region-of-interest approach to develop a reliable parcellation of the OFC into three subdivisions. Focusing on two of the most stable and reliably imaged sulci as anatomical boundaries—olfactory sulcus and lateral orbital sulcus—Nakamura et al. (2008) divided the OFC into three regions of interest: gyrus rectus, middle orbital gyrus, and lateral orbital gyrus.

We recently compared MRI gray matter contributions of the middle orbital gyrus and lateral orbital gyrus to different aspects of social cognition in a sample of healthy adults (Nestor et al., 2013). Subjects also completed a self-report measure of Machiavellian personality traits, along with psychometric tests of social comprehension and declarative episodic memory, all of which we used as proxy measures to examine various features of social cognition. The data pointed to distinct functional-anatomical relationships highlighted by strong correlations of left lateral orbital gyrus and Machiavellian scores and right middle orbital gyrus with social comprehension and declarative episodic memory. In addition, hierarchical regression analyses revealed statistical evidence of a double dissociation between Machiavellian scores and left lateral orbital gyrus, on one hand, and social comprehension with right middle orbital gyrus, on the other hand (Nestor et al., 2013).

Our findings conformed well to those of other studies that have compared the functional roles of lateral and medial OFC subregions in sociality in nonclinical samples (Elliot et al., 2000; Kringelbach, 2005; O'Doherty et al., 2001; Spitzer et al., 2007). These findings suggest that medial and lateral OFC regions can be dissociated, both functionally and anatomically. That is, as Elliot et al. (2000) suggested, the engagement of the medial OFC in reward learning may have an important role in a diversity of learning tasks of higher-order abilities ranging from those that may be described primarily as cognitive to those that extend to social domains related to understanding personal interactions and conforming to social norms. Moreover, the medial OFC has its strongest connections to the hippocampus and associated areas of the cingulate, retrosplenial, and entorhinal cortices and anterior thalamus (Mesulam, 1985; Morecraft et al., 1992; Pandya et al., 1981; Vogt & Pandya, 1987), which would also be consistent with its involvement in higher-order cognition, especially declarative episodic memory. On the other hand, while the lateral OFC also has strong connections to brain regions critical for higher-order cognition, its links to the inferior parietal lobule and dorsolateral prefrontal cortex (Goldman-Rakic, 1987; Fuster, 1997) may suggest a special role in Machiavellian personality traits related to detecting and evaluating social threats to self-interest (Spitzer et al., 2007).

And indeed, the double dissociation of functions in lateral and medial orbital frontal gyri, demonstrated in Nestor et al. (2013), suggests that each of these brain regions may make specific contributions to different aspects of social cognition. For example, Machiavellian personality items tap a broad set of social attitudes and strategies that may be described as reflecting a mixture of selfishness and opportunism. On the Mach IV questionnaire, respondents rate their degree of agreement with twenty statements, such as "It's hard to get ahead without cutting corners here and there." "The best way to deal with people is tell them what they want to hear." Here the current results suggested the left lateral orbital gyrus as a uniquely important source of the OFC contribution to variation in Machiavellian personality traits. Indeed, the results provided evidence of a rather strong and specific relationship of left lateral orbital gyrus and Machiavellian characteristics, with neither the gyrus rectus nor the middle orbital gyrus gray matter volumes contributing to Mach IV scores. By comparison, for the psychometric measures of social comprehension and declarative memory, respondents perform various mental exercises that call for judgment and reasoning about social dilemmas, or learning and remembering new information such as stories, word pairs, and names and faces of people. And here the current results suggested that gray matter volume in the right middle orbital gyrus but not the left lateral orbital gyrus accounted for a unique portion of the variance in social comprehension and declarative memory, as assessed psychometrically (Nestor et al., 2013).

The pattern emerging from these studies is one in which individual differences in left lateral orbital gyrus volume influence social attitudes embodied in Machiavellian personality traits, and variation in right middle orbital gyrus volume corresponds to information-processing abilities related to learning and memory in general as well as reasoning and judgment around social conformity. The neural processes underlying this division of OFC anatomy and social and cognitive functions are, however, unknown. Researchers have emphasized the OFC as a key site, among other regions, in support of reward learning and instrumental conditioning that includes both nonsocial and social content (e.g., Behrens et al., 2009). This may reflect that cognitive and social processes are tightly linked, coevolving to favor a host of vital specialized functional adaptations that advanced fitness by promoting effective human transactions (Duchaine, Cosmides, & Tooby, 2001). That is, from an evolutionary perspective, the mnemonic abilities related to retrieving information about status, personalities, and prior behaviors of individuals may have conferred a selective advantage for solving specific social domain problems, such as perceiving and recalling mental states in predicting the behavior of other people or remembering reputation in detecting cheaters (see, e.g., King-Casas et al., 2005; Duchaine et al., 2001; Wilson, 2007; Nowak & Highfield, 2011).

Sociality of the Orbital Frontal Cortex and Cingulum Bundle in Schizophrenia

We combined neuroimaging with neuropsychological and symptom measures for the purpose of examining the nature of the social brain in schizophrenia (Nakamura et al., 2008; Nestor et al., 2004, 2008, 2010a). We focused on the neuropsychology of motivated decision making using the Iowa Gambling Task (IGT), which has been proposed as a measure that is more closely related to social intelligence than to cognitive intelligence (Bar-On et al., 2003; Bechara et al., 1994). Moreover, converging lines of evidence from systems neuroscience (Knutson et al., 2005; Platt & Glimcher, 1999) and neurobiology (Gold & Shadlen, 2001; Schultz, 2006) have suggested that effective decision making as measured by such tasks as the IGT recruits a set of brain regions that are closely linked to those implicated in social cognition (Körding, 2007). Indeed, findings from numerous studies have converged to show that healthy decision making entails the coordinated activity of orbitofrontal and ventromedial frontal cortex, along with the amygdala for coding of the motivational salience of stimuli, the hippocampus for the formation of new memories, the anterior cingulate cortex for action monitoring and error detection, and the dorsolateral and medial prefrontal cortices for working memory and executive control (Bechara, 2005; Garavan & Stout, 2005). In motivational decisions, these neural processes work in tandem with the central nervous system (CNS) interoceptive system, particularly the insula, which serves to regulate the internal milieu or homeostasis of the organism and to monitor its dynamic physiological, cognitive, and emotional steady state (see Contreras, Ceric, & Torrealba, 2007; Bechara, 2005; Paulus, 2007). Thus, in this systems-level neuroanatomical and cognitive framework, decision making and interoceptive awareness are tightly coupled such that the impact of deciding can either sustain or take individuals into a new homeostatic state of dynamic stability (see Bechara, 2005; Damasio, 1994; Paulus, 2007).

For healthy adults, our data indicated that social decision making, as assessed by the IGT, correlated with MRI gray matter volume of the right middle orbital gyrus, with increased earnings corresponding to larger gray matter volumes (Nakamura et al., 2008). By contrast, for people with schizophrenia, our results showed no significant correlation between any of the OFC subregions and IGT performance (Nakamura et al., 2008).

However, in relation to healthy adults, persons with schizophrenia showed a bilateral reduction in the middle orbital gyrus, with smaller volumes in this subregion correlating with disease-related difficulties in social communication as reflected by increased severity of thought disturbance (Nakamura et al., 2008). Expanding on these findings, we (Nestor et al., 2008, 2010b) subsequently compared neuropsychological performance on the IGT and measures of intelligence and memory with OFC gray matter volume and factional anisotropy of CB white matter integrity. These analyses revealed a number of interesting findings. First, patient and healthy participants showed markedly different patterns of functional-anatomical correlates for CB white matter and OFC gray matter. That is, for healthy participants, OFC gray matter but not CB white matter correlated with both IGT and Wechsler Adult Intelligence Scale (WAIS-III; Wechsler, 1997) IQ measures (Nestor et al., 2010b). For patients, reduced CB white matter integrity correlated significantly with poorer scores in general intelligence as well as for the WAIS-III–derived measure of working memory. However, neither CB nor OFC measures correlated with IGT performance for the patient group (Nestor et al., 2010b). Second, for the patient group, multiple regression analysis indicated that reduced CB white matter but not reduced OFC gray matter predicted lower scores for WAIS-III measures of general intellectual abilities. Surprisingly, even though correlated with WAIS-III IQ, the IGT failed to be linked with either reduced CB white matter or with reduced OFC gray matter in the patient group. For healthy participants, OFC gray matter correlated with both WAIS-III and IGT scores, whereas CB white matter did not. Third, for the patient group only, CB white matter correlated not only with general intelligence but also with visual memory, with a particularly strong association demonstrated between better scores on a task of remembering social scenes and higher right CB fractional anisotropy (Nestor et al., 2008).

In summary, these studies provided direct, head-to-head comparisons within both patient and healthy participant groups of the neuropsychological correlates of the OFC and CB, two key areas that are thought to help form the social brain. The strikingly different pattern of correlations between patient and control groups suggested that schizophrenia may indeed alter the functional organization of the social brain (Burns, 2004, 2006; Crespi & Badcock, 2008). These alterations may be expressed as reduced white matter microstructural integrity of the CB that disrupts long-range axonal communication among widespread networks of brain regions that are vital to cognition and sociality. The disease-related CB white matter disturbance may undermine the role of the ACC in the service of processing dopaminergic "prediction error" signals originating in the striatum that are ultimately used to modify behavior in response to direct feedback (e.g., Dias, Robbins, & Roberts, 1996; Schultz, Dayan, & Montague, 1997). These accumulating and converging findings provide an empirical foundation for the development of a testable and falsifiable hypothesis for a disease-related disturbance in ACC circuitry that is evident, anatomically, by reduced CB white matter integrity; functionally, by abnormalities in prediction-error learning; and neuropsychologically, by diminished general intelligence and disrupted social cognition (see Nestor et al., 2010b).

Social Communication in Schizophrenia

Human interaction and communication is complex, reflecting the dynamic interplay of cognitive, perceptual, motivation, and neural processes that are widely distributed across the social brain. As discussed above, the social brain relies heavily on an all-purpose prediction learning mechanism to guide and direct effective interactions with the world. However, along with making predictions about future behavior on the basis of mental state, the social brain also provides the neural architecture for specialized systems for solving adaptive problems vital for social communication. From an evolutionary perspective, natural selection sculpts abilities that facilitate human social communication from more basic neural systems governing motivation and choice. From these basic functions emerge a complex array of perceptual abilities that are important for judging friend from foe and for deciding whether to approach or avoid, or to engage or withdraw. Haxby et al. (2002), for example, based on their seminal fMRI studies with healthy subjects, proposed distributed neural systems for face perception and social communication. Their model posits that the brain uses basic cues extracted from faces and eyes to access the identity and background of another person; to infer mood, intention, trustworthiness, and motives of others; to share gaze and join in a mutual focus of attention; and to enhance language comprehension (Haxby et al., 2002). These processes may constitute the basic perceptual and neural machinery of social communication, providing a veritable platform for the evolution of important forms of cooperation in domains, such as hunting, trade, warfare, and food sharing (Heinrich et al., 2006).

In schizophrenia, there can be both positive symptoms and negative symptoms, and each may differentially interfere with social communication. First let us consider the most striking and characteristic features of the disorder, the positive (psychotic) symptoms of hallucination and delusions. Hallucinations are defined as false perceptions and are experienced when, for example, patients report hearing people talking about them or hearing their voices spoken aloud (Fletcher & Frith, 2009). These kinds of abnormal perceptions can lead to faulty social inferences disrupting one's ability to communicate with others and to function in the world. In a similar vein, delusions are persistent false and irrational beliefs, often with strong persecutory, paranoid themes, as when patients report being conspired against or harassed in some way. Delusions can also be of utterly bizarre content, as in thought insertion when patients report believing that thoughts that are not their own have been inserted into their minds (Andreasen, Flaum, & Arndt, 1992). In addition to delusions and hallucinations, positive symptoms also include various features of what are referred to as formal thought disorder, such as derailment, which is defined as a pattern of speech in "which ideas slip off track onto ideas obliquely related" (Andreasen et al., 1985, p. 36). The severity of overall formal thought disorder reflects in large part the extent to which it impairs the ability to communicate (Andreasen et al., 1992).

Finally, mentally healthy people can show evidence of positive symptoms, such as delusional beliefs. Indeed, beliefs of being able to communicate with the dead may be seen as bizarre as that of a positive symptom delusion in schizophrenia. But as Fletcher and Frith (2009) pointed out, bizarre claims made by mentally healthy people differ from positive symptoms of schizophrenia on two fronts. First, they do not induce distress and may even be a source of pride or pleasure for mentally healthy people who believe they have these exceptional abilities. Second, and as Fletcher and Frith (2009) so elegantly put it in regards to the favorable social dynamics of these bizarre claims made by mentally healthy persons, in contrast to distress of psychotic symptoms in schizophrenia:

> They may promote rather than prevent social behavior, as they are accepted by a sizeable minority of people who provide each other with support. The latter distinction may be an important one: ultimately, the suffering caused by positive symptoms in patients with schizophrenia may manifest in, and arise from, social difficulties. Social conflict and isolation may be important factors that maintain delusions and modify their expression. (p. 52)

On the other hand, negative symptoms of schizophrenia are defined by the absence of normal functions and reflect diminished levels of motivation, emotional expressivity, social engagement, and social attention (Andreasen et al., 1992). For example, affective flattening or blunting represents a key set of negative symptoms, and these are characterized by unchanging facing expression, decreased spontaneous movements, and a paucity of expressive gestures, poor eye contact, affective nonresponsivity, and lack of vocal inflections (Andreasen et al., 1992). Another important domain of negative symptoms is anhedonia-asociality, rated on the basis of items dealing with recreational interests, sexual activity, ability to feel intimacy and closeness, and relationships with friends (Andreasen et al., 1992). Social inattentiveness also constitutes yet another negative symptom that indexes the degree to which a patient appears uninvolved, unengaged, or "spacey." Overall negative symptoms are notoriously resistant to pharmacological intervention, with some likely surfacing prior to illness onset and often becoming trait-like over the progression of the disease, contributing to the so-called deficit state in chronic schizophrenia. Moreover, negative and positive symptoms may reflect different underlying pathophysiological disorders (Crow, 1980; Liddle, 1987), although the basic mechanisms underlying these disturbances remain to be elucidated.

MRI studies have focused on the anatomy of two structures, the lateral fusiform gyrus (FG) and the superior temporal gyrus (STG), each of which may represent a core system for normal functioning and development of social communication abilities in schizophrenia (Nestor et al., 2007). First let us consider the FG and its role in arguably the most developed visual perceptual skills in humans, face perception. Face perception is fundamental for reading emotions and social signals in the environment (Brothers, 1990; Pinkham et al., 2003). And as Pinkham et al. (2003) noted, facial perception is considered a basic building block of social cognition, a likely first step in the social communication process. Brothers (1990) also described facial recognition as the "lower-level subprocess of social cognition." Neuropsychological studies were perhaps the first to identify a specialized neural system in the human brain for face perception. These investigations documented a condition known as prosopagnosia, characterized by a selective deficit in the ability to recognize familiar faces with relatively spared ability for object recognition. Highlighting a striking dissociation between neural systems that mediate face and object recognition, prosopagnosia is a syndrome caused by lesions in the ventral occipitotemporal cortex that are usually bilateral (Benton, 1980; Damasio et al., 1982; Sergent & Signoret, 1992), although few well-documented cases have been reported in right unilateral lesion patients (deRenzi, 1986; Landis et al., 1986). More recent neurophysiological studies have shown differential bilateral activity in the lateral FG for face perception in comparison to nonsense, control targets or to non-face objects (e.g., Halgren et al., 1999; McCarthy et al., 1997). The specific locus of this regional activity has been replicated across numerous studies so that it is now commonly referred to as the "fusiform face area" or FFA (Kanwisher et al., 1997). This region has been proposed as a neural module specialized for face perception (Kanwisher et al., 1997; McCarthy et al., 1997).

Numerous studies of patients with schizophrenia have pointed to deficits in facial processing, including both facial recognition and recognition of facial expressions. In these reports, patients were shown to perform more poorly than healthy controls on tests of facial recognition memory (Addington & Addington, 1998; Gruzelier et al., 1999; Whittaker et al., 2001). Moreover, findings of these studies have shown that these deficits in facial recognition are stable, suggesting it is trait-like, and there has also been some speculation for its role in misidentification syndromes that are sometimes observed in patients with schizophrenia (Ellis & Lewis, 2001). In addition, structural imaging studies have also investigated the FG in schizophrenia. For example, Palliere-Martinot et al. (2001) investigated gray and white matter volumes in patients with early onset schizophrenia using voxel-based morphometry. They reported significant gray matter reductions in medial frontal gyri, left insula, left parahippocampus, and left FG. Lee et al. (2002) reported bilateral reductions in MRI gray matter volume in the FG that were specific to first-episode schizophrenia in comparison to first-episode affective psychosis.

In light of these findings, several studies have investigated the relationship of FG in face processing in schizophrenia, typically using tasks varying emotional expressions. Findings from some functional imaging studies have suggested reduced FG activation abnormalities and related limbic and paralimbic regions (e.g., Gur et al., 2002; Gur et al., 2007). Other studies, however, have failed to replicate these findings (e.g., Yoon, D'Esposito, & Carter, 2006). The inconsistency of these findings may be due in large part to differences in activation tasks used across these studies as well as to the varying characteristics of the patients and samples studied (see Li et al., 2010). Moreover, in their meta-analysis of functional imaging studies and face processing of emotions in schizophrenia, Li and colleagues (2010) provided strong evidence of reduced activation not only of the FG but also of bilateral amygdala, parahippocampal gyrus, right superior frontal gyrus, and lentiform nucleus.

The most robust effect across studies reflected bilateral reductions in the amygdala (Li et al., 2010), which would be consistent with the fact that these studies mainly used different forms of facial expressions of emotions as their experimental stimuli. Only a few studies have examined FG structural-functional correlates in schizophrenia. For example, in a sample of persons with chronic schizophrenia, we demonstrated that bilateral reductions in the FG gray matter correlated with reduced scores in delayed facial recognition (Onitsuka et al., 2003). In a subsequent study of patients with schizophrenia, Onitsuka et al. (2006) examined the relationship of FG gray matter and event-related potentials elicited to images of faces, cars, and hands. These researchers were especially interested in investigating the relationship between an early occurring, face-sensitive event-related potential, N170, and FG gray matter in their sample of patients with chronic schizophrenia. Their results indicated that patients showed bilateral N170 amplitude reduction in response to images of faces but not to images of other objects, and this N170 amplitude reduction correlated with right posterior FG gray matter volume. The findings of Onitsuka et al. pointed to deficits in the early stages of face perception in schizophrenia, as reflected, functionally, by the N170 amplitude reduction and, anatomically, by smaller FG gray matter volume. This functional-structural correlation suggested that the FG is the site of a defective anatomical substrate for face processing in schizophrenia (Onitsuka et al., 2006).

Superior Temporal Gyrus and Psychosis

Along with the FG, the superior temporal gyrus (STG) may also help to form a network of brain regions important for understanding social communication disturbances in schizophrenia (Nestor et al., 2007). The STG is a relatively large long expanse of the cortex, located along the Sylvian fissure dorsally and the superior temporal sulcus ventrally. Consisting of primary and association auditory cortex (Brodmann's areas 41, 42, and 22), the STG is subdivided into several regions both structurally and functionally. Structurally, the dorsal surface of the STG, also referred to as the superior temporal plane, is situated within the Sylvian fissure, housing Heschl's gyrus, the planum temporale, and the planum polare. Laterally, the STG is positioned on the upper bank of the superior temporal sulcus (STS), which provides extensive connections to parietal, prefrontal, and superior temporal regions that are not found in the lower bank of the STS (Seltzer & Pandya, 1994). In schizophrenia, several MRI studies have reported gray matter volume reductions in the STG (e.g., Barta et al., 1990; Gur et al., 2000; Shenton et al., 1992), although there have also been other studies that have reported negative findings (e.g., Highley et al., 1999; Kulynych et al., 1996; Vita et al., 1995; Zipursky et al., 1994). In addition, McCarley et al. (2002) reported that smaller posterior STG gray matter volume correlated with a disease-related neurophysiological abnormality in the event-related potential known as P300.

Findings from functional imaging studies of healthy participants have suggested that the STG plays an important role in language comprehension. Of particular interest are findings that have demonstrated STG involvement when we correctly attribute the source of auditory stimuli, such as internal speech to our "inner voice" rather than to an external force. For example, Wise et al. (2001) showed across three separate positron emission tomography (PET) studies evidence of differential STG activity for sounds emanating from internal versus external sources. That is, their data suggested greatest activity in the temporal plane for nonspeech and speech sounds, including the sound of a speaker's own voice. By contrast, receptive or heard language, that is, speech coming from an external source, differentially engaged the lateral aspect of the STG. Thus, these results suggested an important role of the STG in answering the "where" and "what" of auditory processing: the temporal plane may support neural computations necessary for discerning the internal source of sound, in recognizing the origins, location, or from "where" an auditory stimulus may arise, whereas the lateral aspect of the STG may facilitate perception and comprehension of the spoken word or in understanding what is being said (Wise et al., 2001). Together, these neural processes may be viewed as basic mechanisms that serve as essential building blocks of social communication, allowing us to naturally and correctly perceive and attribute the source of our inner speech as emanating from within ourselves and not from an external source.

In schizophrenia, there is growing evidence that unusual perceptual experiences that are a hallmark of the psychotic symptom profile of the disease may reflect misattribution of self-generated actions, including inner speech, to others (Allen et al., 2007; Blakemore et al., 2000). For example, several (e.g., Barta et al., 1990) but again not all studies (e.g., Gur et al., 2000) have linked STG volume to various positive, psychotic symptoms in schizophrenia (see Kim et al., 2003; McCarley et al., 1999). Barta et al. (1990) first reported small left anterior STG gray matter volume correlated with heightened auditory hallucination, which other studies have also subsequently demonstrated (Flaum et al., 1995; Levitan et al., 1999; Rajarethinam et al., 2000). In addition, other studies have reported that smaller posterior STG gray matter volume correlated with increased severity of positive symptoms of formal thought disorder and delusions (Barta et al., 1997; Shenton et al., 1992; McCarley et al., 1993; Marsh et al., 1997; Mennon et al., 1995). Moreover, severity of overall positive symptoms has been correlated with smaller gray matter volumes in the left posterior STG (Nestor et al., 2007) as well as whole STG volume (Flaum et al., 1995).

Double Dissociation of Function and Anatomy

Negative symptoms and positive symptoms seem often to dissociate across groups of patients, and the foregoing studies suggest that each may reflect the consequences of different underlying pathophysiology. Thus, in Nestor et al. (2007), we compared the relative contributions of STG and FG to both neuropsychological function and symptoms within a sample of persons with schizophrenia. By examining neuroimaging (MRI), neuropsychology, and symptoms ratings within the same subjects, we aimed to parse the different facets of the well-known heterogeneous phenotype of schizophrenia and to understand better its social and cognitive consequences.

Univariate correlation analyses pointed to a pattern of association reflective of double dissociation of MRI volumes and functions. Follow-up hierarchical regression analyses provided arguably the most rigorous statistical test of our double dissociation hypothesis. And as predicted, the results from the hierarchical regression indicated two distinct dissociable brain structure-function relationships: reduced left STG volume-positive symptoms-executive attention deficits and (2) reduced left FG-negative symptoms-facial memory deficits. Thus, these data pointed to a double dissociation with volume reductions in STG and FG each contributing to distinct aspects of the schizophrenia phenotype. For example, reduced FG gray matter correlated only with poorer neuropsychological scores on a test of facial memory as well as with increased severity of negative symptoms but not with positive symptoms or neuropsychological measures of executive function. An opposite pattern emerged for STG with reduced gray matter volume, for this region correlated only with both increased severity of positive symptoms and poor neuropsychological scores on a measure of executive function but not with negative symptoms or deficits in facial memory. However, the study focused only on these two brain regions in a sample of patients with chronic schizophrenia. Future studies are needed that investigate other brain regions in addition to the STG and FG in samples of patients across different levels of severity and illness course.

Social Information Processing

Information-processing models, heralded as the "microscopes of the mind" (Massaro & Cowan, 1993), employ an array of experimental techniques that are aimed toward elucidating the fundamental operations that characterize the human mind (Posner & McLeod, 1982). More recent applications have begun to focus on what Brothers (1990) refers to as "the mental operations underlying social interactions, which include the human ability to perceive the intentions and dispositions of others" (p. 28). This social information-processing approach has spawned a number of influential experimental paradigms, including those that have examined the effect on performance of manipulating facial features, such as gaze direction, lip movement, and expression. Borrowing from prior studies (e.g., Frischen & Tipper, 2004), we recently adopted an information-processing approach to investigate social attention in schizophrenia (Nestor et al., 2010b).

In contemporary neuroscience models, attention is often divided into two general domains—facilitation and inhibition—each of which entails distinct sets of processes and operations, supported by discrete neural circuitry (Parasuraman, 1998). Within the general domain of attentional inhibition, there exists an experimentally well-established phenomenon, inhibition of return (IOR). IOR is a fundamental mechanism of human perception that biases attentional orienting to novel locations in the environment (Posner & Cohen, 1984). Behaviorally, IOR reflects slower reaction time (RT) to stimuli presented in previously cued locations. Typically in a visual IOR task, a spatial cue flashes at a peripheral location outside of central fixation, signaling an impending target. Subsequent stimuli occurring at or near the cued location are processed faster and more efficiently, but this advantage lasts for only about 300 ms following cue presentation or stimulus-onset asynchrony (SOA), after which there is a slowing of processing for stimuli appearing in the originally cued location (Posner & Cohen, 1984).

This inhibitory aftereffect reflects IOR and is thought to play a major role in healthy cognition, in general, and efficient and adaptive visual search, in particular (Klein, 2000). It prevents attention from being locked into a particular location; it protects against redundant, distracting sensory information; and it presets perception to favor novel locations for foraging and exploration over already sampled, checked, and explored sources that are likely barren. For patients with schizophrenia, normal levels of IOR for standard (Carter et al., 1992; Maruff et al., 1998) as well as for relatively long SOA intervals have been reported (Fuentes & Santiago, 1999; Fuentes et al., 1999). However, other studies have reported delayed (e.g., Huey & Wexler, 1994; Sapir et al., 2001) as well as markedly disturbed (Gouzoulis-Mayfrank et al., 2004) IOR, which has been shown to be independent of medication (Gouzoloulis-Mayfrank, Arnold, & Heekeren, 2006).

This mixed pattern of findings may suggest that visual IOR to peripheral cues is not uniformly and consistently affected by schizophrenia. If this is so, then, would patients with schizophrenia show a similar level of IOR across different types of peripheral cues? We were specifically interested in comparing the effects of nonsocial and social cues on IOR in schizophrenia (Nestor et al., 2010a). Accordingly, we employed a novel IOR paradigm developed by Frischen and Tipper (2004) that allows for within-subject comparisons of two kinds of cues, spatial (via brightening of box) and eye gaze embedded in a face stimulus to signal the location of an impending target. These eye gaze cues provided a test of social attention that could be directly compared with traditional IOR spatial cues. Indeed, eye gaze provided us with an especially salient manipulation with a strong evolutionary basis. For example, Tomasello (2006) has hypothesized that distinctive visible features of the human eye (e.g., white sclera) have evolved to aid joint attention that is a vital building block for the evolution of cooperation and collaboration. In a related vein, other researchers have emphasized the important role eye gaze direction plays in social signaling that governs our basic evolved behavioral tendencies of approach and avoidance (Adams & Kleck, 2003). We therefore reasoned that IOR abnormalities for eye gaze but not spatial cues would be consistent with recent findings failures in social attention in schizophrenia (Sasson et al., 2007). These findings are now often understood within a wider context of disease-related impairments in social motivation, communication, and interaction (e.g., Burns, 2004; Hoffman, 2007).

Our results indicated that for patients with schizophrenia, their RT performance varied as a function of cue type. For nonsocial cues, the patient group showed an IOR effect similar to that of controls. By contrast, for social, eye gaze cues, the patient group showed no evidence of IOR but rather responded faster to targets presented following a delay in previously signaled locations. The patients thus failed to show evidence of an inhibitory aftereffect only for social cues. In addition, IOR to social cues correlated significantly with symptom ratings of attention and bizarre behavior. In both instances, increased symptom severity corresponded with reduced eye gaze IOR. These correlations emerged despite rather overall low levels of severity in positive and negative symptom ratings in this sample of patients with chronic schizophrenia.

These data provide evidence linking social attention abnormalities of encoding gaze direction of human faces with differential symptom expression in schizophrenia. In a similar vein, our data showed these same abnormalities of social attention contributed strongly to neuropsychological impairment in the patient group. Hierarchical regression revealed that social attention abnormalities in this sample of patients with schizophrenia accounted for a significant portion of unique variance across neuropsychological measures of intelligence, working memory, and executive attention. Approximately 24 percent of variance in each of the neuropsychological summary measures, WAIS-II IQ, WAIS-III/Wechsler Memory Scale-III (WMS-III) Working Memory, and Trails B, could be uniquely explained by IOR to eye gaze cues. Higher levels of neuropsychological functioning corresponded with more effective use of gaze cues to guide social attention.

These findings are consistent with studies of healthy participants linking gaze perception to both basic information processes (Sasaki, Ishi, & Gyoba, 2004) and higher-order abilities of memory retrieval and visual attention (Frischen et al., 2007, Frischen & Tipper, 2004), as well as to social cognition, particularly those processes related to disambiguating expressions during face-to-face conversation (Hanna & Brennan, 2007). In addition, for schizophrenia, recent findings have shown that psychometric measures of social and nonsocial cognition each account for a significant portion of unique variance in the disease-related neuropsychological impairment (Nestor et al., 2010b).

To summarize, social attention represents a key human adaptation. As a theoretical construct, it presumably exists within a nomological net of interlocking empirical relationships with other relevant and meaningful behaviors and outcomes. The current findings indicated that, among its multiple empirical indicators, IOR to eye gaze cues may capture a key property of social attention. Indeed, in the current study, persons with schizophrenia showed abnormalities to eye gaze but not spatial cues, with the former strongly associated with disease-related neuropsychological outcomes and symptoms. Future studies are needed to provide additional evidence of construct validity of social attention, which should include measuring eye movement as well as RT along with structural and functional brain imaging.

Conclusions

In this review, we examined through the lens of evolutionary neuroscience the development and expression of schizophrenia, from its putative genetic vulnerability of schizotaxia to its full configuration of positive and negative symptoms. We adopted the perspective that the selective pressures driving the evolution and development of the primate brain are social rather than ecological. From this perspective, we articulated as our principal hypothesis that schizophrenia reflects a disturbance in the development and function of the so-called social brain, defined as a specified network of functionally and anatomically distinct cortical and subcortical regions modulated by particular extrinsic neurotransmitters, such as dopamine, and closely linked to neuropeptides of oxytocin and vasopressin. The orbital frontal cortex, medial frontal cortex, and the adjacent paracingulate cortex, as well posterior temporal sulcus, represent primary sites in the neural circuitry that forms the social brain. In addition, several other structures may play a more secondary role, such as the right parietal cortex, the insular cortex, the basal ganglia, the temporal poles, and the temporal-parietal junction located at the top of the STG. Together, these neural structures define this circumscribed set of brain regions that is dedicated to social cognition. And while functionally diverse and involved in a host of critical computations that need not be unique to social interactions, these structures play a special role in the processing of socially relevant stimuli and thus provide the essential neural architecture of social cognition.

We first reviewed evidence derived from direct head-to-head comparisons within both patient and healthy participant groups of functional correlates of two key areas of the social brain, the OFC and the CB—considered the most prominent white matter tract in the limbic system, as it furnishes both input and output to the dopamine-rich anterior cingulate cortex and lateral frontal sites, as well as to the amygdala, nucleus accumbens, and medial dorsal thalamus (Goldman-Rakic, Selemon, & Schwartz, 1984; Pandya & Seltzer, 1982; Vogt, Rosene, & Pandya, 1979). The results, which revealed a strikingly different pattern of correlations between patient and control groups, suggested to us that schizophrenia may indeed alter the functional organization of the social brain. These alterations may be expressed as reduced white matter microstructural integrity of the CB that may undermine the role of the ACC in the service of processing dopaminergic prediction error signals originating in the striatum that are ultimately used to modify behavior in response to direct feedback (e.g., Dias, Robbins, & Roberts, 1996; Schultz, Dayan, & Montague, 1997). We hypothesize that a disease-related disturbance in ACC circuitry is evident, anatomically, by reduced CB white matter integrity; functionally, by abnormalities in prediction-error learning; and neuropsychologically, by diminished general intelligence and disrupted social cognition (see Nestor et al., 2010b). We acknowledge, however, that the empirical studies that form the basis for this hypothesis are limited to relatively small samples of persons with chronic schizophrenia who have been treated with antipsychotic agents for many years. Moreover, schizophrenia is known for its heterogeneity in both expression and pathophysiology. Thus, independent replication of these findings is needed in samples of patients across different levels of severity and illness course.

Thus, in our model, the social brain relies heavily on an all-purpose prediction learning mechanism to guide and direct effective interactions with the world. However, along with making predictions about future behavior on the basis of mental state, the social brain also provides the neural architecture for specialized systems for solving adaptive problems vital for social communication. From an evolutionary perspective, natural selection sculpts abilities that facilitate human social communication from more basic neural systems governing motivation and choice. From these basic functions emerge a complex array of perceptual abilities that are important for social learning perception and judgment. These basic functions are supported by the core of a distributed neural system that is dedicated to the visual analysis of faces and housed in the occipital-temporal regions in the extrastriate visual cortex (Haxby et al., 2002). We suggest that positive and negative symptoms may be understood as reflecting disturbances in this core system, a conjecture that is supported by our findings that pointed to a double dissociation in neural structures, as measured by gray matter volumes in the FG and the STG, and function, as measured by symptoms and neuropsychology. These findings, we submit, help to delineate the social brain in schizophrenia as characterized by distinct dissociable structure-function relationships: (1) reduced left STG volume-positive symptoms-executive attention deficits and (2) reduced left FG-negative symptoms-facial memory deficits.

In conclusion, schizophrenia exacts an often debilitating cognitive and social toll on those afflicted with the disorder. As a brain disorder, it can create new and compelling experiences, unconstrained by reality, rich in emotional connotations, psychically distressing, and often socially toxic—a phenomenology perhaps unlike any other known brain disorder. The research program presented here, rooted in evolutionary neuroscience of the social brain, provides a first step toward uniting the mental and physical in studies of schizophrenia, as reflected in the integration of multimodal methods of information processing, neuropsychology, symptom ratings, and structural neural imaging.

References

Adams, R. B., Jr., & Kleck, R. E. (2003). Perceived gaze direction and the processing of facial displays of emotion. *Psychological Science, 14*(6), 644–647.

Addington, J., & Addington, D. (1998). Facial affect recognition and information processing in schizophrenia and bipolar disorder. *Schizophrenia Research, 32*(3), 171–181.

Adolphs, R. (2003). Cognitive neuroscience of human social behaviour. *Nature Reviews Neuroscience, 4*(3), 165–178.

Allen, P., Amaro, E., Fu, C. Y., Williams, S. R., Brammer, M. J., . . . McGuire, P. K. (2007). Neural correlates of the misattribution of speech in schizophrenia. *British Journal of Psychiatry, 190*(2), 162–169.

Amodio, D. M., & Frith, C. D. (2006). Meeting of minds: The medial frontal cortex and social cognition. *Nature Reviews Neuroscience, 7*(4), 268–277.

Andreasen, N. C. (1985). *Comprehensive assessment of symptoms and history (CASH)*. Iowa City, Iowa: The University of Iowa.

Andreasen, N. C., Flaum, M. C., & Arndt, S. (1992). The comprehensive assessment of symptoms and history (CASH): An instrument for assessing diagnosis and psychopathology. *Archives of General Psychiatry, 49*(8), 615–623.

Armstrong, R. A., Myers, D., & Smith, C. U. (1995). What determines the size frequency distribution of beta-amyloid (A beta) deposits in Alzheimer's disease patients? *Neuroscience Letters, 187*(1), 13–16.

Bar-On, R., Tranel D., Denburg, N. L., & Bechara A. (2003). Exploring the neurological substrate of emotional and social intelligence. *Brain, 126*(8), 1790–1800.

Barta, P. E., Pearlson, G. D., Powers, R. E., & Richards, S. S. (1990). Auditory hallucinations and smaller superior temporal gyral volume in schizophrenia. *American Journal of Psychiatry, 147*(11), 1457–1462.

Barta, P. E., Powers, R. E., Aylward, E. H., & Chase, G. A. (1997). Quantitative MRI volume changes in late onset schizophrenia and Alzheimer's disease compared to normal controls. *Psychiatry Research: Neuroimaging, 68*(2–3), 65–75.

Baumgartner, T., Heinrichs, M., Vonlanthen, A., Fischbacher, U., & Fehr, E. (2008). Oxytocin shapes the neural circuitry of trust and trust adaptation in humans. *Neuron, 58*(4), 639–650.

Bechara, A. (2005). Decision making, impulse control and loss of willpower to resist drugs: A neurocognitive perspective. *Nature Neuroscience, 8*(11), 1458–1463.

Bechara, A., Damasio, A. R., Damasio, H., & Anderson, S. W. (1994). Insensitivity to future consequences following damage to human prefrontal cortex. *Cognition, 50*(1–3), 7–15.

Behrens, T. J., Hunt, L. T., & Rushworth, M. S. (2009). The computation of social behavior. *Science, 324*(5931), 1160–1164.

Behrens, T. E. J., Hunt, L. T., Woolrich, M. W., & Rushworth, M. F. S. (2008). Associative learning of social value. *Nature, 456*(7129), 245–249.

Benton, A. (1980). The neuropsychology of facial recognition. *American Psychologist, 35*(2), 176–186.

Blakemore, S., Smith, J. J., Steel, R. R., Johnstone, E. C., & Frith, C. D. (2000). The perception of self-produced sensory stimuli in patients with auditory hallucinations and passivity experiences: Evidence for a breakdown in self-monitoring. *Psychological Medicine, 30*(5), 1131–1139.

Bleuler, E. (1924). *Textbook of psychiatry.* New York: Macmillan.

Botvinick, M. M., Cohen, J. D., & Carter, C. S. (2004). Conflict monitoring and anterior cingulate cortex: An update. *Trends in Cognitive Sciences, 8*(12), 539–546.

Brothers, L. (1990). The social brain: a project for integrating primate behavior and neurophysiology in a new domain. *Concepts in Neuroscience, 1*, 27–51.

Burns, J. (2004). An evolutionary theory of schizophrenia: Cortical connectivity, metarepresentation, and the social brain. *Behavioral and Brain Sciences, 27*(6), 831–885.

———. (2006). Psychosis: A costly by-product of social brain evolution in *Homo sapiens. Progress in Neuro-Psychopharmacology & Biological Psychiatry, 30*(5), 797–814.

Bush, G., Luu, P., & Posner, M. I. (2000). Cognitive and emotional influences in anterior cingulate cortex. *Trends in Cognitive Sciences, 4*(6), 215–222.

Carter, C. S., Braver, T. S., Barch, D. M., Botvinick, M. M., Noll, D., & Cohen, J. D. (1998). Anterior cingulate cortex, error detection, and the online monitoring of performance. *Science, 280*(5364), 747–749.

Carter, C. S., Robertson, L. C., Chaderjian, M. R., Celaya, L. J., & Nordahl, T. E. (1992). Attentional asymmetry in schizophrenia: Controlled and automatic processes. *Biological Psychiatry, 31*(9), 909–918.

Chapman, L. J., Edell, W. S., & Chapman, J. P. (1980). Physical anhedonia, perceptual aberration, and psychosis proneness. *Schizophrenia Bulletin, 6*(4), 639–653.

Chiavaras, M. M., & Petrides, M. (2000). Orbitofrontal sulci of the human and macaque monkey brain. *Journal of Comparative Neurology, 422*(1), 35–54.

Contreras, M., Ceric, F., & Torrealba, F. (2007). Inactivation of the interoceptive insula disrupts drug craving and malaise induced by lithium. *Science, 318*(5850), 655–658.

Crespi, B., & Badcock, C. (2008). Psychosis and autism as diametrical disorders of the social brain. *Behavioral and Brain Sciences, 31*(3), 241–261.

Crow, T. J. (1980). Molecular pathology of schizophrenia: More than one disease process? *British Medical Journal, 280*(6207), 66–68.

Damasio, A. (1994) *Descartes' error: Emotion, reason, and the human brain.* New York: Putnam & Sons.

Damasio, A. R., Damasio, H., & Van Hoesen, G. W. (1982). Prosopagnosia: Anatomical basis and neurobehavioral mechanism. *Neurology, 32*, 331–341.

Damasio, H., Grabowski, T., Frank, R., Galaburda, A. M., & Damasio, A. R. (1994). The return of Phineas Gage: clues about the brain from the skull of a famous patient. *Science, 264*(5162), 1102–1105.

deRenzi, E. (1986). Current issues on prosopagnosia. In H. D. Ellis, M. A. Jeeves, F. G. Newcombe, & A. Young (Eds.), *Aspects of face processing* (pp. 243–252). Dordrecht, the Netherlands: Martinus Nijhoff.

Dias, R., Robbins, T. W., & Roberts, A. C. (1996). Dissociation in prefrontal cortex of affective and attentional shifts. *Nature, 380*(6569), 69–72.

Donaldson, Z. R., & Young, L. J. (2008). Oxytocin, vasopressin, and the neurogenetics of sociality. *Science, 322*(5903), 900–904.

Duchaine, B., Cosmides, L., & Tooby, J. (2001). Evolutionary psychology and the brain. *Current Opinion in Neurobiology, 11*(2), 225–230.

Dunbar, R. I. M., & Shultz, S. (2007). Evolution in the social brain. *Science, 317*(5843), 1344–1347.

Duvernoy, H. M. (1999). *The human brain: Surface, three-dimensional sectional anatomy with MRI, and blood supply.* New York, NY: Springer, Wien.

Eisenberger, N. I., Lieberman, M. D., & Williams, K. D. (2003). Does rejection hurt? An fMRI study of social exclusion. *Science, 302*, 290–292.

Elliot, R., Dolan, R. J., & Frith, C. (2000). Dissociable functions in the medial and lateral orbitofrontal cortex: Evidence from human neuroimaging studies. *Cerebral Cortex, 10*(3), 308–317.

Ellis, H. D., & Lewis, M. B. (2001). Capgras delusion: A window on face recognition. *Trends in Cognitive Sciences, 5*(4), 149–156.

Emery, N. J. (2000). The eyes have it: The neuroethology, function, and evolution of social gaze. *Neuroscience and Biobehavioral Reviews, 24*(6), 581–604.

Ferguson, J. N., Aldag, J. M., Insel, T. R., & Young, L. J. (2001). Oxytocin in the medial amygdala is essential for social recognition in the mouse. *Journal of Neuroscience, 21*(20), 8278–8285.

Flaum, M., O'Leary, D. S., Swayze, V. W., & Miller, D. D. (1995). Symptom dimensions and brain morphology in schizophrenia and related psychotic disorders. *Journal of Psychiatric Research, 29*(4), 261–276.

Fletcher, P. C., & Frith, C. D. (2009). Perceiving is believing: A Bayesian approach to explaining the positive symptoms of schizophrenia. *Nature Reviews Neuroscience, 10*(1), 48–58.

Frischen, A., Bayliss, A. P., & Tipper, S. P. (2007). Gaze cueing of attention: Visual attention, social cognition, and individual differences. *Psychological Bulletin, 133*(4), 694–724.

Frischen, A., & Tipper, S. P. (2004). Orienting attention via observed gaze shift evokes longer-term inhibitory effects: Implications for social interactions, attention and memory. *Journal of Experimental Psychology General, 133*(4), 516–533.

Frith, C. (2007). The social brain? *Philosophical Transactions of the Royal Society B: Biological Sciences, 362*(1480), 671–678.

Frith, U., & Frith, C. (2010). The social brain: allowing humans to boldly go where no other species has been. *Philosophical Transactions of the Royal Society B: Biological Sciences, 365*(1537), 165–176.

Fuentes, L. J., & Santiago, E. (1999). Spatial and semantic inhibitory processing in schizophrenia. *Neuropsychology, 13*(2), 259–270.

Fuentes, L. J., Vivas, A. B., & Humphreys, G. W. (1999). Inhibitory mechanisms of attentional networks: Spatial and semantic inhibitory processing. *Journal of Experimental Psychology: Human Perception and Performance, 25*(4), 1114–1126.

Fuster, J. M. (1997). *The prefrontal cortex: Anatomy, physiology, and neuropsychology of the frontal lobe.* Philadelphia, PA: Lippincott-Raven.

Garavan, H., & Stout, J. C. (2005). Neurocognitive insights into substance abuse. *Trends in Cognitive Sciences, 9*(4), 195–201.

Gold, J. I., & Shadlen, M. N. (2001). Neural computations that underlie decisions about sensory stimuli. *Trends in Cognitive Sciences, 5*(1), 10–16.

Goldman-Rakic, P. S. (1987). Development of cortical circuitry and cognitive function. *Child Development, 58*(3), 601–622.

Goldman-Rakic, P. S., Selemon, L. D., & Schwartz, M. L. (1984). Dual pathways connecting the dorsolateral prefrontal cortex with the hippocampal formation and parahippocampal cortex in the rhesus monkey. *Neuroscience, 12*(3), 719–743.

Gouzoulis-Mayfrank, E., Arnold, S., & Heekeren, K. (2006). Deficient inhibition of return in schizophrenia—further evidence from an independent sample. *Progress in Neuro-Psychopharmacology & Biological Psychiatry, 30*(1), 42–49.

Gouzoulis-Mayfrank, E., Heekeren, K., Voss, T., Moerth, D., Thelen, B., & Meincke, U. (2004). Blunted inhibition of return in schizophrenia—evidence from a longitudinal study. *Progress in Neuro-Psychopharmacology & BiologicalPsychiatry, 28*(2), 389–396.

Gruzelier, J. H., Wilson, L., Liddiard, D., Peters, E., & Pusavat, L. (1999). Cognitive asymmetry patterns in schizophrenia: Active and withdrawn syndromes and sex differences as moderators. *Schizophrenia Bulletin, 25*(2), 349–362.

Gur, R. E., Loughead, J., Kohler, C. G., Elliott, M. A., Lesko, K., Ruparel, K., . . . Gur, R. C. (2007). Limbic activation associated with misidentification of fearful faces and flat affect in schizophrenia. *Archives of General Psychiatry, 64*(12), 1356–1366.

Gur, R. E., McGrath, C., Chan, R. M., Schroeder, L., Turner, T., . . . Gur, R. C. (2002). An fMRI study of facial emotion processing in patients with schizophrenia. *American Journal of Psychiatry, 159*(12), 1992–1999.

Gur, R. E., Turetsky, B. I., Cowell, P. E., Finkelman, C., Maany, V., . . . Gur, R. C. (2000). Temporolimbic volume reductions in schizophrenia.*Archives of General Psychiatry, 57*(8), 769–775.

Halgren, E., Dale, A. M., Sereno, M. I., Tootell, R. H., Marinkovic, K., & Rosen, B. R. (1999). Location of human face-selective cortex with respect to retinotopic areas. *Human Brain Mapping, 7*(1), 29–37.

Hanna, J. E., & Brennan, S. E. (2007). Speakers' eye gaze disambiguates referring expressions early during face-to-face conversation. *Journal of Memory and Language, 57*(4), 596–615.

Haxby, J. V., Hoffman, E. A., & Gobbini, M. (2002). Human neural systems for face recognition and social communication. *Biological Psychiatry, 51*(1), 59–67.

Henrich, J., McElreath, R., Barr, A., Ensminger, J., Barrett, C., . . . Ziker, J. (2006). Costly punishment across human societies. *Science, 312*(5781), 1767–1770.

Herrmann, E., Call, J., Hernández-Lloreda, M., Hare, B., & Tomasello, M. (2007). Humans have evolved specialized skills of social cognition: The cultural intelligence hypothesis. *Science, 317*(5843), 1360–1366.

Herrmann, E., Hernández-Lloreda, M., Call, J., Hare, B., & Tomasello, M. (2010). The structure of individual differences in the cognitive abilities of children and chimpanzees. *Psychological Science, 21*(1), 102–110.

Highley, J., McDonald, B., Walker, M. A., Esiri, M. M., & Crow, T. J. (1999). Schizophrenia and temporal lobe asymmetry: A post-mortem stereological study of tissue volume. *British Journal of Psychiatry, 175,* 127–134.

Hoffman, R. E. (2007). A social deafferentation hypothesis for induction of active schizophrenia. *Schizophrenia Bulletin, 33*(5), 1066–1070.

Huey, E. D., & Wexler, B. E. (1994). Abnormalities in rapid, automatic aspects of attention in schizophrenia: Blunted inhibition of return. *Schizophrenia Research, 14*(1), 57–63.

Humphrey, N. K. (1976). The social function of intellect. In P. P. G. Bateson & R. A. Hinde, (Eds.), *Growing points in ethology* (pp. 303–317). Cambridge, UK: Cambridge University Press.

Kanwisher, N., McDermott, J., & Chun, M. M. (1997). The fusiform face area: A module in human extrastriate cortex specialized for face perception. *Journal of Neuroscience, 17*(11), 4302–4311.

Kim, J., Crespo-Facorro, B., Andreasen, N. C., O'Leary, D. S., Magnotta, V., & Nopoulos, P. (2003). Morphology of the lateral superior temporal gyrus in neuroleptic naïve patients with schizophrenia: relationship to symptoms. *Schizophrenia Research, 60*(2–3), 173–181.

King-Casas, B., Tomlin, D., Anen, C., Camerer, C. F., Quartz, S. R., & Montague, P. R. (2005). Getting to know you: Reputation and trust in a two-person economic exchange. *Science, 308*(5718), 78–83.

Kirsch, P., Esslinger, C., Chen, Q., Mier, D., Lis, S., Siddhanti, S., . . . Meyer-Lindenberg, (2005). Oxytocin modulates neural circuitry for social cognition and fear in humans. *Journal of Neuroscience, 25*(49), 11489–11493.

Klein, R. M. (2000). Inhibition of return. *Trends in Cognitive Sciences, 4*(4), 138–147.

Kling, A. S., & Brothers, L. A. (1992). The amygdala and social behaviour. In J. P. Aggleton (Ed.), *The amygdala: Neurobiological aspects of emotion, memory, and mental dysfunction* (pp. 353–378). New York: Wiley-Liss.

Knight, R. T. (2007). Neural networks debunk phrenology. *Science, 316*(5831), 1578–1579.

Knutson, B., Taylor, J., Kaufman, M., Peterson, R., & Glover, G. (2005). Distributed neural representation of expected value. *Journal of Neuroscience, 25*(19), 806–4812.

Koch, K., Schachtzabel, C., Wagner, G., Reichenbach, J. R., Sauer, H., & Schlösser, R. (2008). The neural correlates of reward-related trial-and-error learning: An fMRI study with a probabilistic learning task. *Learning & Memory, 15*(10), 728–732.

Körding, K. (2007). Decision theory: What 'should' the nervous system do? *Science, 318*(5850), 606–610.

Kosfeld, M., Heinrichs, M., Zak, P. J., Fischbacher, U., & Fehr, E. (2005). Oxytocin increases trust in humans. *Nature, 435*(7042), 673–676.

Kraepelin, E. (1919). *Dementia praecox and paraphrenia* (R. M. Barclay, G. M. Robertson, Trans.). Edinburgh, Scotland: L and S Livingstone.

Kretschmer, A. A. (1934). *A text-book of medical psychology*. Oxford, England: Oxford University Press.

Kringelbach, M. L. (2005). The human orbitofrontal cortex: Linking reward to hedonic experience. *Nature Reviews Neuroscience, 6*(9), 691–702.

Krueger F., Parasuraman, R., Iyengar V., Thornburg, M., Weel, J., Lin, M., . . . Lipsky, R. (2012). Oxytocin receptor genetic variation promotes human trust behavior. *Frontiers in Human Neuroscience, 6*(4), 1–9.

Kulynych, J. J., Vladar, K., Jones, D. W., & Weinberger, D. R. (1996). Superior temporal gyrus volume in schizophrenia: A study using MRI morphometry assisted by surface rendering. *American Journal of Psychiatry, 153*(1), 50–56.

Kwapil, T. (1998). Social anhedonia as a predictor of the development of schizophrenia-spectrum disorders. *Journal of Abnormal Psychology, 107*(4), 558–565.

Landis, T., Cummings, J. L., Christen, L., Bogen, J. E., & Imhof, H. G. (1986). Are unilateral right posterior cerebral lesions sufficient to cause prosopagnosia?

Clinical and radiological findings in six additional patients. *Cortex,* 22(2), 243–252.

Lee, C. U., Shenton, M. E., Salisbury, D. F., Kasai, K., Onitsuka, T., Dickey, C. C., . . . McCarley, R. W. (2002). Fusiform gyrus volume reduction in first episode schizophrenia: A magnetic resonance imaging study. *Archives of General Psychiatry,* 59, 775–778.

Lee, H. J., Macbeth, A. H., Pagani, J. H., & Young, W. S. (2009). Oxytocin: The great facilitator of life. *Progress in Neurobiology,* 88(2), 127–151.

Levitan, C., Ward, P. B., & Catts, S. V. (1999). Superior temporal gyral volumes and laterality correlates of auditory hallucinations in schizophrenia. *Biological Psychiatry,* 46(7), 955–962.

Li, H., Chan, R. K., McAlonan, G. M., & Gong, Q. (2010). Facial emotion processing in schizophrenia: A meta-analysis of functional neuroimaging data. *Schizophrenia Bulletin,* 36(5), 1029–1039.

Liddle, P. F. (1987). The symptoms of chronic schizophrenia: A re-examination of the positive-negative dichotomy. *British Journal of Psychiatry,* 151, 145–151.

Marsh, L., Harris, D., Lim, K. O., Beal, M., Hoff, A. L., Minn, K., . . . Pfefferbaum, A. (1997). Structural magnetic resonance imaging abnormalities in men with severe chronic schizophrenia and an early age at clinical onset. *Archives of General Psychiatry,* 54(12), 1104–1112.

Maruff, P., Danckert, J. J., Pantelis, C. C., & Currie, J. J. (1998). Saccadic and attentional abnormalities in patients with schizophrenia. *Psychological Medicine,* 28(5), 1091–1100.

Massaro, D. W., & Cowan, N. (1993). Information processing models: Microscopes of the mind. *Annual Review of Psychology,* 44, 383–425.

McCarley, R. W., Salisbury, D. F., Hirayasu, Y., Yurgelun-Todd, D. A., Tohen, M., . . . Shenton, M. E. (2002). Association between smaller left posterior superior temporal gyrus volume on magnetic resonance imaging and smaller left temporal P300 amplitude in first-episode schizophrenia. *Archives of General Psychiatry,* 59(4), 321–331.

McCarley, R. W., Shenton, M. E., O'Donnell, B. F., Faux, S. F., Kikinis, R., Nestor, P. G., & Jolesz, F. A. (1993). Auditory P300 abnormalities and left posterior superior temporal gyrus volume reduction in schizophrenia. *Archives of General Psychiatry,* 50(3), 190–197.

McCarley, R. W., Wible, C. G., Frumin, M., Hirayasu, Y., Levitt, J. J., Fisher, I. A., & Shenton, M. E. (1999). MRI anatomy of schizophrenia. *Biological Psychiatry,* 45(9), 1099–1119.

McCarthy, G., Puce, A., Gore, J. C., & Allison, T. (1997). Face-specific processing in the human fusiform gyrus. *Journal of Cognitive Neuroscience,* 9(5), 605–610.

Meehl, P. E. (1962). Schizotaxia, schizotypy, schizophrenia. *American Psychologist,* 17(12), 827–838.

———. (1975). Hedonic capacity: Some conjectures. *Bulletin of the Menninger Clinic,* 39, 295–307.

———. (1989). Schizotaxia revisited. *Archives of General Psychiatry,* 46(10), 935–944.

Meehl, P. E. (1990). Toward an integrated theory of schizotaxia, schizotypy, and schizophrenia. *Journal of Personality Disorders, 4*(1), 1–99.

Mennon, R. R., Barta, P. E., Aylward, E. H., & Richards, S. S. (1995). Posterior superior temporal gyrus in schizophrenia: Grey matter changes and clinical correlates. *Schizophrenia Research, 16*(2), 127–135.

Mesulam, M. M. (1985). *Principles of behavioral and cognitive neurology.* Philadelphia: F. A. Davis.

Morecraft, R. J., Geula, C., & Mesulam, M. M. (1992). Cytoarchitecture and neural afferents of orbitofrontal cortex in the brain of the monkey. *Journal of Comparative Neurology, 323*(3), 341–358.

Morris, G., Nevet, A., Arkadir, D., Vaadia, E., & Bergman, H. (2006). Midbrain dopamine neurons encode decisions for future action. *Nature Neuroscience, 9*(8), 1057–1063.

Mukamel, R., Ekstrom, A. D., Kaplan, J., Iacoboni, M., & Fried, I. (2010). Single-neuron responses in humans during execution and observation of actions. *Current Biology, 20,* 750–756.

Murray, R., Lappin, J., & Di Forti, M. (2008). Schizophrenia: From developmental deviance to dopamine dysregulation. *European Neuropsychopharmacology, 18*(Suppl. 3), S129–S134.

Nakamura, M., Nestor, P. G., Levitt, J. J., Cohen, A. S., Kawashima, T., . . . McCarley, R. W. (2008). Orbitofrontal volume deficit in schizophrenia and thought disorder. *Brain, 31*(1), 180–195.

Nakamura, M., Nestor, P. G., McCarley, R. W., Levitt, J. J., Hsu, L., Kawashima, T., . . . Shenton, M. E. (2007). Altered orbitofrontal sulcogyral pattern in schizophrenia. *Brain, 130*(3), 693–707.

Nestor, P. G., Klein, K., Pomplun, M., Niznikiewicz, M., & McCarley, R. W. (2010a). Gaze cueing of attention in schizophrenia: Individual differences in neuropsychological functioning and symptoms. *Journal of Clinical and Experimental Neuropsychology, 32*(3), 281–288.

Nestor, P. G., Kubicki, M., Gurrera, R. J., Niznikiewicz, M., Frumin, M., McCarley, R. W., & Shenton, M. E. (2004). Neuropsychological correlates of diffusion tensor imaging in schizophrenia. *Neuropsychology, 18*(4), 629–637.

Nestor, P. G., Kubicki, M., Nakamura, M., Niznikiewicz, M., McCarley, R. W., & Shenton, M. E. (2010b). Comparing prefrontal gray and white matter contributions to intelligence and decision making in schizophrenia and healthy controls. *Neuropsychology, 24*(1), 121–129.

Nestor, P. G., Kubicki, M., Niznikiewicz, M., Gurrera, R. J., McCarley, R. W., & Shenton, M. E. (2008). Neuropsychological disturbance in schizophrenia: A diffusion tensor imaging study. *Neuropsychology, 22*(2), 246–254.

Nestor, P. G., Nakamura, M., Niznikiewicz, M., Thompson, E., Levitt, J. J., Choate, V., Shenton, M. E., & McCarley, R. W. (2013). In search of the functional neuroanatomy of sociality: MRI subdivisions of orbital frontal cortex and social cognition. *Social Cognitive and Affective Neuroscience, 8*(4), 460–467.

Nestor, P. G., Onitsuka, T., Gurrera, R. J., Niznikiewicz, M., Frumin, M., Shenton, M. E., & McCarley, R. W. (2007). Dissociable contributions of MRI volume reductions of superior temporal and fusiform gyri to symptoms and neuropsychology in schizophrenia. *Schizophrenia Research, 91*(1–3), 103–106.

Nestor, P. G., Valdman, O., Niznikiewicz, M., Spencer, K., McCarley, R. W., & Shenton, M. E. (2006). Word priming in schizophrenia: Associational and semantic influences. *Schizophrenia Research, 82*(2–3), 139–142.

Nishimori, K., Takayanagi, Y., Yoshida, M., Kasahara, Y., Young, L. J., & Kawamata, M. (2008). New aspects of oxytocin receptor function revealed by knockout mice: Socio sexual behaviour and control of energy balance. *Progress in Brain Research, 170*, 79–90.

Nowak, M. A., & Highfield, R. (2011). *Super cooperators: altruism, evolution, and why we need each other to succeed.* New York, NY: Free Press.

O'Doherty, J., Kringelbach, M. L., Rolls, E. T., Hornak, J., & Andrews, C. (2001). Abstract reward and punishment representations in the human orbitofrontal cortex. *Nature Neuroscience, 4*(1), 95–102.

Onitsuka, T., Niznikiewicz, M. A., Spencer, K. M., Frumin, M., Kuroki, N., Lucia, L. C., . . . McCarley, R. W. (2006). Functional and structural deficits in brain regions subserving face perception in schizophrenia. *American Journal of Psychiatry, 163*(3), 455–462.

Onitsuka, T., Shenton, M. E., Kasai, K., Nestor, P. G., Toner, S. K., . . . McCarley, R. W. (2003). Fusiform gyrus volume reduction and facial recognition in chronic schizophrenia. *Archives of General Psychiatry, 60*(4), 349–355.

Ono, M., Kubik, S. & Abernathy, C. D. (1990). *Atlas of the cerebral sulci.* New York, NY: Thieme Medical.

Pailliere-Martinot, M. L., Caclin, A., Artiges, E. Poline, J. B., Joliot, M., Mallet, L., . . . Martinot, J. L. (2001). Cerebral gray matter and white matter reductions and clinical correlates in patients with early onset schizophrenia. *Schizophrenia Research, 50*, 19–26.

Pandya, D. N., & Seltzer, B. (1982). Intrinsic connections and architectonics of posterior parietal cortex in the rhesus monkey. *Journal of Comparative Neurology, 204*, 196–210.

Pandya, D. N., Van Hoesen, G. W., & Mesulam, M. M. (1981). Efferent connections of the cingulate gyrus in the rhesus monkey. *Experimental Brain Research, 42*(3–4) 319–330.

Parasuraman, R. (1998). *The attentive brain.* Cambridge, MA: MIT Press.

Paulus, M. P. (2007). Decision-making dysfunctions in psychiatry—altered homeostatic processing? *Science, 318*(5850), 602–606.

Perrett, D. I., Hietanen, J. K., Oram, M. W., & Benson, P. J. (1992). Organization and functions of cells responsive to faces in the temporal cortex. In V. Bruce, A. A. Cowey, A. W. Ellis, & D. I. Perrett (Eds.), *Processing the facial image* (pp. 23–30). New York, NY: Clarendon/Oxford University Press.

Petrovic, P., Kalisch, R., Singer, T., & Dolan, R. J. (2008). Oxytocin attenuates affective evaluations of conditioned faces and amygdala activity. *Journal of Neuroscience, 28*(26), 6607–6615.

Pinkham, A. E., Penn, D. L., Perkins, D. O., & Lieberman, J. (2003). Implications for the neural basis of social cognition for the study of schizophrenia. *American Journal of Psychiatry, 160*(5), 815–824.

Platt, M. L., & Glimcher, P. W. (1999). Neural correlates of decision variables in parietal cortex. *Nature, 400*(6741), 233–238.

Plaut, D. C. (1995). Double dissociation without modularity: Evidence from connectionist neuropsychology. *Journal of Clinical and Experimental Neuropsychology, 17*(2), 291–321.

Posner, M. I., & Cohen, Y. (1984). Components of visual orienting. In H. Bouma & D. G. Bowhui (Eds.), *Attention and performance* (pp. 531–556). Hillsdale, NJ: Erlbaum.

Posner, M. I., & McLeod, P. (1982). Information processing models: in search of elementary operations. *Annual Review of Psychology, 33,* 477–514.

Premack, D., & Woodruff, G. (1978). Does the chimpanzee have a theory of mind. *Behavioral and Brain Sciences, 1*(4), 515–526.

Rajarethinam, R. P., DeQuardo, J. R., Nalepa, R., & Tandon, R. (2000). Superior temporal gyrus in schizophrenia: A volumetric magnetic resonance imaging study. *Schizophrenia Research, 41*(2), 303–312.

Rakic, P. (1988). Defects of neuronal migration and the pathogenesis of cortical malformations. *Progress in Brain Research, 73,* 15–37.

Raleigh, M. J., & Steklis, D. (1981). Effects of orbitofrontal and temporal neocortical lesions on the affiliative behavior of vervet monkeys. *Experimental Neurology, 73*(2), 378–389.

Rizzolatti, G., Fadiga, L., Gallese, V., & Fogassi, L. (1996). Premotor cortex and the recognition of motor actions. *Cognitive Brain Research, 3,* 131–141.

Sallet, J., Mars, R. B., Noonan, M. P., Andersson, J. L., O'Reilly, J. X., Jbabdi, S., . . . Rushworth, M. F. S. (2011). Social network size affects neural circuits in macaques. *Science, 334*(697), 697–700.

Sapir, A., Henik, A., Dobrusin, M., & Hochman, E. (2001). Attentional asymmetry in schizophrenia: Disengagement and inhibition of return deficits. *Neuropsychology, 15*(3), 361–370.

Sasaki, H., Ishii, H., & Gyoba, J. (2004). Effects of gaze perception on response to location or feature. *Psychologia, 47*(2), 104–112.

Sasson, N., Tsuchiya, N., Hurley, R., Couture, S. M., Penn, D. L., . . . Piven, J. (2007). Orienting to social stimuli differentiates social cognitive impairment in autism and schizophrenia. *Neuropsychologia, 45*(11), 2580–2588.

Schultz, W. (2006). Behavioral theories and the neurophysiology of reward. *Annual Review of Psychology, 57,* 87–115.

Schultz, W., Dayan, P., & Montague, P. (1997). A neural substrate of prediction and reward. *Science, 275*(5306), 1593–1599.

Seltzer, B., & Pandya, D. N. (1994). Parietal, temporal, and occipital projections to cortex of the superior temporal sulcus in the rhesus monkey: A retrograde tracer study. *Journal of Comparative Neurology, 343*(3), 445–463.

Sergent, J., & Signoret, J. (1992). Varieties of functional deficits in prosopagnosia. *Cerebral Cortex, 2*(5), 375–388.

Shenton, M. E., Kikinis, R., Jolesz, F. A., & Pollak, S. D. (1992). Abnormalities of the left temporal lobe and thought disorder in schizophrenia: A quantitative magnetic resonance imaging study. *New England Journal of Medicine, 327*(9), 604–612.

Shenton, M. E., Kikinis, R., Jolesz, F. A., Pollak, S. D., Lemay, M., . . . Mc-
Carley, R. W. (1992). Left temporal lobe abnormalities in schizophrenia and
thought disorder: A quantitative MRI study. *New England Journal of Medicine, 27,* 604–612.

Somerville, L. H., Heatherton, T. F., & Kelley, W. M. (2006). Anterior cingulate
cortex responds differentially to expectancy violation and social rejection. *Nature Neuroscience, 9*(8), 1007–1008.

Spitzer, M., Fischbacher, U., Hermberger, B., Groen, G., & Fehr, E. (2007). The
neural signature of social norm compliance. *Neuron, 56,* 185–196.

Teuber, H. L. (1955). Physiological psychology. *Annual Review of Psychology, 6,*
267–296.

Tomasello, M. (2006). Acquiring linguistic constructions. In D. Kuhn, R. S. Siegler, W.
Damon, & R. M. Lerner (Eds.), *Handbook of child psychology: Vol 2. Cogni-
tion, perception, and language* (6th ed., pp. 255–298). Hoboken, NJ: John
Wiley.

van Schaik, C. P., Isler, K., & Burkart, J. M. (2012). Explaining brain size variation: From social to cultural brain. *Trends in Cognitive Sciences, 16*(5),
277–284.

Vita, A., Dieci, M., Giobbio, G., & Caputo, A. (1995). Language and thought disorder in schizophrenia: Brain morphological correlates. *Schizophrenia Research, 15*(3), 243–251.

Vogt, B. A., & Pandya, D. N. (1987). Cingulate cortex of the rhesus monkey: II.
Cortical afferents. *Journal of Comparative Neurology, 262*(2), 271–289.

Vogt, B. A., Rosene, D. L., & Pandya, D. N. (1979). Thalamic and cortical afferents differentiate anterior from posterior cingulate cortex in the monkey.
Science, 204(4389), 205–207.

Yoon, J. H., D'Esposito, M., & Carter, C. S. (2006). Preserved function of the
fusiform face area in schizophrenia as revealed by fMRI. *Psychiatry Research:
Neuroimaging, 148*(2–3), 205–216.

Walter, H., Kammerer, H., Frasch, K., Spitzer, M., & Abler, B. (2009). Altered reward functions in patients on atypical antipsychotic medication in line with
the revised dopamine hypothesisof schizophrenia. *Psychopharmacology (Berl),
206*(1), 121–132.

Walum, H., Westberg, L., Henningsson, S., Neiderhiser, J. M., Reiss, D., Igl, W., . . .
Lichtenstein, P. (2008). Genetic variation in the vasopressin receptor 1a gene
(AVPR1A) associates with pair-bonding behavior in humans. *Proceedings of
the National Academy of Sciences of the United States of America, 105*(37),
14153–14156.

Wechsler, D. (1997). *Wechsler Adult Intelligence Scale–Third Edition.* San Antonio,
TX: The Psychological Corporation.

Whalen, P. J., Bush, G., McNally, R. J., Wilhelm, S., McInerney, S. C., Jenike, M. A., &
Rauch, S. L. (1998). The emotional counting Stroop paradigm: A functional
magnetic resonance imaging probe of the anterior cingulate affective division.
Biological Psychiatry, 44(12), 1219–1228.

Whittaker, J. F., Deakin, J. W., & Tomenson, B. B. (2001). Face processing in schizophrenia: Defining the deficit. *Psychological Medicine, 31*(3), 499–507.

Wilson, D. S. (2007). *Evolution for everyone: How Darwin's theory can change the way we think about our lives*. New York, NY: Delacorte.

Wise, R. J. S., Scott, S. K., Blank, S. C., Mummery, C. J., & Warburton, E. (2001). Identifying separate neural sub-systems within Wernicke's area. *Brain, 124*, 83–95.

Zipursky, R. B., Marsh, L., Lim, K. O., & DeMent, S. (1994). Volumetric MRI assessment of temporal lobe structures in schizophrenia. *Biological Psychiatry, 35*(8), 501–516.

5.

Social Neuroscience and Psychopathology

Identifying the Relationship between Neural Function, Social Cognition, and Social Behavior

Christine I. Hooker

SOCIAL CONTACT IS a fundamental human need, crucial for health and well-being. Indeed, the desire for social relationships is so universal that forced deprivation, such as solitary confinement, is a form of punishment worldwide, and commercial products aimed at improving relationships are a driving economic force. However, as a quick glance of self-help books will demonstrate, the desire for social relationships and the ability to develop and maintain them varies widely across individuals. Extremes on either end of the distribution indicate the risk and/or expression of mental illness. Excessive dependence on others and fear of interpersonal rejection are associated with social anxiety, depression, and borderline personality features, whereas disinterest in social relationships, lack of close friends, and deficits in social skills are associated with autism- and schizophrenia-spectrum disorders.

Social problems are especially harmful for psychiatrically vulnerable populations. Compromised social support systems expose vulnerable individuals to the negative impact of stressful life events (Horan et al., 2006; Penn et al., 2004). Social deficits can also irritate other people and exacerbate interpersonal conflict (King, 2000). The potential consequences of these negative interactions are significant since interpersonal conflicts, especially those characterized by criticism and hostility, precipitate the onset, relapse, or exacerbation of psychiatric symptoms (Hooker et al., 2014; Hooley, 2007; also see Hooley, Chapter 9, this volume).

Yet, although social relationships are central to the human experience, relatively little is known about the neural systems that support social behavior, and this limited knowledge hinders the development of interventions to improve social deficits. The complexity of social behavior—a dynamic process in which multiple social and emotional skills influence relationships over time—creates several research challenges.

This chapter is a selective review, with an emphasis on research challenges and methodological strategies, of (1) the neural systems that support social behavior; (2) how these neural systems are compromised in mental illness, particularly schizophrenia-spectrum disorders; and (3) how this information can facilitate treatment of social deficits.

The Neuroscience of Social Functioning: What Are the Challenges?

A tenet of scientific research is to isolate the process under investigation and control for all other variables; yet, social behavior is not an isolated process. Interpersonal interactions are dynamic, reciprocal, and context-dependent events in which the behavior of one individual is influenced by the other. Research on neural systems of social behavior must account for and/or examine the influence of these variables. Research must also account for potential discrepancies between social ability and social motivation. Ability is usually assessed with laboratory tests of social cognition, such as ability to accurately recognize pictures of facial expressions or identify the intentions of different people in a social scenario (see Lee, Horan, & Green, Chapter 7, this volume). However, just because someone has the capacity to understand complex mental states and interpersonal dynamics does not mean that he or she will apply those skills equally in all relationships or use those skills with prosocial intentions. So, while the laboratory offers the benefits of tightly controlled experiments, the information gained from them is limited, if it doesn't apply to real-life behavior.

Although social psychologists have sophisticated methods to measure interpersonal dynamics, the main tools of neuroscientists, such as functional magnetic resonance imaging (fMRI) and other neuroimaging techniques, have unique constraints. Participants in an fMRI experiment, for example, are squeezed into a tight horizontal tube with their head restrained and body immobilized; the room is dark, the scanner loud, and behavioral responses are often confined to a button press—five buttons at most. This is a difficult environment to identify social phenomena that are even remotely ecologically valid. Social neuroscience requires new and creative methods to connect neural function to real-life social behavior. Thus far, research in social neuroscience has focused on, and effectively established, the neural systems that are involved in core, laboratory-based skills for processing social and emotional information, such as face perception, emotion recognition, emotion regulation, and other aspects of social cognition. Moving forward will require the integration of multiple methods to capture the complexity of social behavior and offer an ecologically valid model of brain-behavior relationships.

Research on the social neuroscience of psychopathology faces additional challenges. People with severe disorders, such as schizophrenia and autism, have deficits in multiple (nonsocial) cognitive skills that can contribute to poor performance on social cognitive tasks and obscure associated neural systems. The most severe psychiatric patients may not be able to complete certain social cognition tasks at all, raising concerns about how well results generalize to the entire patient population. Alternatively, those individuals with intact cognitive skills may recruit brain regions normally dedicated to nonsocial processes to compensate for dysfunction in social systems. Cultural background, socioeconomic status, and stigma associated with mental illness can also influence social cognitive processes and associated brain mechanisms (Chiao & Mathur, 2010; Hackman et al., 2010; Krabbendam et al., 2014). Moreover, neural dysfunction can manifest in a number of ways. Hypoactivity can indicate neuropathology preventing activity or problems employing a psychological strategy that engages activity, whereas hyperactivity can indicate inefficient neural processing or additional effort (Callicott et al., 2003). These different manifestations of neural dysfunction can vary across individuals, effectively canceling out group differences when comparing individuals with and without the disorder. Failure to account for these limitations and potential confounds can lead to faulty conclusions about which brain areas are supporting a specific social behavior. Since information about neural mechanisms of social behavior is used to guide treatment development, faulty conclusions can be costly mistakes.

Several methodological strategies can be used to address these challenges. First and foremost, interpretation of brain function is greatly enhanced if neural measures are tied to behavior (i.e., variation in neural structure or function should predict variation in the target social behavior). While this sounds obvious, combining fMRI and behavioral methods effectively requires careful consideration of experimental design so that appropriate variation is elicited in each domain. One strategy is to first isolate a targeted brain function using controlled laboratory-based experiments and then investigate whether it predicts more ecologically valid measures of social behavior. The latter measures include experience sampling methods (ESMs) in which people are prompted to report on their thoughts, feelings, and behaviors at various times during the normal course of their day (Hooker et al., 2014; Hooker et al., 2010a) or video-recordings of real-life social interactions that are subsequently coded for specific social behaviors. This multimethod approach optimizes sensitivity of both neural and social measures.

A technique, often used in psychopathology research, is to manipulate or statistically control for behavioral performance on fMRI tasks in order to minimize confounds associated with different skill levels. For example, although participants with schizophrenia usually perform worse than healthy controls on social cognitive tasks, an experimenter might adjust task difficulty or require a performance criterion prior to scanning, so that both groups perform the task equally well (Manoach, 2003; Thermenos et al., 2005). Thus, hyperactivity in the schizophrenia group can be interpreted as neural inefficiency since more neural resources are required to achieve the same level of performance as controls. Another strategy to reduce confounds related to psychiatric illness is to study social neuroscience processes in individuals at risk for developing the disorder, such as first-degree relatives, or with a specific vulnerability related to the disorder, such as high levels of personality traits related to psychopathology. Examples of these strategies are described below.

The Building Blocks of Social Functioning

From a neural systems perspective, the core social and emotional processes can be grouped into four broad categories based on the network of brain regions that are preferentially recruited to support the process. (1) Social perception, the accurate perception and interpretation of social cues, including the perception of socially relevant stimuli, such as face identity, gaze direction, and communicative gestures. Neural regions involved in social perception include the fusiform gyrus, superior temporal sulcus, and the lateral occipital cortex. (2) Emotion processing, including emotional experience, expression, recognition, and learning. Neural regions involved in emotion processing include the amygdala, ventral and orbital prefrontal cortex, insula, somatosensory cortices, and subcortical structures, such as the striatum and thalamus. (3) Self-regulation, including the regulation of internal emotional states as well as the influence of social and emotional information on behavior. Neural regions involved in self-regulation include regions typically associated with cognitive control, such as the lateral prefrontal cortex (LPFC) and anterior cingulate cortex (ACC). (4) Mental state attribution, referred to as theory of mind (ToM) or mentalizing, which broadly includes the understanding and reasoning about one's own mental state and the mental states of others. Neural regions involved in ToM include the superior temporal cortex (STC), temporoparietal junction (TPJ), medial prefrontal cortex (MPFC), precuneus, and the temporal poles (see review articles: Adolphs, 2009; Barrett et al., 2007; Calder & Young, 2005; Heatherton, 2011; Lieberman, 2007; Ochsner & Gross, 2005). The social processes and associated networks listed here are neither exhaustive nor exclusive. Social behavior is psychologically complex and draws upon multiple interacting brain regions depending on the combination of psychological processes involved. Emotion regulation, for example, includes both emotion processing and self-regulation and could be listed in either category above. Other important social processes (not listed here), such as empathy, attributional style, attachment, and social dominance, involve multiple behavioral processes and neural systems. (See Lee, Horan, and Green, Chapter 7, this volume, for additional discussion on empathy and attributional style.)

Emotion Processing in Social Contexts: Role of the Amygdala

An immense body of research demonstrates that the amygdala is involved in emotional experience and emotional learning. Most data are from classical conditioning paradigms. In classical conditioning, an individual is presented with a neutral stimulus followed by a reward or punishment, and, afterward, the stimulus (i.e., the conditioned stimulus) evokes the same emotional response as the reward or punishment. For example, a neutral tone is followed by electric shock, and, afterward, the tone alone evokes fear associated with electric shock. The amygdala is active when directly experiencing rewards and punishments but is more critically involved in learning the stimulus-emotion association (i.e., learning the predictive value of the cue) (for reviews, see LaBar & Cabeza, 2006; LeDoux, 2000; Phelps, 2004, 2006).

Importantly, emotional learning can occur through direct experience with reward and punishment (as in classical conditioning) or by observing the experience of others, referred to as "observational" or "social" learning. Behavioral studies demonstrate that social learning is an effective and efficient avenue for learning about potential dangers and rewards. Children are more likely to avoid an object after observing their mother's fearful response to it and more likely to approach an object after witnessing their mother's joyful response (Campos et al., 1994). Monkeys raised in captivity with no exposure to or fear of snakes develop a fear response to snakes after observing another monkey's fearful reaction (Mineka & Cook, 1993; Mineka et al., 1984). Although classical conditioning is one of the most studied phenomena in neuroscience, there is virtually no research on the neural basis of social learning.

In a series of experiments, my colleagues and I used a classical conditioning framework to investigate the neural mechanisms of social learning and how these neural mechanisms contribute to psychopathology. Since emotional learning from direct experience with reward and punishment relies on amygdala function, our hypothesis was that emotional learning from observation also relies on amygdala function.

There were several challenges to testing this hypothesis. The amygdala is active in response to emotional facial expressions during almost any social cognitive task, including passive viewing, emotion matching, and emotion recognition (Sergerie et al., 2008). This activity appears to facilitate emotion recognition ability, since degree of amygdala correlates with emotion recognition accuracy and amygdala lesions cause emotion recognition deficits (Adolphs, 2010). However, facial expressions communicate information about another person's internal emotional state as well as emotionally relevant objects or events in the external environment. Thus, amygdala activity could reflect the attempt to learn associations between the observed emotional expression and a stimulus in the environment. Indeed, amygdala response tends to be the most robust in response to fearful expressions. One interpretation is that fear communicates a threat in the environment but not what it is or where it is. This ambiguity regarding the stimulus-emotion association is thought to drive maximal amygdala response, which increases arousal and vigilance and thereby enhances detection and processing of the environmental threat (Whalen, 1998, 2007). However, emotional facial expressions can act as a predictive cue as well as a primary reinforcement. A beautiful woman's smiling face is inherently pleasing and activates reward-processing regions (O'Doherty et al., 2003; Spreckelmeyer et al., 2009); similarly, fear and other negative expressions evoke unpleasant feelings in the observer (Hooker et al., 2014; Sergerie et al., 2008).

Identifying whether amygdala response to emotional expressions reflects activity related to emotional learning or activity related to emotional experience requires a direct comparison of learning from emotional faces to perceiving those same faces without learning. We developed a novel experiment to examine this comparison (Hooker et al., 2006). In the association learning (AL) condition, participants saw a woman's neutral face in the center of the screen with an unfamiliar (neutral) object on either side. At the beginning of the trial, a fixation cross appeared underneath one of the objects and the participant predicted whether the woman was going to have a fearful or neutral reaction to that object. Once he or she made the prediction, the woman turned to look at the object and had either a fearful or neutral reaction. In another block of trials, participants predicted whether the woman was going to have a happy or neutral reaction. Thus, participants learned the threat or reward value of a previously neutral object from the emotional expression of someone else. In the expression only (EO) condition, the woman's face appeared on the screen, but there were no objects. Participants predicted whether she would have a fearful versus neutral (or happy versus neutral) expression, but there was no association to learn. The main analysis compared the AL condition to the EO condition (see Plate 1).

Results showed that the amygdala was significantly more active when learning the emotional value (including both threat and reward value) of an object from another person's facial expression than it was to perceiving the same facial expressions (fearful and happy) when presented alone. These findings suggest that amygdala activity in response to facial expressions reflects an attempt to learn emotionally relevant (and survival-relevant) information from them.

These findings highlight an even greater need to understand the influence of social context. What, exactly, do we learn from other people? And, what characteristics of the observer, the communicator, and the environment influence what we learn and how we learn it?

Social Learning and Psychopathology

Although learning to avoid danger and approach reward is crucial for survival, an exaggerated response to perceived danger can lead to maladaptive fear, including anxiety disorders (Mineka & Ohman, 2002), and exaggerated response to reward can lead to reward-seeking behaviors, including addiction disorders (LaLumiere & Kalivas, 2007). Nonetheless, most neuroscience research on maladaptive learning is conducted within a classical conditioning framework, and the social context is rarely considered. It is well known that symptoms of certain psychiatric disorders are influenced by social learning. For example, posttraumatic stress disorder (PTSD) can develop after direct experience of fear or after witnessing the fear of someone else (Mineka & Zinbarg, 1996; Ohman & Mineka, 2001). Similarly, drug addiction can accelerate (or decelerate) depending on the amount of drug use in the person's immediate social environment (Leshner, 1997).

Personality traits, such as neuroticism, are associated with the vulnerability to develop maladaptive stimulus-reinforcement associations, particularly fear associations. Neuroticism is characterized by an increased sensitivity to punishments and a tendency to feel negative affect (John &
Srivastava, 1999). Individuals with high levels of neuroticism have a greater
risk for developing anxiety disorders (Bienvenu et al., 2007). Although it has
been proposed that increased sensitivity to punishment in people with high
neuroticism causes enhanced fear learning (Eysenck, 1967; Gray, 1982),
behavioral studies do not consistently show this pattern (Matthews &
Gilliland, 1999), and, at the point of this experiment, there was no information about the influence of neuroticism in social learning.

We tested the idea that the effect of neuroticism in maladaptive learning
is mediated by exaggerated amygdala response to fear and punishment
(Hooker et al., 2008b). This hypothesis arose from a neurodevelopmental
framework. Prior research indicates that people with the short allele of the
5-HTT polymorphism (serotonin transporter gene), compared to those
without the allele, have more amygdala activity to fearful faces (Hariri et al.,
2005; Hariri et al., 2006), higher neuroticism (Lesch et al., 1996), and
greater risk for mood and anxiety disorders (Lesch, 2007). One possibility
is that self-reported neuroticism in adolescence or adulthood (which is measured with questions like "I'm worried that the worst will happen") may
be the consequence of increased sensitivity of the amygdala in response to
negative information. And it is this neural activity, in the context of fearful
experiences, that contributes to the development of maladaptive fear.

We tested healthy adult participants with varying levels of neuroticism.
Using healthy participants who vary on a personality trait associated with
vulnerability to the disorder minimizes research confounds associated
with established illness, including medication effects, generalized cognitive
deficits, internalized stigma, and compensatory neural processes. To best
understand the relevance of social learning to anxiety disorders, we investigated each stage of social learning: acquisition of object-emotion associations, subsequent expression of learned emotional value, and enhanced
memory for emotion associated objects. We then investigated whether
these processes were modulated by neuroticism.

The experiment used a similar paradigm as before (see Plate 2). A woman's face appears on the screen with two unrecognizable objects—one on
either side. Participants predict whether she will respond fearfully or neu-
trally to the object, and they learn the emotional value of the object by
observing the woman's response. Immediately after learning, participants
performed a recognition task in which objects were presented (one at a
time), including the just learned fear object and neutral object as well as

new objects. Participants were asked, "Is this an object that was presented before?" Neural response to the objects presented alone provided the opportunity to test whether the emotion object had acquired neurally represented emotional value from the woman's emotional reaction. After scanning, participants completed a surprise memory posttest in which they viewed objects seen in the experiment and identified whether or not the object had been presented to the woman (Hooker et al., 2008b).

As expected, we found that, across all participants, the amygdala–hippocampal complex was more active when learning object-fear associations from someone else's fearful expression than it was to learning object-neutral associations from someone else's neutral expressions. After learning, the amygdala was more active to fear (vs. neutral) associated objects when these objects were presented alone. In addition, greater amygdala-hippocampal activity during fear learning predicted better long-term memory for objects with a learned association (i.e., both fear objects and neutral objects from the fear learning experiment). Moreover, higher levels of neuroticism predicted greater neural activity in the amygdala–hippocampal complex during fear (vs. neutral) learning (Hooker et al., 2008b) (see Plates 2 and 3).

These findings show that social learning has a lasting effect on an individual's response to his or her environment. Amygdala activity when observing someone else's fearful reaction "tagged" that object with emotional value, such that the object evoked an amygdala response when presented alone after learning. In addition, the degree of amygdala activity during the fear learning experience predicted memory for everything in the environment (i.e., the object associated with threat as well as the object associated with safety). This is consistent with data showing that amygdala activity during encoding of emotional stimuli, such as emotional words or pictures, predicts later memory for those stimuli (Hamann & Canli, 2004; Hamann et al., 1999) and suggests that amygdala response to emotional arousal modulates encoding and consolidation processes (LaBar & Cabeza, 2006; Phelps, 2006). Because people with high neuroticism have a higher degree of amygdala activity during learning, they may be more susceptible to developing problematic fear responses. More specifically, high amygdala activity could assign exaggerated threat value to the learned object, so that future encounters with the learned object would elicit an unnecessarily high level of fear and arousal. The learned object may also be encoded more deeply, which could contribute to longer lasting and more intrusive memories. These types of responses after a fear experience are characteristic of anxiety disorder symptoms, including those related to PTSD, simple phobia, and social phobia.

Knowing that the social context is a potential risk factor provides the opportunity for individuals to communicate their needs and vulnerabilities to partners and family members. An emotionally reactive spouse or friend can magnify the risk of maladaptive learning. Fearful reactions to small, arguably inconsequential events, such as a spider on the wall, could cause considerable distress for a person with elevated neuroticism. In extreme circumstances, like an uncontrollable natural disaster, the fearful reactions of others potentiate the fear experience and could contribute to the onset of an anxiety disorder, such as PTSD. If significant others in the social environment can reasonably contain their fear reactions, it could reduce the risk of maladaptive learning.

Self-Regulation

Self-regulation, including the regulation of emotion and behavior, is achieved through a variety of strategies that use cognitive skills, such as attention and inhibition, to control emotional experience and behavioral reactions (Brown et al., 2006; Ochsner & Gross, 2005). Stressful events, including interpersonal conflicts and other social stressors, provoke negative affect and require recruitment of regulatory skills to cope effectively. Failure to regulate emotion after a stressful event results in persistent negative mood and potentially self-destructive responses, such as rumination or substance use, which can trigger a downward spiral and ultimately impair functioning (Ayduk et al., 2001; Li & Sinha, 2008; Nolen-Hoeksema, 2000). Poor self-regulation is not only a common problem in psychiatric disorders but also a primary cause of symptom exacerbation after stressful event (Hooley, 2007; Monroe et al., 2001; Muscatell et al., 2009).

Effective self-regulation relies on a network of neural regions, including the lateral prefrontal cortex (LPFC), that support cognitive control and related processes (Ochsner & Gross, 2005). The LPFC, particularly the ventral portion (VLPFC), facilitates emotion regulation by, automatically or effortfully, engaging strategies that employ cognitive skills, such as attentional control and reappraisal, to control the influence of emotional information on subjective experience (Lieberman, 2007; Ochsner & Gross, 2005). The reappraisal task is a common experimental measure of emotion regulation (Ochsner et al., 2002), frequently used with psychiatric populations (Modinos et al., 2010). While undergoing fMRI, participants view pictures of negative scenes and are instructed to either reappraise (i.e., reevaluate or reinterpret) the scene to decrease their negative affect or view the scene without attempting to regulate emotional response. The LPFC is more active during reappraisal than passive viewing, and greater LPFC is related to less amygdala activity as well as less distress from the negative picture, suggesting that LPFC activity controls the experience of negative affect by inhibiting amygdala response (Ochsner et al., 2002; Ochsner et al., 2004).

A limitation of this and similar approaches is that emotion regulation is treated as an isolated experience, removed from social context. In addition, the negative stimuli used to provoke negative affect are used as a proxy for a real-life affective challenge, and it is assumed that behavioral and neural responses observed in the scanner represent what they would do in real life. This is a shaky assumption, since the experimental context is a highly structured environment in which participants are instructed to regulate their emotion and given a strategy to do it. Just because an individual is capable of employing LPFC-mediated regulatory strategies does not mean that he or she will do so in daily life.

To address these limitations, my colleagues and I used a combination of fMRI and experience sampling methods to test whether LPFC control-related functions predicted the ability to regulate emotion and behavior after an interpersonal conflict with a romantic partner (Hooker et al., 2010a). Couples in a committed relationships participated in an fMRI experiment in which they viewed pictures of their partner displaying interpersonally relevant positive (e.g., happy, caring), negative (e.g., angry, disappointed), and neutral expressions. Viewing the partner's negative expression was the affective challenge meant to elicit control-related LPFC activity. There were no instructions to regulate emotional response with the idea that a person's natural tendency to regulate in the scanner would be the best predictor of regulation in real life. After the scan, participants completed an online daily diary in which, each evening for twenty-one days, they reported whether or not they had a conflict with their partner and rated the extent to which they felt positive and negative mood, as well as engaged in rumination and substance use.

Measuring mood and behavior each day is more accurate than most social functioning assessments that rely on retrospective accounts over weeks or months. And, the repeated assessments over twenty-one days provides the opportunity to investigate day-to-day changes—specifically, whether an interpersonal conflict on one day caused an increase in negative mood and maladaptive behaviors the next day.

Results showed that LPFC activity to a partner's negative (vs. neutral) expression predicted ability to recover from an interpersonal conflict with that person. Although everyone had a more negative mood the day of the conflict, LPFC activity significantly predicted mood and behavior the day after the conflict, such that people with low LPFC activity to their partner's negative expression had higher levels of negative mood, destructive thought patterns (rumination), and substance use (see Plate 4).

Interestingly, LPFC activity to positive (vs. neutral) expressions also predicted emotion regulation after conflict. Specifically, VLPFC activity to positive expressions was related to upregulation of positive mood (e.g., happy, accepted, supported) but not downregulation of negative mood (e.g., sad, disappointed, angry) after conflict. These findings suggest that LPFC recruitment when processing positive social signals is a valence-specific trait that predicts regulation of positive emotion in interpersonal contexts.

The results, overall, have important implications for psychopathology as they suggest that LPFC deficits could be a vulnerability factor that interacts with social stressors to predict mood and behavior problems (Hooker et al., 2010a).

Self-Regulation and Psychopathology

Social stress is a well-known risk factor for the onset and relapse of psychiatric disorders, including major depressive disorder, schizophrenia, borderline personality disorder, and others. Deficits in LPFC regulatory functions are also common to these disorders and may be a vulnerability factor for the exacerbation of symptoms from interpersonal conflict and other social stressors (see Hooley, Chapter 9, this volume, for additional discussion).

Although most emotion regulation research in basic science and psychiatry has focused on the downregulation of negative emotion, research on the upregulation of positive emotion is also important. Individuals at risk for or suffering from schizophrenia-spectrum disorders have behavioral deficits in the experience, expression, and regulation of positive emotion (Kring & Elis, 2013). Social anhedonia (SA), defined as diminished pleasure from social relationships, is a personality trait associated with schizophrenia-spectrum pathology. SA is present prior to the onset of psychosis, persists despite antipsychotic treatment, and contributes to functional disability (Blanchard et al., 1998; Horan et al., 2008). Abnormally high SA is evident in first-degree relatives of people with schizophrenia (Laurent et al., 2000; Schurhoff et al., 2003) and, in young adults, prospectively predicts schizophrenia-spectrum disorders five to ten years later (Gooding et al., 2005; Gooding et al., 2007; Kwapil, 1998). Combined with irrefutable evidence of LPFC dysfunction in schizophrenia liability and illness (Barch, 2005; MacDonald et al., 2009), the data indicate that SA may be caused by LPFC deficits upregulating positive emotion from social relationships.

We used fMRI and daily diary methods (similar to the couples study described above) to test whether healthy adults with high SA had reduced LPFC activity to positive social signals and, if so, whether these LPFC deficits predicted daily ratings of mood and schizophrenia-spectrum symptoms as well as the exacerbation of mood and symptoms after an interpersonal conflict (Hooker et al., 2014).

During fMRI, participants viewed videos of interpersonally relevant positive, negative, and neutral facial expressions. After the scan, in an online daily diary, they rated the severity of schizophrenia-spectrum symptoms every evening for twenty-one days. Results showed that, compared to low SA, high SA participants had less VLPFC activity to positive versus neutral expressions. Analysis with the daily diary ratings revealed that the interaction of SA and VLPFC activity to positive expressions predicted the daily experience of schizophrenia-spectrum symptoms. Specifically, participants with both high SA and low VLPFC activity had worse cognition, paranoia, psychomotor retardation, and motivation. In addition, among high SA participants, VLPFC activity predicted the daily relationship between conflict distress and paranoia. High SA participants with low VLPFC activity had worse paranoia on days of high-conflict distress compared to days of low-conflict distress.

These findings indicate that SA, as measured by behavioral reports of diminished pleasure from social relationships, is related to reduced VLPFC engagement when processing positive social signals, and among high SA individuals, those with lower VLPFC engagement are especially susceptible to the negative impact of interpersonal conflict. Moreover, even though people can experience high SA for multiple reasons, including social rejection or medication side effects, our results indicate that the combination of high SA and low LPFC function may be specifically related to schizophrenia-spectrum pathology and a possible marker of psychosis-vulnerability.

Theory of Mind, Simulation, and Empathy

"Theory of mind" (ToM)—also known as "mental state attribution" or "mentalizing"—is the ability to infer the mental states of others, including their beliefs, goals, intentions, and emotions, and the understanding of how those mental states motivate behavior (Frith & Frith, 2006a, 2006b; Saxe et al., 2004). Mental states can be inferred through "mental state decoding"—which involves decoding observable nonverbal social cues (e.g., facial expressions, gaze direction, and body posture), as well as "mental state reasoning," which involves integrating information from multiple sources and engaging in high-level reasoning about mental states and how they influence a person's actions and reactions (Baron-Cohen, 1995; Frith & Frith, 2005; Saxe, 2005). These ToM skills contribute to empathy, particularly the cognitive component of empathy (Shamay-Tsoory et al., 2003; Shamay-Tsoory et al., 2005), and help deepen interpersonal relationships (see Lee, Horan, and Green, Chapter 7, this volume, for further discussion of mental state attribution and different facets of empathy).

ToM processing, especially mental state reasoning, recruits a network of regions, including both dorsal (D) and ventral (V) MPFC, as well as the TPJ, STS, posterior cingulate, and precuneus. This neural system supports multiple psychological processes that facilitate ToM skills. A main process is *simulation*—which involves using one's own experience as a basis for inferring the experience of others. Simulation includes both automatic and effortful processes. An example of effortful simulation is when an individual tries to understand another person's experience by consciously imagining (or "simulating") how he or she would feel or behave in the same situation. This often involves remembering a similar experience of his or her own and using this as a reference for understanding the other person. Evidence suggests that the MPFC, particularly the VMPFC, supports simulation through self-referential processing, which includes integrating information about the self, constructing self-identity, and facilitating the comparison between self and others (Amodio & Frith, 2006; Rudebeck et al., 2008; van der Meer et al., 2010).

"Mirroring" the actions and emotions of others is a form of automatic simulation that is supported by the mirror neuron system. The mirror neuron system includes the ventral premotor cortex and inferior parietal lobe and spans both primary and secondary motor and somatosensory cortices (Gallese & Goldman, 1998; Gallese et al., 2004). Data show that observing another person's action activates the neural region associated with the execution of that action. For example, observing someone else waving his or her hand activates the *observer's* hand region of the motor cortex (Iacoboni et al., 2005). This mirror neuron activity generates an internal representation of the other person's action, which facilitates an understanding of that person's goals and intentions (Gallese, 2007; Gallese et al., 2004; Hooker et al., 2008a; Hooker et al., 2010b; Keysers & Gazzola, 2007; Keysers et al., 2004).

Theory of Mind and Psychopathology

Several neurological and psychological disorders have deficits in ToM, particularly mental state reasoning, as well as structural and functional abnormalities in brain regions supporting ToM. These disorders include autism, schizophrenia, and frontotemporal dementia, and for all of these disorders, deficits in ToM skills are related to poor interpersonal relationships and compromised quality of life (Baron-Cohen, 1995; Brune, 2005; Snowden et al., 2003). However, each of these disorders is also associated with severe cognitive deficits, such as attention and memory deficits, making it difficult to identify the specific neural problem associated with ToM deficits and associated social difficulties.

ToM deficits are a major cause of social dysfunction in schizophrenia, yet identifying the neural basis of ToM deficits, separate from the confounding influence of general cognitive deficits associated with schizophrenia, is especially difficult. Individuals with schizophrenia have poor behavioral performance on advanced ToM tasks, such as recognizing a social faux pas (Bora et al., 2009). These impairments are observable prior to illness onset, remain when psychotic symptoms are remitted (Pickup, 2006), and predict social functioning, even when controlling for the influence of general cognition (Couture et al., 2006; Pijnenborg et al., 2009; Roncone et al., 2002). Thus, revealing specific neural mechanisms contributing to ToM difficulties may help identify a neurocognitive processes for which remediation and treatment could have functional benefits.

We conducted a study to identify a potential relationship between VMPFC abnormalities and ToM ability (Hooker et al., 2011). VMPFC functions are crucial for mental state reasoning and cognitive empathy (Shamay-Tsoory, 2011; Shamay-Tsoory & Aharon-Peretz, 2007). Schizophrenia is associated with both structural and functional abnormalities in the VMPFC (Honea et al., 2005; Williams, 2008). However, previous research on the relationship between VMPFC dysfunction and ToM ability in schizophrenia has produced conflicting results. Although several ToM studies demonstrate the predicted pattern of less activity in the VMPFC and other ToM regions in schizophrenia versus healthy participants (Brunet et al., 2003), other studies report that schizophrenia participants have abnormally high activity in ToM regions or recruit non-ToM regions to complete the ToM task (Benedetti et al., 2009; Marjoram et al., 2006).

These findings highlight methodological challenges of using fMRI to investigate a social cognitive skill that is difficult for people with schizophrenia. Task-related neural activity is hard to interpret—hypoactivity can reflect lack of attention and hyperactivity can reflect additional effort (Callicott et al., 2000; Callicott et al., 2003). Furthermore, performance-based ToM tasks may not provide the most ecologically valid and clinically useful assessment, since they do not account for the motivation or success in using these skills to enhance social relationships. The day-to-day use of ToM skills may be better evaluated with self-report, experience sampling, observation, or interview-based functional assessments.

We addressed these methodological challenges by investigating the relationship between neural structure, specifically gray matter volume (GMV), and three different behavioral assessments of ToM processing. ToM measures included (1) behavioral performance on an advanced ToM task in which participants read a short social vignette and identified whether or not a character in the story made a social faux pas, (2) self-reported tendency to engage in perspective taking (e.g., "Before criticizing somebody, I try to imagine how *I* would feel if I were in their place"), and (3) an interview-based assessment of the capacity and tendency to consider the perspectives and emotions of other people, such as family and friends, in their real-life relationships. Each measure assesses the ability to integrate both cognitive and affective components of ToM processing in the service of understanding others. Using three different behavioral methods provides converging evidence that the observed relationship between brain structure and behavioral assessment reflects the true relationship between brain structure and ToM processing—that is, the core construct under investigation—and not an epiphenomenon of the assessment method.

Indeed, we found that among schizophrenia patients, three different measures of advanced ToM skills were significantly related to VMPFC GMV (see Plate 5). In addition, when controlling for general cognition among schizophrenia participants, the relationship between ToM task performance (the faux pas task) and VMPFC GMV was reduced slightly, but the relationship between self-reported and interview-rated ToM and VMPFC GMV remained strong. These findings suggest that the laboratory-based faux pas task shared some common "test-taking" features with the standard neuropsychological tasks used to assess cognition, including the ability to sustain attention and/or tolerate explicit performance assessments. However, the fact that self-report and interview-based ToM measures demonstrated a strong and significant relationship with VMPFC, even when controlling for general cognitive abilities, suggests that, in schizophrenia, GMV loss in the VMPFC is particularly associated with deficits using ToM skills to enhance social relationships in daily life (Hooker et al., 2011).

Given prior evidence that VMPFC facilitates ToM through the processes related to self-reflection, self-monitoring, and comparing the self to others (Rudebeck et al., 2008; van der Meer et al., 2010), our findings indicate that in schizophrenia, VMPFC structural and functional abnormalities are related to deficits in monitoring and using information relevant to the self in the service of understanding others. If future research verifies this interpretation, it suggests that interventions aimed at improving ToM processing, specifically VMPFC support of ToM, in schizophrenia could employ exercises that encourage self-reflection and the evaluation of one's own experience relative to others.

Conclusion

The purpose of this chapter was not to provide a comprehensive review of the neural mechanisms involved in social behavior. Rather, the goal was to illustrate some of the challenges of social neuroscience research and a few initial methods for addressing them. Capturing the complexity of social behavior will require the continued development of new and creative methods. Ultimately, identifying how specific brain regions support social cognitive skills and the use of those skills in daily life can facilitate the prevention and treatment of mental illness.

References

Adolphs, R. (2009). The social brain: Neural basis of social knowledge. *Annual Review of Psychology, 60,* 693–716.

———. (2010). What does the amygdala contribute to social cognition? *Annals of the New York Academy of Sciences,* 1191, 42–61.

Amodio, D. M., & Frith, C. D. (2006). Meeting of minds: The medial frontal cortex and social cognition. *Nature Reviews Neuroscience, 7,* 268–277.

Ayduk, O., Downey, G., & Kim, M. (2001). Rejection sensitivity and depressive symptoms in women. *Personality and Social Psychology Bulletin, 27,* 868–877.

Barch, D. M. (2005). The cognitive neuroscience of schizophrenia. *Annual Review of Clinical Psychology,* 1, 321–353.

Baron-Cohen, S. (1995). *Mindblindness: An essay on autism and theory of mind.* Cambridge, MA: MIT Press.

Barrett, L. F., Mesquita, B., Ochsner, K. N., & Gross, J. J. (2007). The experience of emotion. *Annual Review of Psychology,* 58, 373–403.

Benedetti, F., Bernasconi, A., Bosia, M., Cavallaro, R., Dallaspezia, S., Falini, A., et al. (2009). Functional and structural brain correlates of theory of mind and empathy deficits in schizophrenia. *Schizophrenia Research,* 114, 154–160.

Bienvenu, O. J., Hettema, J. M., Neale, M. C., Prescott, C. A., & Kendler, K. S. (2007). Low extraversion and high neuroticism as indices of genetic and environmental risk for social phobia, agoraphobia, and animal phobia. *American Journal of Psychiatry,* 164, 1714–1721.

Blanchard, J. J., Mueser, K. T., & Bellack, A. S. (1998). Anhedonia, positive and negative affect, and social functioning in schizophrenia. *Schizophrenia Bulletin,* 24, 413–424.

Bora, E., Yucel, M., & Pantelis, C. (2009). Theory of mind impairment in schizophrenia: Meta-analysis. *Schizophrenia Research,* 109, 1–9.

Brown, S. M., Manuck, S. B., Flory, J. D., & Hariri, A. R. (2006). Neural basis of individual differences in impulsivity: Contributions of corticolimbic circuits for behavioral arousal and control. *Emotion,* 6, 239–245.

Brune, M. (2005). "Theory of mind" in schizophrenia: a review of the literature. *Schizophrenia Bulletin,* 31, 21–42.

Brunet, E., Sarfati, Y., Hardy-Bayle, M. C., & Decety, J. (2003). Abnormalities of brain function during a nonverbal theory of mind task in schizophrenia. *Neuropsychologia,* 41, 1574–1582.

Calder, A. J., & Young, A. W. (2005). Understanding the recognition of facial identity and facial expression. *Nature reviews Neuroscience,* 6, 641–651.

Callicott, J. H., Bertolino, A., Mattay, V. S., Langheim, F. J., Duyn, J., Coppola, R., et al. (2000). Physiological dysfunction of the dorsolateral prefrontal cortex in schizophrenia revisited. *Cerebral Cortex,* 10, 1078–1092.

Callicott, J. H., Mattay, V. S., Verchinski, B. A., Marenco, S., Egan, M. F., Weinberger, D. R. (2003). Complexity of prefrontal cortical dysfunction in schizophrenia: More than up or down. *American Journal of Psychiatry,* 160, 2209–2215.

Campos, J. J., Mumme, D. L., Kermoian, R., & Campos, R. G. (1994). A functionalist perspective on the nature of emotion. *Monographs in Social Research and Child Development,* 59, 284–303.

Chiao, J. Y., & Mathur, V. A. (2010). Intergroup empathy: How does race affect empathic neural responses? *Current Biology,* 20, R478–R480.

Couture, S. M., Penn, D. L., & Roberts, D. L. (2006). The functional significance of social cognition in schizophrenia: A review. *Schizophrenia Bulletin,* 32, S44–S63.

Eysenck, H. J. (1967). *The biological basis of personality.* Springfield, IL: Charles C. Thomas.

Frith, C., & Frith, U. (2005). Theory of mind. *Current Biology,* 15, R644–R646.

———. (2006a). How we predict what other people are going to do. *Brain Research,* 1079, 36–46.

———. (2006b). The neural basis of mentalizing. *Neuron,* 50, 531–534.

Gallese, V. (2007). Embodied simulation: from mirror neuron systems to interpersonal relations. *Novartis Foundation Symposia,* 278, 3–12; discussion 12–19, 89–96, 216–221.

Gallese, V., & Goldman, A. (1998). Mirror neurons and the simulation theory of mind-reading. *Trends in Cognitive Sciences,* 2, 493–501.

Gallese, V., Keysers, C., & Rizzolatti, G. (2004). A unifying view of the basis of social cognition. *Trends in Cognitive Sciences,* 8, 396–403.

Gooding, D. C., Tallent, K. A., & Matts, C. W. (2005). Clinical status of at-risk individuals 5 years later: Further validation of the psychometric high-risk strategy. *Journal of Abnormal Psychology,* 114, 170–175.

———. (2007). Rates of avoidant, schizotypal, schizoid and paranoid personality disorders in psychometric high-risk groups at 5-year follow-up. *Schizophrenia Research,* 94, 373–374.

Gray, J. A. (1982). *Neuropsychology of anxiety.* New York: Oxford University Press.

Hackman, D. A., Farah, M. J., & Meaney, M. J. (2010). Socioeconomic status and the brain: Mechanistic insights from human and animal research. *Nature Reviews Neuroscience,* 11, 651–659.

Hamann, S., & Canli, T. (2004). Individual differences in emotion processing. *Current Opinion in Neurobiology,* 14, 233–238.

Hamann, S. B., Ely, T. D., Grafton, S. T., & Kilts, C. D. (1999). Amygdala activity related to enhanced memory for pleasant and aversive stimuli. *Nature Neuroscience,* 2, 289–293.

Hariri, A. R., Drabant, E. M., Munoz, K. E., Kolachana, B. S., Mattay, V. S., Egan, M. F., et al. (2005). A susceptibility gene for affective disorders and the response of the human amygdala. *Archives of General Psychiatry,* 62, 146–152.

Hariri, A. R., Drabant, E. M., & Weinberger, D. R. (2006). Imaging genetics: Perspectives from studies of genetically driven variation in serotonin function and corticolimbic affective processing. *Biological Psychiatry,* 59, 888–897.

Heatherton, T. F. (2011). Neuroscience of self and self-regulation. *Annual Review of Psychology,* 62, 363–390.

Honea, R., Crow, T. J., Passingham, D., & Mackay, C. E. (2005). Regional deficits in brain volume in schizophrenia: a meta-analysis of voxel-based morphometry studies. *American Journal of Psychiatry,* 162, 2233–2245.

Hooker, C. I., Benson, T. L., Gyurak, A., Yin, H., Tully, L. M., & Lincoln, S. H. (2014). Neural activity to positive expressions predicts daily experience of schizophrenia-spectrum symptoms in adults with high social anhedonia. *Journal of Abnormal Psychology,* 123, 190–204.

Hooker, C. I., Bruce, L., Lincoln, S. H., Fisher, M., & Vinogradov, S. (2011). Theory of mind skills are related to gray matter volume in the ventromedial prefrontal cortex in schizophrenia. *Biological Psychiatry,* 70, 1169–1178.

Hooker, C. I., Germine L. T., Knight, R. T., & D'Esposito, M. (2006). Amygdala response to facial expressions reflects emotional learning. *Journal of Neuroscience,* 26, 8915–8922.

Hooker, C. I., Gyurak, A., Verosky, S. C., Miyakawa, A., & Ayduk, O. (2010a). Neural activity to a partner's facial expression predicts self-regulation after conflict. *Biological Psychiatry,* 67, 406–413.

Hooker, C. I., Verosky, S. C., Germine, L. T., Knight, R. T., & D'Esposito, M. (2008a). Mentalizing about emotion and its relationship to empathy. *Social Cognition and Affective Neuroscience,* 3, 204–217.

———. (2010b). Neural activity during social signal perception correlates with self-reported empathy. *Brain Research,* 1308, 100–113.

Hooker, C. I., Verosky, S. C., Miyakawa, A., Knight, R. T., & D'Esposito, M. (2008b). The influence of personality on neural mechanisms of observational fear and reward learning. *Neuropsychologia,* 46, 2709–2724.

Hooley, J. M. (2007). Expressed emotion and relapse of psychopathology. *Annual Review of Clinical Psychology,* 3, 329–352.

Horan, W. P., Blanchard, J. J, Clark, L. A., & Green, M. F. (2008). Affective traits in schizophrenia and schizotypy. *Schizophrenia Bulletin,* 34, 856–874.

Horan, W. P., Subotnik, K. L., Snyder, K. S., & Nuechterlein, K. H. (2006). Do recent-onset schizophrenia patients experience a "social network crisis"? *Psychiatry*, 69, 115–129.

Iacoboni, M., Molnar-Szakacs, I., Gallese, V., Buccino, G., Mazziotta, J. C., & Rizzolatti, G. (2005). Grasping the intentions of others with one's own mirror neuron system. *PLoS Biology*, 3, e79.

John, O. P., & Srivastava, S. (1999). The Big Five trait taxonomy: History, measurement, and theoretical perspectives In O. P. John & L. A. Pervin (Eds.), *Handbook of personality: Theory and research* (pp. 102–38). New York: Guilford.

Keysers, C., & Gazzola, V. (2007). Integrating simulation and theory of mind: From self to social cognition. *Trends in Cognitive Sciences*, 11(5), 194–196.

Keysers, C., Wicker, B., Gazzola, V., Anton, J. L., Fogassi, L., & Gallese, V. (2004). A touching sight: SII/PV activation during the observation and experience of touch. *Neuron*, 42, 335–346.

King, S. (2000). Is expressed emotion cause or effect in the mothers of schizophrenic young adults? *Schizophrenia Research*, 45, 65–78.

Krabbendam, L., Hooker, C. I., & Aleman, A. (2014). Neural effects of the social environment. *Schizophrenia Bulletin*, 40, 248–251.

Kring, A. M., & Elis, O. (2013). Emotion deficits in people with schizophrenia. *Annual Review of Clinical Psychology*, 9, 409–433.

Kwapil, T. R. (1998). Social anhedonia as a predictor of the development of schizophrenia-spectrum disorders. *Journal of Abnormal Psychology*, 107, 558–565.

LaBar, K. S., & Cabeza, R. (2006). Cognitive neuroscience of emotional memory. *Nature Reviews Neuroscience*, 7, 54–64.

LaLumiere, R. L., & Kalivas, P. W. (2007). Reward and drugs of abuse In R. P. Kesner & J. L. Martinez (Eds.), *Neurobiology, learning, memory* (pp. 459–482). Salt Lake City, UT: Elsevier.

Laurent, A., Biloa-Tang, M., Bougerol, T., Duly, D., Anchisi, A. M., Bosson, J. L., et al. (2000). Executive/attentional performance and measures of schizotypy in patients with schizophrenia and in their nonpsychotic first-degree relatives. *Schizophrenia Research*, 46, 269–283.

LeDoux, J. E. (2000). Emotion circuits in the brain. *Annual Review of Neuroscience*, 23, 155–184.

Lesch, K. P. (2007). Linking emotion to the social brain: The role of the serotonin transporter in human social behaviour. *EMBO Reports*, 8(Special No.), S24–S29.

Lesch, K. P., Bengel, D., Heils, A., Sabol, S. Z., Greenberg, B. D., Petri, S., et al. (1996). Association of anxiety-related traits with a polymorphism in the serotonin transporter gene regulatory region. *Science*, 274, 1527–1531.

Leshner, A. I. (1997). Addiction is a brain disease, and it matters. *Science*, 278, 45–47.

Li, C. S., & Sinha, R. (2008). Inhibitory control and emotional stress regulation: Neuroimaging evidence for frontal-limbic dysfunction in psycho-stimulant addiction. *Neuroscience Biobehavioral Review*, 32, 581–597.

Lieberman, M. D. (2007). Social cognitive neuroscience: A review of core processes. *Annual Review of Psychology, 58*, 259–289.

MacDonald, A. W., III, Thermenos, H. W., Barch, D. M., & Seidman, L. J. (2009). Imaging genetic liability to schizophrenia: Systematic review of FMRI studies of patients' nonpsychotic relatives. *Schizophrenia Bulletin, 35*, 1142–1162.

Manoach, D. S. (2003). Prefrontal cortex dysfunction during working memory performance in schizophrenia: Reconciling discrepant findings. *Schizophrenia Research, 60*, 285–298.

Marjoram, D., Job, D. E., Whalley, H. C., Gountouna, V. E., McIntosh, A. M., Simonotto, E., et al. (2006). A visual joke fMRI investigation into Theory of Mind and enhanced risk of schizophrenia. *Neuroimage, 31*, 1850–1858.

Matthews, G., & Gilliland, K. (1999). The personality theories of H. J. Eysenck and J. A. Gray: A comparative review. *Personality and Individual Differences, 26*, 583–626.

Mineka, S., & Cook, M. (1993). Mechanisms involved in the observational conditioning of fear. *Journal of Experimental Psychological Genetics, 122*, 23–38.

Mineka, S., Davidson, M., Cook, M., & Keir, R. (1984). Observational conditioning of snake fear in rhesus monkeys. *Journal of Abnormal Psychology, 93*, 355–372.

Mineka, S., & Ohman, A. (2002). Born to fear: Non-associative vs associative factors in the etiology of phobias. *Behavioral Research and Therapy, 40*, 173–184.

Mineka, S., & Zinbarg, R. (1996). Conditioning and ethological models of anxiety disorders: Stress-in-dynamic-context anxiety models. *Nebraska Symposium on Motivation, 43*, 135–210.

Modinos, G., Ormel, J., & Aleman, A. (2010). Altered activation and functional connectivity of neural systems supporting cognitive control of emotion in psychosis proneness. *Schizophrenia Research, 118*, 88–97.

Monroe, S. M., Harkness, K., Simons, A. D., & Thase, M. E. (2001). Life stress and the symptoms of major depression. *Journal of Nervous and Mental Disease, 189*, 168–175.

Muscatell, K. A., Slavich, G. M., Monroe, S. M., & Gotlib, I. H. (2009). Stressful life events, chronic difficulties, and the symptoms of clinical depression. *Journal of Nervous and Mental Disease, 197*, 154–160.

Nolen-Hoeksema, S. (2000). The role of rumination in depressive disorders and mixed anxiety/depressive symptoms. *Journal of Abnormal Psychology, 109*, 504–511.

Ochsner, K. N., Bunge, S. A., Gross, J. J., & Gabrieli, J. D. (2002). Rethinking feelings: An FMRI study of the cognitive regulation of emotion. *Journal of Cognitive Neuroscience, 14*, 1215–1229.

Ochsner, K. N., Ray, R. D., Cooper, J. C., Robertson, E. R., Chopra, S., et al. (2004). For better or for worse: Neural systems supporting the cognitive down- and up-regulation of negative emotion. *Neuroimage 23*, 483–499.

Ochsner, K. N., & Gross, J. J. (2005). The cognitive control of emotion. *Trends in Cognitive Sciences, 9*, 242–249.

O'Doherty, J., Winston, J., Critchley, H., Perrett, D., Burt, D. M., & Dolan, R. J. (2003). Beauty in a smile: the role of medial orbitofrontal cortex in facial attractiveness. *Neuropsychologia, 41*, 147–155.

Ohman, A., & Mineka, S. (2001). Fears, phobias, and preparedness: Toward an evolved module of fear and fear learning. *Psychological Review,* 108, 483–522.

Penn, D. L., Mueser, K. T., Tarrier, N., Gloege, A., Cather, C., Serrano, D., et al. (2004). Supportive therapy for schizophrenia: possible mechanisms and implications for adjunctive psychosocial treatments. *Schizophrenia Bulletin, 30,* 101–112.

Phelps, E. A. (2004). Human emotion and memory: Interactions of the amygdala and hippocampal complex. *Current Opinion in Neurobiology, 14,* 198–202.

———. (2006). Emotion and cognition: insights from studies of the human amygdala. *Annual Review of Psychology, 57,* 27–53.

Pickup, G. J. (2006). Theory of mind and its relation to schizotypy. *Cognitive Neuropsychiatry, 11,* 177–192.

Pijnenborg, G. H., Withaar, F. K., Evans, J. J., van den Bosch, R. J., Timmerman, M. E., & Brouwer, W. H. (2009). The predictive value of measures of social cognition for community functioning in schizophrenia: Implications for neuropsychological assessment. *Journal of the International Neuropsychological Society,* 15, 239–247.

Roncone, R., Falloon, I. R., Mazza, M., De Risio, A., Pollice, R., Necozione, S., et al. (2002). Is theory of mind in schizophrenia more strongly associated with clinical and social functioning than with neurocognitive deficits? *Psychopathology,* 35, 280–288.

Rudebeck, P. H., Bannerman, D. M., & Rushworth, M. F. (2008). The contribution of distinct subregions of the ventromedial frontal cortex to emotion, social behavior, and decision making. *Cognitive, Affective & Behavioral Neuroscience, 8,* 485–497.

Saxe, R. (2005). Against simulation: the argument from error. *Trends in Cognitive Sciences, 9,* 174–179.

Saxe, R., Carey, S., & Kanwisher, N. (2004). Understanding other minds: Linking developmental psychology and functional neuroimaging. *Annual Review of Psychology,* 55, 87–124.

Schurhoff, F., Szoke, A., Bellivier, F., Turcas, C., Villemur, M., Tignol, J., et al. (2003). Anhedonia in schizophrenia: A distinct familial subtype? *Schizophrenia Research,* 61, 59–66.

Sergerie, K., Chochol, C., Armony, J. L. (2008). The role of the amygdala in emotional processing: A quantitative meta-analysis of functional neuroimaging studies. *Neuroscience and Biobehavioral Reviews, 32,* 811–830.

Shamay-Tsoory, S. G. (2011). The neural bases for empathy. *Neuroscientist, 17,* 18–24.

Shamay-Tsoory, S. G., Aharon-Peretz, J., & Levkovitz, Y. (2007). The neuroanatomical basis of affective mentalizing in schizophrenia: Comparison of patients with schizophrenia and patients with localized prefrontal lesions. Schizophr. Res. 90, 274–83.

Shamay-Tsoory, S. G., Tomer, R., Berger, B. D., & Aharon-Peretz, J. (2003). Characterization of empathy deficits following prefrontal brain damage: the role of the right ventromedial prefrontal cortex. *Journal of Cognitive Neuroscience,* 15, 324–337.

Shamay-Tsoory, S. G., Tomer, R., Berger, B. D., Goldsher, D., & Aharon-Peretz, J. (2005). Impaired "affective theory of mind" is associated with right ventromedial prefrontal damage. *Cognitive and Behavioral Neurology,* 18, 55–67.

Snowden, J. S., Gibbons, Z. C., Blackshaw, A., Doubleday, E., Thompson, J., Craufurd, D., et al. (2003). Social cognition in frontotemporal dementia and Huntington's disease. *Neuropsychologia,* 41, 688–701.

Spreckelmeyer, K. N., Krach, S., Kohls, G., Rademacher, L., Irmak, A., Konrad, K., et al. (2009). Anticipation of monetary and social reward differently activates mesolimbic brain structures in men and women. *Social Cognitive and Affective Neuroscience,* 4, 158–165.

Thermenos, H. W., Goldstein, J. M., Buka, S. L., Poldrack, R. A., Koch, J. K., et al. (2005). The effect of working memory performance on functional MRI in schizophrenia. Schizophr. Res. 74:179–194.

van der Meer, L., Costafreda, S., Aleman, A., & David, A. S. (2010). Self-reflection and the brain: a theoretical review and meta-analysis of neuroimaging studies with implications for schizophrenia. *Neuroscience and Biobehavioral Reviews,* 34, 935–946.

Whalen, P. J. (1998). Fear, vigilance, and ambiguity: Initial neuroimaging studies of the human amygdala. *Current Directions in Psychological Science,* 7, 177–188.

———. (2007). The uncertainty of it all. *Trends in Cognitive Sciences,* 11, 499–500.

Williams, L. M. (2008). Voxel-based morphometry in schizophrenia: Implications for neurodevelopmental connectivity models, cognition and affect. *Expert Review of Neurotherapeutics,* 8, 1049–1065.

THE SOCIAL MIND

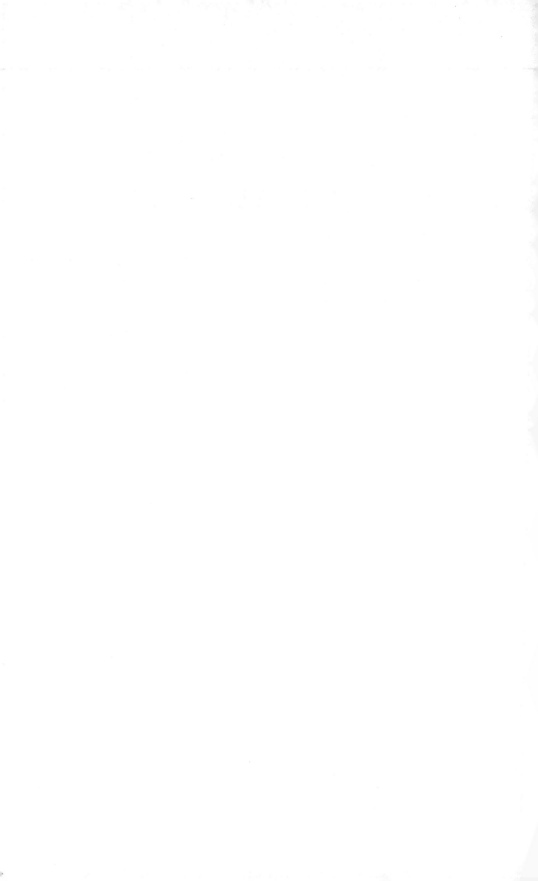

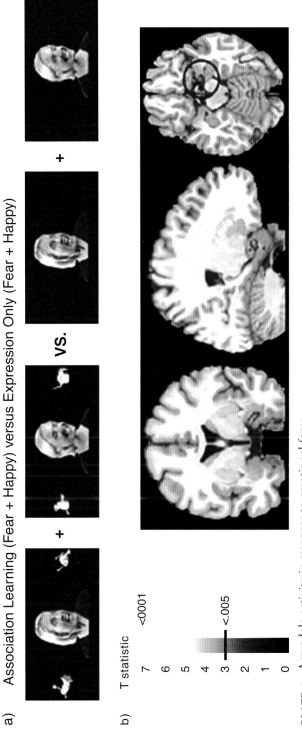

PLATE 1. Amygdala activity in response to emotional faces.

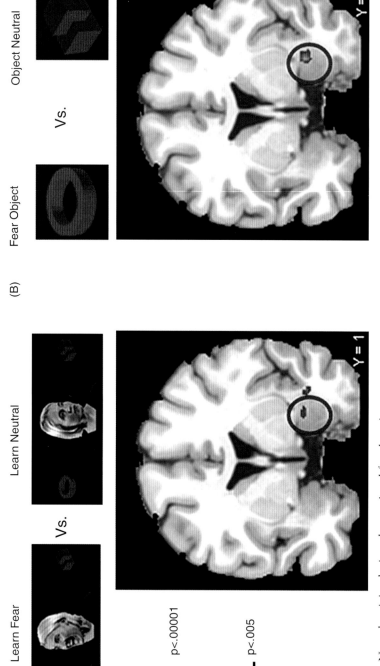

PLATE 2. Neural activity during observational fear learning.

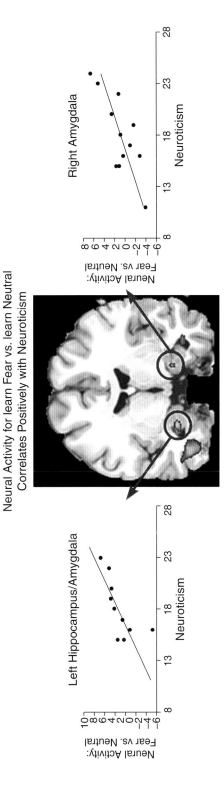

PLATE 3. Amygdala activity, fear learning, and neuroticism.

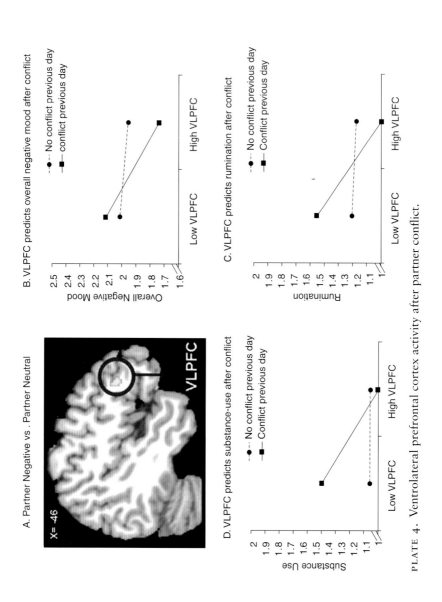

PLATE 4. Ventrolateral prefrontal cortex activity after partner conflict.

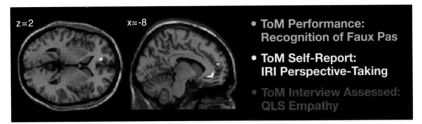

PLATE 5. Theory-of-mind skills and gray matter volume in schizophrenia.

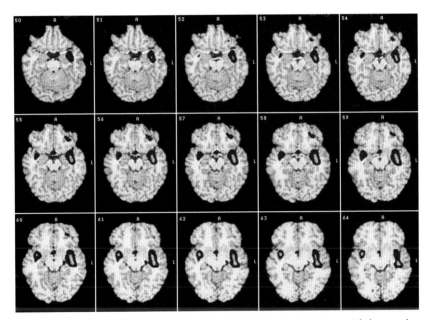

PLATE 6. Statistical Parametric Mapping maps showing regions with lower glucose metabolism in the early deprivation group compared to age-matched pediatric epilepsy controls, superimposed onto a representative magnetic resonance imaging scan in standardized space. Left side of the image represents the right side of the brain. Regions in red and yellow represent significant ($p < 0.05$) areas of decreased activity in the deprived group compared to controls.

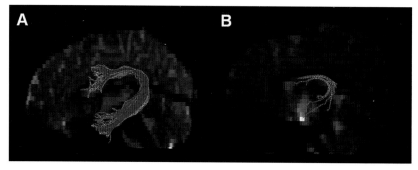

PLATE 7. Image showing the left arcuate fasciculus in (A) a child with a history of early deprivation and (B) a typically developing, nonadopted control.

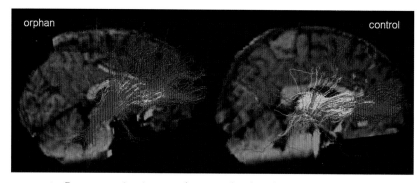

PLATE 8. Representative images showing the distribution of probabilistic fiber tracks originating from a region in the right head of the caudate nucleus in a child with a history of early deprivation (left) and a healthy nonadopted child (right). Fibers that reach the cortical mantel (2 cm depth) are rendered in red, and fibers not reaching the cortex are rendered in green. Note that the children with histories of early deprivation have a fiber pattern that appears more diffuse, possibly due to a disruption of the neuronal pruning process.

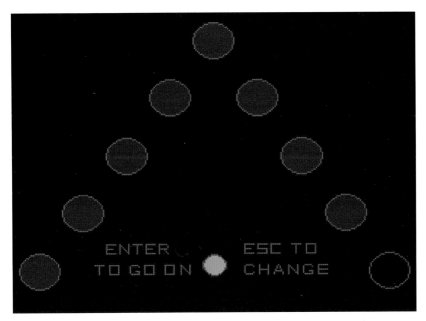

PLATE 9. Example attention training exercise using cognitive enhancement therapy: attention reaction conditioner.

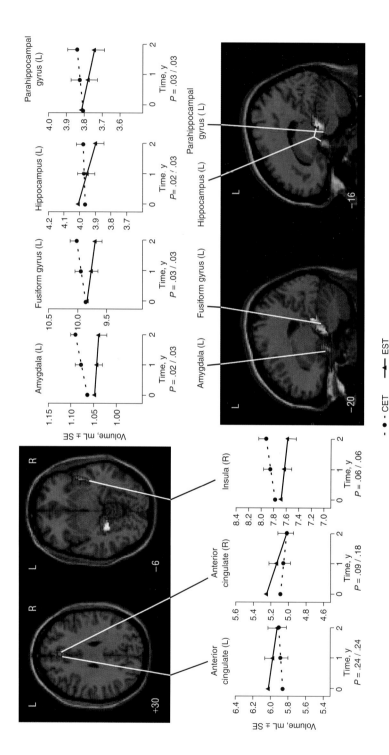

PLATE 10. Two-year effects of cognitive enhancement therapy (CET) and enriched supportive therapy (EST) on gray matter change in early course schizophrenia. Source: Eack et al. (2010b).

6.

The Mind and Social Cognition

Larry J. Seidman

W E TAKE as a given that human beings are social animals and that the long human gestational period lays a special foundation with the biological mother that is subsequently expressed in attachment and rearing primarily by nuclear families across cultures and across human history (Bowlby, 1969). During this extended development, babies, infants, toddlers, and teenagers turn into adults shaped by their genes and by many environmental factors, especially their families. The fact that there is individual plasticity and considerable variation in rearing practices across cultures and historical time periods does not strongly challenge this basic fact (Aries, 1962). The family rearing practices are necessary but not sufficient to stimulate cognition optimally. Formal education and informal education by the broader social world of peers, extended family, and acquaintances, as well as by all forms of media ranging from books to Internet to television, also have an important impact on the development of cognition.

The work by Behen and Chugani (Chapter 12, this volume) provides strong, if not tragic, evidence that somewhat like the disturbances in the development of the cat visual cortex induced by blocking visual input (Hubel & Weisel, 1963), suggesting a "critical period" for visual stimulation, there may be analogous critical periods for social development requiring nurturance and love for normal social development to occur. These would include appropriate touch, movement, auditory and visual input, smell, and other stimuli coming directly from loving caretakers, who also provide reasonable and consistent external regulation for the child when he or she cannot. These caretaker interactions are likely to be regulated by hormones and the cognitive and social-emotional capacities of the parents, as well as by the neural capacities of the developing child, that interact with the parents in an extended dance over one, two, or more decades, at least in modern Western society (Arnett, 2004). These caretakers must protect the infant or child from physical harm, whether it be from infection, war, or starvation, as well as from socioemotional harm, from abuse, neglect, and trauma. The development of sophisticated studies of development in humans and in nonhuman primates, particularly the great apes, our closest neighbors in evolution (McEwen, 2000), provides very clear examples of how intrinsic biological development and social environment are intertwined. Of course, this leaves plenty of room for determining just how much of the variance is accounted for by nature and nurture on any given dimension or situation. Nevertheless, the evidence suggests that the simplistic silos of past conceptualization emphasizing the separateness of these processes ought to be left in the dustbin of history.

This book, a multidisciplinary effort to provide a framework for this broad perspective, addresses a number of issues, partly stimulated by derailments of normal social development, manifest in certain psychiatric disorders such as schizophrenia. We have identified with the biopsychosocial perspective (Engel, 1977), in which the three components of biology, psychology, and the social world must be studied together. For example, the problems of social interaction experienced by a majority of individuals with schizophrenia, a neuropsychiatric disorder of the brain and mind affecting roughly 1 percent of the human population, has stimulated a great deal of research into the origin, nature, and development of these difficulties. Mostly, this push is driven by the desire to help improve these problems, through innovative and nonharmful treatments, as reflected in the inspiring work of Eack and Keshavan (Chapter 15, this volume). This search has led into many areas, especially of cognition, including neurocognitive and, more recently, social cognitive processes. Thus, our book encapsulates a time-honored tradition in medicine in which an understanding of abnormal behavior and psychopathology leads back to an understanding of what it means to be human and what is necessary for normal function to occur.

In this chapter, I provide some historical context and framework for a number of chapters in the book, especially those dealing with social cognition, family environments, brain function, and psychiatric disorders. These chapters provide eloquent examples of the importance of the relatively new domain of social cognition and the impact of the environment (criticism and "expressed emotion") on such disorders such as schizophrenia and depression. Before doing so, a brief history of dominant trends in the field of cognition and mental disorders is presented to provide a context for this focus.

History and Origins of the Study of Intellectual Function

In the scientific field of psychology, the idea of the "psyche" constitutes the total human mind. The word, originally derived from Greek, dates back to ancient times. The study of mind goes back to antiquity and perhaps earlier. Many philosophers and scholars from ancient civilizations, Chinese, Hebraic, Hindu, and others, wrote about their understandings of mind and existence, often embodied in classic religious or philosophical texts. However, in the origins of Western civilization, explorations in intellectual function were taken to perhaps their most influential level by the Greeks more than two millennia ago, whose interest in the mind was embodied in the ideas of Socrates, Plato, and Aristotle. Their thinking about the mind was foundational in Western intellectual thought, and their philosophical influence continued throughout the Middle Ages, when religious thought dominated. Interestingly, Aristotle carried out empirical studies more than 2,000 years ago on perception and memory. Thus, the subsequent scientific discipline of psychology has its roots in his ideas, and this history is addressed thoroughly by Gardner (1983, 1985).

The later European periods of the Enlightenment and Renaissance ushered in a period where empirical data began to be integrated with philosophical thought in a more systematic way. According to Gardner (1985), the period of the Industrial Revolution ushered in a variety of "new sciences and philosophical specialties, several of which purported to deal with the nature of the human mind" (p. 4). This interest accelerated in the nineteenth century, with the advent of empirical data collection in England (Galton) and Germany (Wundt), in-depth psychological models (Freud, James), and the beginnings of modern behavioral neurology (Broca, Wernicke). The modern era of the discipline of psychology, which typically covers development, social psychology, cognition, and clinical and neuroscientific domains, is dominated by experimental methodology (Glass & Holyoak, 1986).

Neurocognition and Social Cognition

The earlier modes of understanding the mind provided a foundation for the modern "cognitive science" that has grown tremendously in the past fifty years. The word *cognition* originates from the Latin "cognosco" and the Greek "gnosko," basically, to know. Cognition typically has comprised the study of a group of mental processes, including attention, learning and memory, reasoning, problem solving, and language (Glass & Holyoak, 1986). The concept of "executive functions," higher-order aspects of cognition that regulate other functions, has emerged in the past fifty years as knowledge of the prefrontal cortex, with which it is inextricably linked, has grown. Noticeably absent from the above description is the term *social cognition*, which has become an increasingly important part of cognitive science over the past few decades. One can say that social cognition, at least for humans, is the cognitive process relating to information about other humans and involves a variety of processes, including perception, encoding, and storage and retrieval of socially relevant information. As noted by Schutt, Seidman, and Keshavan (Chapter 1, this volume), humans are social beings who benefit from and are benefited by having capacities or skills for understanding other people's feelings ("empathy"; Brothers, 1989) or intentions ("theory of mind"; Baron-Cohen, 1995; Baron-Cohen et al., 2001), and yet social cognition is a relatively late development in the "cognitive revolution." Why might this be the case? Perhaps this "delay" was associated with the inevitable link with emotions, which themselves have also received more intensive scientific study only more recently, perhaps because better measures have been developed and because knowledge of the neural substrates underlying emotion has grown (LeDoux, 2000). Or, perhaps this field, which had been more strongly associated with social psychology, did not have many measures in common clinical use, which indirectly undercut the salience of the field. And of course, the advent of cognitive neuroscience and the use of functional magnetic resonance imaging (fMRI) in the early 1990s, a tool that allowed scientists to peer into the human brain while the mind was at work, have facilitated the field of social cognition. Once specific neural networks underlying forms of social cognition were identified, as described by Hooker (Chapter 5, this volume), the field of social cognition was given strong validation. Thus, the new experimental field linking mind and brain, "cognitive neuroscience," while focusing first on traditional "cold" modules of the mind, such as learning and memory, has spurred interest in the important forms of "hot" cognition that deal with emotion and social function and have helped them develop as accepted scientific domains. For the most part, the modules of the mind or "intelligences," as Gardner (1983) termed it, did not initially include emotional experience or behavior. Social cognition, in part because it deals with the human world, rather than the world of objects, is more closely linked with emotions, now an established area of focus in human neuroscience and certainly a key part of our evolutionary history (MacLean, 1990).

As depicted in Figure 6.1, the field of cognitive studies is wide ranging and can be divided for heuristic purposes into "nonsocial" ("cold") cognition and social ("hot") cognition. Nonsocial or neurocognition includes traditional realms of cognitive study, such as components of learning and memory, language, and so forth. These domains are typically studied at molar levels, often in tests used in battery format by clinical neuropsychologists (Seidman, 1997; Seidman & Toomey, 1999; Seidman, Bruder, & Giuliano, 2008). An example of this application to clinical research is the MATRICS (Measurement and Treatment Research in Cognition in Schizophrenia) Consensus Cognitive Battery (Nuechterlein et al., 2008). Splitting the domains into more elemental components of cognitive processing, such as in psycholinguistic analysis of language, or as in the CENTRACS battery (Cognitive Neuroscience Test Reliability and Clinical Applications for schizophrenia; Carter & Barch, 2007), is aimed at delineating the cognitive processes underlying deficits in disorders such as schizophrenia.

The field of social cognition, described in considerable detail in this volume (Addington & Barbato, Chapter 8; Hooker, Chapter 5; Lee, Horan, & Green, Chapter 7; Nestor, Choate, & Shirai, Chapter 4) has emerged in the last two decades as a very useful complement to neurocognition and is largely independent of neurocognition.

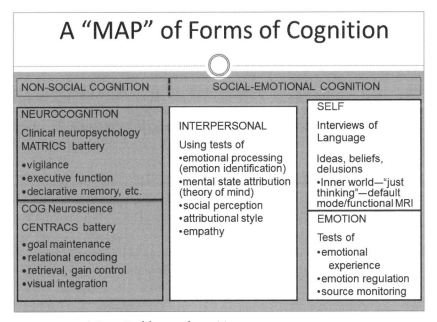

FIGURE 6.1. A "map" of forms of cognition.

Behaviorism vs. Cognition

The cognitive revolution, which originated in the 1940s and 1950s, was a dramatic departure from two previous trends: introspection and behaviorism. "Introspection," as documented in Gardner (1985), was the scientific method used by many psychologists until the twentieth century, when its approach was challenged by the science of "behaviorism," an approach favored mainly in the United States. The behaviorists "put forth two related propositions. First of all, those researchers interested in a science of behavior ought to restrict themselves to public methods of observation, which any scientist could apply. Second, those interested in a science of behavior ought to focus exclusively on behavior: researchers ought assiduously to eschew such topics as mind, thinking, or imagination and such concepts as plans, desires, or intentions" (Gardner, 1985, p. 11). While it seems hard to believe now that such ideas dominated human psychology in the first half of the twentieth century, behaviorism was an empirical science that led to a great deal of useful research for lower animals and corrected some of the problems of introspection. Clinically, it laid a foundation for a variety of forms of behavior therapy and was useful for applied fields such as education. Nevertheless, the inability of behaviorism to address human aspects of cognition, such as language, fantasy, planning, decision making, and so on, led to its demise as the central method for understanding human behavior. The rigorous methods of experimental cognitive science and the development of functional magnetic resonance imaging (MRI) have cemented cognitive neuroscience as a rigorous scientific discipline, in which social cognition is playing an increasingly important role. Functional MRI studies of people solving tasks and "just thinking" (Buckner et al., 2008) have opened up the inner world of cognition to rigorous experimental study, as documented in a number of chapters in this book (see Hooker, Chapter 5; Keshavan, Chapter 2).

Modules of the Mind vs. "G," General Intelligence, and "Mass Action"

One final issue to take up briefly is the degree to which these domains of cognition, social cognition included, are truly separable domains. The issue of multiple intelligences versus "g" or general intelligence, has been the source of debate in psychology since the early part of the twentieth century, with various scientists ("splitters" vs. "lumpers") associated with different sides of the debate regarding elements of cognition as well as specialization of the brain (cf. Gardner, 1983). "G" is typically represented by the intelligence quotient (IQ) or the first factor in factor analysis, a statistical technique that is used to identify the underlying factor structure of a group of tests given to a large number of participants. While IQ has been misused for racist reasons and misunderstood by the public and scientists alike (cf. Gould, 1981), it can be used effectively as an estimate of general cognitive ability.

To some extent, this scientific debate was driven by those studying lower animals such as rats (Lashley, 1931), who tended to see "mass action" or equipotentiality among brain regions, in contrast to those studying primates, especially humans, who tended to identify specializations of the human brain. Brain structure, especially the cortex, is increasingly differentiated from lower mammals to humans (cf. Turner, Chapter 3; Nestor, Choate, & Shirai, Chapter 4; Keshavan, Chapter 2, all this volume). Over time, and particularly with the advent of functional MRI in the early 1990s, the empirical data supporting specialized areas for processing information have gained the ascendant position. However, more recently, cognitive and clinical neuroscientists have increasingly moved toward a neural systems approach to understanding cognitive function in the brain (Makris et al., 2009). Where clinical neuroscience focused initially on localizing structural abnormalities and the function of individual brain areas or structures, it has moved to examine networks and pathways. The goal has been increasingly to understand the neural systems of normal and abnormal behavior with the rise of new techniques of brain structure (diffusion tensor MRI to measure white matter pathways) and function (functional connectivity). Thus, as described by Hooker (Chapter 5, this volume), social cognitive processes are linked to networks of structures, contributing different elements. Nevertheless, the task of fully understanding how disparate regions of the brain work together in real time is a major challenge to the field.

Relationship to Psychopathology

We now turn more specifically to chapters in the book that address social cognition and related processes. In the chapter by Lee, Horan, and Green (Chapter 7, this volume), the authors address definitions of social cognition and its relationship to schizophrenia. One of the key issues characterizing individuals with schizophrenia is significant impairment in social and role functioning and how to help understand it and treat it. Social cognition has emerged as very important, in part, to help explain social and role impairments (Green et al., 2008). Research on social cognition has expanded substantially over the past ten years, commonly focusing on four broad domains: emotional processing, mental state attribution, social perception, and attributional style. Lee et al. also address aspects of empathy behaviorally and through functional MRI studies. Their comprehensive review demonstrates that a significant impairment in most social cognitive domains has been observed at the first episode of psychosis as well as in more chronic stages of illness (Green et al., 2012). They demonstrate that social cognition is an important mediator through which disturbances in early visual perception and neurocognition ultimately lead to poor functioning in schizophrenia. Their work models in a sophisticated way, early visual processing measured during functional MRI, and how this early processing difficulty plays out in more complex social cognitive processes and ultimately with real-world deficits.

Addington and Barbato (Chapter 8, this volume) take the work of Lee et al. to an earlier phase of psychotic illness, a period when individuals may be developing psychosis, the so-called clinical high-risk (CHR) or "prodromal" phase. The CHR phase of illness is a research-based classification that has drawn considerable interest over the past decade as a focus on early intervention and prevention of psychosis has developed. The "subclinical" signs and symptoms that a person experiences prior to the onset of a full-blown syndrome characterize the CHR phase (Yung, Phillips, Yuen, & McGorry, 2004). The CHR phase, like the focus on mild cognitive impairment (MCI) as a stage possibly preceding the onset of Alzheimer disease, offers a potential window for early treatment. The question addressed by the authors is whether the social cognitive impairments are observed in first-episode schizophrenia are present in the CHR phase. The authors carefully review the extant literature on studies that are derived from different approaches to identification of high risk for psychosis. They point out that studies are currently relatively few, the samples are largely on the small side, and only limited social cognitive domains have been assessed. Nevertheless, the results are promising, particularly in facial affect perception, in which individuals at CHR show difficulties comparable to those in first-episode psychosis (Addington et al., 2012). Thus, the evidence suggests that measures of social cognition are relevant to the preonset period prior to manifestation of full-blown psychosis. It remains to be determined how extensive these impairments are across the domains of social cognition.

Hooker (Chapter 5, this volume) focuses more on understanding the brain mechanisms of social cognition. She reviews the literature identifying the relationship between neural function, social cognition, and social behavior, mainly through functional MRI studies. She selectively reviews social neuroscience research focused on identifying the neural basis of social behavior. Hooker describes the networks of brain structures that are preferentially recruited to support the four processes that she describes as part of social cognition: social perception, emotion processing, self-regulation, and mental state attribution. The neural networks are not simple to summarize because, as Hooker notes, "The social processes and associated networks listed here are neither exhaustive nor exclusive. Social behavior is psychologically complex and draws upon multiple interacting brain regions depending on the combination of psychological processes involved." Hooker also focuses on how specific methodologies may be employed to integrate social context into experiments. Her work highlights how social neuroscience research can move beyond the individual to the dyad to better understand human behavior. In work of her own, Hooker et al. (2010) showed that the activity of the lateral prefrontal cortex, in response to a partner's negative expression, predicted ability to recover from an interpersonal conflict with a partner. This chapter highlights the challenge in trying to understand brain function in an ecologically valid manner, with social context taken into account.

Hooley (Chapter 9, this volume) takes a different tack in understanding a form of social cognition in the origin of some forms of mental illness in her review of "Criticism and the Course of Mental Disorders." According to Hooley, "Expressed emotion (EE) reflects the extent to which the key relative of a psychiatric patient speaks about that patient in a critical, hostile, or emotionally overinvolved way during the course of a private interview with a researcher." Thus, high EE is a putative environmental risk factor and a robust predictor of relapse and other poor clinical outcomes in people with various forms of mental disorders (Hooley, 2007). She summarizes that "when patients with schizophrenia or mood disorders live in family environments that are characterized by criticism, hostility, or high levels of EOI, they are at significantly increased risk of early relapse compared to patients who do not live in such family environments." However, she also indicates that "expressed emotion" is not a single, unidirectional process emanating from family members that causes a mental illness. Rather, she paints it as part of a complex field of stress sensitivities experienced by some persons with mental illness. In elegant neuroimaging research of her own, she demonstrates that persons in a remitted state after recovering from depression process criticism differently than do healthy comparison subjects (Hooley et al., 2005). The criticism is induced in the functional MRI experiment when subjects hear personally relevant criticisms from their own mothers. Individuals with a history of depression show different activation patterns in the amygdala and dorsolateral prefrontal cortex than do controls (Hooley et al., 2009). This work highlights the importance of the interaction between biological vulnerability and the environment.

Conclusions

The field of social cognition has grown remarkably over the past two decades and complements the increasingly important role of neuropsychology in psychiatry and neurology. The growth of applications to neurodevelopmental disorders, such as schizophrenia and autism, which are characterized by substantial impairments in social functioning and in social cognition, is likely to lead to improved treatments for these disorders. Already, major advances in social cognitive treatment, as described by Eack and Keshavan (Chapter 15, this volume), foreshadow an improving future for disorders in which social cognitive dysfunctions are central. Moreover, an increased emphasis on the developmental aspects of social cognition (Saxe et al., 2004) may lead to preventative strategies in which environmental modifications are made to protect and optimize social cognition and neurocognition in high-risk children.

References

Addington, J., Piskulic, D., Perkins, D., Woods, S. W., Liu, L., & Penn, D. L. (2012). Affect recognition in people at clinical high risk of psychosis. *Schizophrenia Research, 140,* 87–92.

Aries, P. (1962). *Centuries of childhood: A social history of family life.* New York: Vintage.

Arnett, J. J. (2004). *Emerging adulthood: The winding road from late teens through the twenties.* New York: Oxford University Press.

Baron-Cohen, S. (1995). *Mindblindness: An essay on autism and theory of mind.* Cambridge, MA: MIT Press.

Baron-Cohen, S., Wheelwright, S., Hill, J., Raste, Y., & Plumb, I. (2001). The "Reading the mind in the eyes" test revised version: A study with normal adults, and adults with Asperger syndrome or high-functioning autism. *Journal of Child Psychology & Psychiatry & Allied Disciplines, 42,* 241–251.

Bowlby, J. (1969). *Attachment* (Vol. I). New York: Basic Books.

Brothers, L. (1989). A biological perspective on empathy. *American Journal of Psychiatry, 146,* 10–19.

Buckner, R. L., Andrews-Hanna, J. R., & Schacter, D. L. (2008). The brain's default network: Anatomy, function, and relevance to disease. *Annals of the New York Academy of Sciences, 1124,* 1–38.

Carter, C. S., & Barch, D. M. (2007). Cognitive neuroscience-based approaches to measuring and improving treatment effects on cognition in schizophrenia: The CNTRICS initiative. *Schizophrenia Bulletin, 33,* 1131–1137.

Engel, G. L. (1977). The need for a new medical model: a challenge for biomedicine. *Science, 196,* 129–136.

Gardner, H. (1983). *Frames of mind: The theory of multiple intelligences.* New York: Basic Books.

———. (1985). *The mind's new science: A history of the cognitive revolution.* New York: Basic Books.

Glass, A. J., & Holyoak, K. J. (1986). *Cognition* (2nd ed.). New York: Random House.

Gould, S. J. (1981). *The mismeasure of man.* New York: W. W. Norton.

Green, M. F., Bearden, C. E., Cannon, T. D., Fiske, A. P., Hellemann, G. S., Horan, W. P., Kee, K., Kern, R. S., Lee, J., Sergi, M. J., Subotnik, K. L., Sugar, C. A., Ventura, J., Yee, C. M., & Nuechterlein, K. H. (2012). Social cognition in schizophrenia, Part 1: Performance across phase of illness. *Schizophrenia Bulletin, 38,* 854–864.

Green, M. F., Penn, D. L., Bentall, R., Carpenter, W. T., Gaebel, W., Gur, R. C., Kring, A. M., Park, S., Silverstein, S. M., & Heinssen, R. (2008). Social cognition in schizophrenia: An NIMH workshop on definitions, assessment, and research opportunities. *Schizophrenia Bulletin, 34,* 1211–1220.

Hooker, C. I., Gyurak, A., Verosky, S. C., Miyakawa, A., & Ayduk, O. (2010). Neural activity to a partner's facial expression predicts self-regulation after conflict. *Biological Psychiatry, 67,* 406–413.

Hooley, J. M. (2007). Expressed emotion and relapse of psychopathology. *Annual Review of Clinical Psychology, 3,* 329–352.

Hooley, J. M., Gruber, S. A., Parker, H., Guillaumot, J., Rogowska, J., & Yurgelun-Todd, D. A. (2009). Cortico-limbic response to personally-challenging emotional stimuli after complete recovery from major depression. *Psychiatry Research: Neuroimaging, 171,* 106–119.

Hooley, J. M., Gruber, S. A., Scott, L. A., Hiller, J. B., & Yurgelun-Todd, D. A. (2005). Activation in dorsolateral prefrontal cortex in response to maternal criticism and praise in recovered depressed and healthy control participants. *Biological Psychiatry, 57,* 809–812.

Hubel, D. H., & Weisel, T. N. (1963). Single cell responses in striate cortex of kittens deprived of vision in one eye. *Journal of Neurophysiology, 26,* 1003–1017.

Lashley, K. S. (1931). Mass action in cerebral function. *Science, 73,* 245–254.

LeDoux, J. E. (2000). Emotion circuits in the brain. *Annual Review of Neuroscience, 23,* 155–184.

MacLean, P. D. (1990). *The triune brain in evolution: Role of paleocerebral functions.* New York: Plenum.

Makris, N., Biederman, J., Monuteaux, M. C., & Seidman, L. J. (2009). Towards conceptualizing a neural systems-based anatomy of attention-deficit/hyperactivity disorder. *Developmental Neuroscience, 21,* 36–49.

McEwen, B. S. (2000). Effects of adverse experiences for brain structure and function. *Biological Psychiatry*, 48, 721–731.

Nuechterlein, K. H., Green, M. F., Kern, R. S., Baade, L. E., Barch, D. M., Cohen, J. D., Essock, S., Fenton, W. S., Frese, F. J., Gold, J. M., Goldberg, T., Heaton, R. K., Keefe, R. S. E, Kraemer, H., Mesholam-Gately, R., Seidman, L. J., Stover, E., Weinberger, D., Young, A. S., Zalcman, S., Marder, S. R. (2008). The MATRICS Consensus Cognitive Battery: Part 1. Test selection, reliability, and validity. *American Journal of Psychiatry*, 165, 203–213.

Saxe, R., Carey, S., & Kanwisher, N. (2004). Understanding other minds: linking developmental psychology and functional neuroimaging. *Annual Review of Psychology*, 55, 87–124.

Seidman, L. J. (1997). Neuropsychological testing. In A. Tasman, J. Kay, & J. Lieberman (Eds.), *Psychiatry* (pp. 498–508). Philadelphia: WB Saunders.

Seidman, L. J., Bruder, G., & Giuliano, A. J. (2008). Neuropsychological testing and neurophysiological assessment. In A. Tasman, J. Kay, J. A. Lieberman, M. B. First, & M. Maj (Eds.) *Psychiatry* (3rd ed., pp. 556–569). London: John Wiley.

Seidman, L. J., & Toomey, R. (1999). The clinical use of psychological and neuropsychological tests. In A. Nicholi (Ed.), *The Harvard guide to psychiatry* (3rd ed., pp. 40–65). Cambridge, MA: Harvard University Press.

Yung, A. R., Phillips, L. J., Yuen, H. P., & McGorry, P. D. (2004). Risk factors for psychosis in an ultra high-risk group: Psychopathology and clinical features. *Schizophrenia Research*, 67, 131–142.

7.

Social Cognition in Schizophrenia

Where We Are and Where We Are Going

Junghee Lee, William P. Horan,
and Michael F. Green

H UMANS ARE social beings: we interact with others and form meaningful relationships with others in everyday life. Without being taught explicitly, young children can understand the feelings of others simply by looking at their faces or hearing their voices. As adults, we know when others are telling the truth, lying to be polite, or being sarcastic. We can also feel others' pain/exuberance and understand what others are experiencing in situations of remarkable diversity (e.g., a friend being in an accident, a friend passing the bar exam). These processes occur very naturally; however, despite the apparent ease of using them, they actually involve very complex underlying abilities. These abilities, referred as social cognition, include how we recognize and respond to the emotions, intentions, and dispositions of others (Adolphs, 2001). Because these abilities underlie effective social behavior, social cognition has received much attention in studies on mental disorders that are marked by social dysfunction, including schizophrenia.

Schizophrenia is a chronic, debilitating mental illness, affecting approximately 1 percent of the general population around the world. In addition to psychotic symptoms, such as hallucinations and delusions, individuals with schizophrenia exhibit high levels of disability in several areas of functioning, including independent living, social relationships, and work. Considerable effort has been devoted to identifying key determinants of poor functioning in schizophrenia. Over the past decade, there has been rapid growth in research on social cognition, which appears to play a unique role among the many factors that contribute to poor functioning in schizophrenia. In this chapter, we survey three aspects of social cognitive research in schizophrenia. First, we review the areas of social cognition that have been most commonly studied in schizophrenia, focusing on four social cognitive domains. Second, we examine recently emerging translational research efforts that apply concepts and methods from social cognitive and affective neuroscience to schizophrenia. For this section, we will use research on empathy as an example. Third, we review recent efforts to develop and test models of how social cognition interacts with other predictors of outcome, including neurocognition, perception, and motivation, to ultimately determine functional outcome in schizophrenia. To conclude this chapter, we discuss several remaining challenges associated with the recent growth in knowledge of social cognition in schizophrenia to be addressed in future studies.

The Current State of Social Cognitive Research in Schizophrenia

Using behavioral paradigms, as well as neuroimaging methods (e.g., functional magnetic resonance imaging [fMRI] and electroencephalography [EEG]), studies of social cognition in schizophrenia have commonly focused on four broad domains (Green et al., 2005; Green et al., 2008): emotional processing, mental state attribution, social perception, and attributional style. We will discuss each one briefly.

Emotional Processing

Emotional processing involves diverse aspects of perceiving and utilizing emotion to facilitate adaptive functioning. The broad term of *emotional processing* can be subdivided into three key aspects: emotion identification, emotional experience, and emotion regulation. Emotion identification, or affect recognition, is the most extensively studied aspect of social cognition in schizophrenia. Individuals with schizophrenia consistently show impairments in identifying or discriminating among visual emotional cues displayed in still photographs or videos showing emotional faces or body gestures (Kohler et al., 2010). In addition to the visual modality, individuals with schizophrenia also have difficulty identifying auditory emotional cues in vocalizations or videotaped monologues (Hoekert et al., 2007;

Leitman et al., 2007; Gold et al., 2012). Although some studies found more severe impairments for certain negative emotions (e.g., fear, disgust) than positive emotions (Kohler et al., 2003; Edwards et al., 2001), findings of valence-modulated impairments are not consistent (Silver et al., 2009; Kee et al., 2003). Overall, the magnitude of impairment in schizophrenia is large: meta-analytic reviews of diverse affect recognition tasks reported an overall effect size of .89 to .94 for individuals with schizophrenia versus healthy controls (Savla et al., 2012; Kohler et al., 2010). In addition, meta-analytic reviews of fMRI studies indicate hypoactivation in several brain areas, including the amygdala, fusiform gyrus, and right superior frontal gyrus, during facial affect recognition (Li et al., 2010; Taylor et al., 2012; Anticevic et al., 2012). (See also Hooker, Chapter 5, this volume, for a detailed explanation of the amygdala and emotion processing.) Impaired vocal affect recognition in schizophrenia has been associated with reduced activation in the superior temporal and inferior frontal gyri (Leitman et al., 2011).

Another aspect of emotional processing that is studied in schizophrenia is emotional experience, which involves how affected individuals respond to emotionally evocative stimuli in terms of their subjective experiences and physiological responses. Individuals with schizophrenia report elevated anhedonia on self-report questionnaires and clinical assessments (Horan et al., 2006). Anhedonia refers to diminished experience of pleasure from activities that most individuals find pleasurable (e.g., hobbies, spending time with family or friends). Despite these impairments, studies using laboratory tasks consistently indicate that individuals with schizophrenia report experiencing emotional reactions that are similar to healthy individuals when they are exposed to both positive and negative stimuli (e.g., pictures, foods, films) (Cohen & Minor, 2010). Studies using EEG and fMRI also indicate generally intact neural responses to emotionally evocative stimuli in individuals with schizophrenia (Ursu et al., 2011; Horan et al., 2010; Dowd & Barch, 2010). Thus, converging evidence suggests that individuals with schizophrenia actually have an intact capacity to experience emotions in response to evocative stimuli. It should be noted, though, that individuals with schizophrenia tend to report higher levels of unpleasant emotions in response to positive and neutral stimuli compared to healthy individuals (Cohen & Minor, 2010) and that other aspects of emotional experience, such as anticipating or recalling emotions, may be disturbed in schizophrenia (Gard et al., 2007; Herbener, 2008; Wynn et al., 2010a).

A third aspect, emotion regulation, has received little attention in schizophrenia until recently. Emotion regulation refers to the processes that enable us to influence which emotions we experience, as well as when and how intensely we experience and express them (Gross, 1998). Two of the

most extensively studied emotion regulation strategies are cognitive reappraisal and behavioral suppression. Reappraisal involves construing an
emotion-eliciting situation in a way that changes its meaning and emotional
impact (e.g., thinking of a medical procedure as highly beneficial for one's
long-term health instead of focusing on its immediate physical discomfort).
Suppression involves intentionally diminishing outward expressions of one's
emotional reactions (e.g., maintaining a "poker face"). With self-report
questionnaires assessing habitual use of these strategies, studies have shown
inconsistent findings: some found lower use of reappraisal (Livingstone
et al., 2009; van der Meer et al., 2009; Horan et al., 2013) or greater use
of suppression in schizophrenia (van der Meer et al., 2009), whereas others
found no group difference (Henry et al., 2008; Badcock et al., 2011; Perry
et al., 2011). Other approaches for emotion regulation show more consistent deficits in schizophrenia. For example, the "Managing Emotions"
component of the Mayer-Salovey-Caruso Emotional Intelligence Test
(MSCEIT) asks individuals to rate the effectiveness of potential strategies
for emotion regulation after reading vignettes describing emotional responses
in diverse interpersonal situations. Individuals with schizophrenia show
lower accuracy in judging the effectiveness of emotion regulation strategies that could be used in diverse situations (Kee et al., 2009; Green et al.,
2012a). In addition, an fMRI study found that individuals with schizophrenia also show reduced ventrolateral prefrontal cortex activation as
well as reduced coupling between the prefrontal cortex and amygdala while
regulating negative emotions through reappraisal (Morris et al., 2012).
Consistent with this neuroimaging finding, a recent EEG study found that
individuals with schizophrenia demonstrated abnormal appraisal-related
modulation of event-related potential (ERP) responses to negative stimuli
(Horan et al., 2013).

Mental State Attribution

Mental state attribution (also known as theory of mind or mentalizing) refers to the ability to infer intentions, dispositions, and beliefs of others
(Baron-Cohen et al., 2001; Frith, 1992). Mental state attribution is centrally
involved in social processes such as understanding others' perspectives, hints,
intentions, deception, and nonliteral language use (e.g., sarcasm, meta-
phors) in everyday life. Studies on mental state attribution in schizophrenia
have traditionally relied heavily on paper-and-pencil measures, including
simple stories, sequential picture sets of simple drawings, and pictures of
eyes (Frith & Corcoran, 1996; Corcoran et al., 1995; Baron-Cohen et al.,

2001; Langdon et al., 1997; Happe, 1994). For example, false belief tasks evaluate first-order false beliefs, which refer to understanding that people can have different beliefs about the same situation (e.g., What does John think? I know this teapot contains coffee, but when John sees this teapot, he will think there is tea in it) or more complex second-order false beliefs (e.g., What does John think that Mary will think? Because John thinks this teapot has tea in it, he thinks Mary will want to have tea when she asks him to pass the teapot). Other paradigms using picture stimuli ask subjects to arrange cartoon panels in a coherent fashion using knowledge about the mental states of the characters depicted in the pictures (e.g., intention to deceive) (Brune, 2003) or the emotional state of the characters in pictures only showing their eyes (Kettle et al., 2008).

In addition to paper-and-pencil tests, alternative paradigms using dynamic stimuli have been applied to assess mental state attribution in schizophrenia. When observing short animation clips that depict dynamic "interactions" among geometric shapes, individuals with schizophrenia are significantly less likely than controls to spontaneously attribute social meaning to the animations (Horan et al., 2009; Pedersen et al., 2012; Koelkebeck et al., 2010). Another task, the Awareness of Social Inference Test, measures how well individuals make inferences about others' intentions (e.g., detecting sarcasm and lies) using video clips of interactions between two adults. Individuals with schizophrenia show an impaired ability to detect lies and sarcasm on this task compared to healthy controls (Kern et al., 2009; Chung et al., 2011; Sparks et al., 2010). The magnitude of impaired mental state attribution is large. Meta-analytic studies showed effect sizes of .96 to 1.25 for individuals with schizophrenia compared to controls across highly diverse paradigms (Bora et al., 2009; Sprong et al., 2007; Savla et al., 2012).

Despite the numerous behavioral studies on mental state attribution in schizophrenia, there are much fewer studies on the neural mechanisms of impaired mental state attribution. Most studies using fMRI indicate that individuals with schizophrenia show reduced activation in several brain regions involved in mental state attribution, including the temporal-parietal junction, the medial prefrontal cortex, and the superior temporal gyrus (Lee et al., 2011a; Das et al., 2012; Brune et al., 2011; Walter et al., 2009). A study using magnetoencephalography (MEG) showed reduced activation in relevant brain regions, including the posterior superior temporal sulcus, right temporal-parietal junction, and the right inferior parietal lobule in the first 200 to 600 ms when individuals with schizophrenia performed a mental state attribution task (Vistoli et al., 2011).

Social Perception

Social perception involves the ability to judge social cues and understand roles, rules, and goals that typically characterize different types of social situations or social relationships (Corrigan & Green, 1993; Corrigan et al., 1992). In a typical social perception task such as the Profile of Nonverbal Sensitivity (PONS) (Rosenthal et al., 1979), individuals need to process verbal, paraverbal, and/or nonverbal cues to understand complex or ambiguous social situations (e.g., identifying interpersonal features such as intimacy, status, mood state, and veracity). Using the PONS, studies showed impaired social cue perception in individuals with schizophrenia (Sergi et al., 2006; Wynn et al., 2010b). Another task, the Relationships across Domains test, assesses social relationship perception by asking individuals to judge the appropriateness of social interactions using brief vignettes describing a female-male dyad interaction in particular situations. Individuals with schizophrenia perform more poorly than healthy controls on this task, presumably because they have difficulty assessing the types of relationships that the dyads illustrate (Sergi et al., 2009; Green et al., 2012a). A recent meta-analysis of 13 studies reported a large impairment (effect size of 1.04) in schizophrenia (Savla et al., 2012). In contrast to behavioral studies on social perception, we are unaware of any studies that examined the neural correlates of social perception in schizophrenia.

Attributional Style

Attributional style refers to how one characteristically explains the causes of positive and negative events in his or her everyday life. Attribution style can be divided into three categories: external personal attribution (i.e., causes attributed to other people), external situational attribution (i.e., causes attributed to situational factors), and internal attribution (i.e., causes due to oneself). Compared to other domains of social cognition, there are relatively few assessment measures for attributional style. The few existing studies have tended to focus on the relationship between self-reported attributional style and delusions. When explaining negative events, individuals with persecutory delusions have been found to report elevated levels of external personal attributions rather than situational attributions (known as "personalizing bias") (Bentall, 2001; Garety & Freeman, 1999) and to perceive more hostility for ambiguous situations (An et al., 2010; Combs et al., 2009). Findings on the attributional style of individuals with schizophrenia who do not show severe persecutory delusions are not consistent: findings range from an attributional style similar to controls (Combs et al., 2009) to more internal (Mizrahi et al., 2008) or external (Janssen et al., 2006). A recent meta-analysis also confirms negligible differences (effect size of 0.17) between individuals with schizophrenia and controls for personalizing bias (Savla et al., 2012). Similar to social perception, little is known about neural structures or correlates of attribution style in schizophrenia.

Emerging Social Cognitive and Affective Neuroscience Translational Research: Empathy and Its Applications to Schizophrenia

Research on social cognition in schizophrenia has historically focused on the four domains reviewed above. However, social cognition is a broad field (Lieberman, 2007; Ochsner, 2008), and recent advances in social cognitive and affective neuroscience have provided a rich foundation for translational research into other types of domains that are likely relevant to schizophrenia (e.g., empathy, self-referential processing, social reward processing). In this section, we will describe recently emerging work on empathic processing in healthy individuals and schizophrenia as an example of translational efforts from social cognitive and affective neuroscience to schizophrenia research.

Empathy in Healthy Individuals

Empathy—an ability to share and understand the unique emotional experiences of other people—is involved in virtually all aspects of social interaction and is crucial for successful relationships (Eisenberg & Miller, 1987). Empathy is a complex, multifaceted psychological construct (Singer & Lamm, 2009; Decety & Jackson, 2004), and we will focus on three components of empathy: trait empathy, emotional empathy, and cognitive empathy.

Trait empathy refers to one's own beliefs about his or her empathic characteristics and can be measured by asking individuals to endorse items on self-report questionnaires about their thoughts or feelings in diverse situations. For instance, the widely used Interpersonal Reactivity Index (IRI) (Davis, 1983) characterizes one's beliefs about empathic abilities in four areas: fantasy, empathic concern, perspective taking, and personal distress. Compared to individuals with low scores in trait empathy, people with high scores are more sensitive to socially relevant information (van den Brink et al., 2012; Hofelich & Preston, 2012) and show more prosocial behaviors (O'Connell et al., 2013).

Emotional empathy refers the innate, relatively automatic tendency to share in the emotional experiences of other people (Decety & Meyer, 2008). Emotional empathy has been studied by measuring "resonance" between individuals either behaviorally, such as the tendency to mimic others' gestures, body position, or emotional facial expressions (i.e., emotional contagion), or physiologically through neuroimaging paradigms. The mirror neuron system, including the pars opercularis, adjacent ventral premotor cortex, and anterior parietal lobule, is proposed as a key neural substrate for resonance between individuals (Iacoboni & Dapretto, 2006). For example, increased blood-oxygen-level dependent (BOLD) activation in the mirror neuron system is observed when participants imitate behaviors of others (e.g., finger movement, facial movement) (Molenberghs et al., 2009) or merely observe others displaying these behaviors (Pfeifer et al., 2008). The mirror neuron system in humans has also been examined through EEG methods. For example, modulation of a 8- to 12-Hz rhythm (i.e., μ suppression) over the sensory motor cortex using EEG is an established index of mirror neuron system activity, which is suppressed during both simple action execution and observation (Arnstein et al., 2011) and is sensitive to the degree of social interaction depicted in visual stimuli (Oberman et al., 2007).

A third component is cognitive empathy or emotional attribution, which refers to the ability to make explicit attributions about the emotional states of another person (e.g., I think he is sad). Cognitive empathy involves deliberate inferential processing concerning the affective state of another person while considering situational and other contextual information as opposed to emotional empathy, which involves relatively automatic processes. As such, it can be thought of as a type of mental state attribution that focuses on the emotional state of other people. Neural regions associated with cognitive empathy are distinct from brain areas involved in emotional empathy. For instance, when inferring the affective states of another person (i.e., cognitive empathy), increased activation is found in the dorsomedial prefrontal cortex and superior temporal sulcus (Schnell et al., 2011) as well as in the lateral orbital frontal gyrus (Hynes et al., 2006). A recent meta-analytic review also showed increased activations in the left anterior midcingulate cortex and the left orbitofrontal cortex on cognitive empathy tasks (Fan et al., 2011).

All three aspects of empathy are likely to contribute to empathic behavior in everyday life. Recent studies on empathic accuracy—the ability to accurately judge the amount and kind of emotion another person is experiencing (Levenson & Ruef, 1992; Ickes et al., 1990)—illustrates two key points on how the components of empathy interact with each other to generate efficient empathic behavior. First, accurate empathic judgment appears to involve both emotional empathy and cognitive empathy. For example, while performing an empathic accuracy task, individuals show increased activations in the sensorimotor cortex of the mirror neuron network, as well as the superior temporal sulcus and the medial prefrontal cortex, which have been implicated in emotion attribution (Zaki et al., 2009). Second, empathic judgment relies on characteristics of both the person empathizing (a "perceiver") and the person being empathized with (a "target"). For example, individuals show more accurate empathic judgment when the target is perceived as being more emotionally expressive (e.g., more social cues) (Zaki et al., 2008; Flury et al., 2009; Snodgrass et al., 1998). Further, when judging the affective states of highly expressive targets, individuals with high trait empathy were more accurate than individuals with low trait empathy (Zaki et al., 2008).

To summarize, we reviewed recent studies on three components of empathy and empathic accuracy, and these findings strongly suggest that all three components are critical for empathic understanding in everyday life. However, it should be noted that empathy is a complex and multifaceted construct, and we did not cover all the components involved in empathy. Further, it should also be noted that less is known about the exact mechanism through which each component is involved in empathic understanding. On a related note, empathy is closely related to other social cognitive domains. For example, emotional processing, including emotion recognition and emotional experience, is related to emotional empathy (Shamay-Tsoory, 2011; Decety & Jackson, 2004). Mental state attribution is integral for accurate empathic understanding (Zaki et al., 2009). Given the critical involvement of these social cognitive domains in empathy, further studies are needed to determine the nature of the relationship between empathy and other social cognitive domains.

Recent Studies on Empathy in Schizophrenia

As described above, social cognitive and affective neuroscience has identified multiple components of empathy that need to be coordinated to facilitate adaptive social functioning. It has also provided valid methods for probing the integrity of, and coordination among, these components in clinical populations such as schizophrenia. We will briefly review findings on trait, emotional, and cognitive empathy in schizophrenia.

Regarding trait empathy, individuals with schizophrenia generally report lower empathic ability on self-report questionnaires (Derntl et al., 2009; Montag et al., 2007; Shamay-Tsoory et al., 2007; Sparks et al., 2010; Bora et al., 2008). On the IRI, individuals with schizophrenia tend to show lower scores on the Perspective Taking and Empathic Concern scales. Further, individuals with schizophrenia with lower self-reported empathic ability show worse community functioning (Smith et al., 2012).

Regarding emotional empathy, only a few studies have examined this construct in schizophrenia. Compared to healthy controls, individuals with schizophrenia show less involuntary mimicking when watching videos of people yawning or laughing (Haker & Rossler, 2009) and when viewing images of angry and happy facial expressions (Varcin et al., 2010). Although these findings suggest a dysfunctional mirror neuron network in schizophrenia, a few studies using EEG and fMRI have produced mixed findings. When observing the hand motions of other people, one study showed decreased mu rhythm suppression in individuals with schizophrenia (McCormick et al., 2012), whereas another showed comparable mu suppression in individuals with schizophrenia and controls (Horan et al., 2014b). Similarly, using fMRI, one study showed an abnormal mirror neuron network system in schizophrenia during observation of complex finger movements (Thakkar et al., 2014), whereas the other study failed to find any group difference when observing simple hand movements and faces expressing emotions (Horan et al., 2014a). Thus, further studies will be needed to determine to what extent the mirror neuron system is aberrant in schizophrenia.

In contrast to emotional empathy, individuals with schizophrenia consistently show impaired performance and aberrant neural activity during cognitive empathy tasks. For example, when attributing emotions to characters depicted in photos of people interacting in daily life situations, individuals with schizophrenia showed worse performance than did healthy controls (Smith et al., 2014). Using similar paradigms, other studies showed reduced neural activations in individuals with schizophrenia in several brain regions, including the superior temporal gyrus, temporal parietal junction, middle temporal gyrus, and precuneus (Benedetti et al., 2009; Derntl et al., 2012), or hyperactivation in the insula (Lee et al., 2010).

Recent studies on empathic accuracy have shed light on how these components contribute to impaired empathic behavior in schizophrenia. Individuals with schizophrenia were less accurate than healthy controls on an empathic accuracy task in which participants judge transient changes of emotional states of other people describing autobiographic events (Lee et al., 2011b). Further, empathic accuracy was differentially modulated by the expressivity of the targets across the groups: healthy controls showed higher empathic accuracy when judging the affective states of highly expressive targets versus less expressive targets, but the empathic accuracy of individuals with schizophrenia was less affected by the expressivity of a target. A subsequent fMRI study (Harvey et al., 2012) showed that individuals with schizophrenia hypoactivated the precuneus, middle frontal gyrus, and thalamus compared to healthy controls, suggesting that blunted activations in these areas are related to poor empathic accuracy in schizophrenia. Further, the emotional expressivity of targets modulated activations in several brain regions, such as the medial prefrontal cortex, lateral prefrontal cortex, and inferior parietal lobule in healthy controls, but no such changes were noted in individuals with schizophrenia. Thus, individuals with schizophrenia show impaired empathic accuracy across behavioral and neural levels, which may reflect an inability to incorporate the informational value of social cues that are emitted by social targets.

Pathways from Social Cognition to Functioning in Schizophrenia

The rapid growth of social cognition research in schizophrenia described above has been largely motivated by the expectation that social cognition will provide a clearer understanding of the causes of social disability associated with this disorder. Considerable research now supports the theorized link between social cognitive impairments and functional outcome. Social cognitive deficits show consistently strong relations to poor functioning in schizophrenia. A recent meta-analytic review (Fett et al., 2011) revealed strong relationships between functional outcome and three social cognitive domains: mental state attribution = 0.48, social perception = 0.41, and emotion perception = 0.31. In addition, the association between social cognition and functional outcome is stronger than the association with some other known determinants of functional outcome. For example, social cognition explained an average of 16 percent of the variance in functioning, which was significantly larger than the 6 percent of the variance accounted by nonsocial neurocognition (Fett et al., 2011). Furthermore, social cognition can explain variance in functioning beyond that provided by nonsocial cognition alone (Brekke et al., 2005; Roncone et al., 2002; Poole et al., 2000).

Moving beyond the association between social cognition and functional outcome, emerging work is examining how social cognition interacts with other known factors that affect functional outcome (e.g., neurocognition, perception, negative symptoms). First, social cognition serves as a mediator in the relationships among neurocognition, social cognition, and functional outcome, as evidenced by a recent review (Schmidt et al., 2011). Specifically, social cognition has significant relationships to nonsocial neurocognition, on one hand, and to community functioning, on the other, and the direct relationships between neurocognition and outcome are reduced or eliminated when social cognition is added to a model. This review also found that about 25 percent of the variance in outcome is explained by mediation models (Schmidt et al., 2011). Second, social cognition similarly mediates a relationship between early visual perception and functional outcome in schizophrenia. Deficits in early visual perception are strong correlates of poor functioning in schizophrenia (Green et al., 2011), and this relationship is fully mediated by social cognition (Sergi et al., 2006). These findings suggest that social cognition is an important mechanism through which disturbances in early visual perception and neurocognition ultimately lead to poor functioning in schizophrenia.

Third, motivational factors appear to be an intervening factor in the relationship between social cognition and functioning. Similar to social cognition, motivational disturbances/negative symptoms show consistent relations to impaired functional outcome in schizophrenia (Blanchard et al., 2011). A key question has been whether social cognition and motivation act independently upon functional outcome (Bowie et al., 2006; Bowie et al., 2008) or whether they are part of a single path in which impaired social cognition reduces motivation, which in turn affects poor functioning (Grant & Beck, 2009). Using structural equation modeling (SEM) with a relatively large sample of individuals with schizophrenia, we recently evaluated an integrative model with key determinants of functional outcome in schizophrenia, including visual perception, social cognition, defeatist beliefs, and experiential negative symptoms (Green et al., 2012b). Defeatist beliefs refer to overly generalized negative beliefs about one's ability to successfully perform tasks (Beck et al., 2009). Experiential negative symptoms include avolition/apathy and anhedonia/asociality (Blanchard et al., 2011). As shown in Figure 7.1, a streamlined, single pathway best explained the data. This pathway runs from perception to social cognition to defeatist beliefs to experiential negative symptoms to community functioning. In other words, impaired social cognition can lead to poor community functioning through motivational factors (e.g., defeatist beliefs and negative symptoms). Thus, as the research described in this section demonstrates, social cognition plays a crucial role in accounting for poor community functioning in schizophrenia.

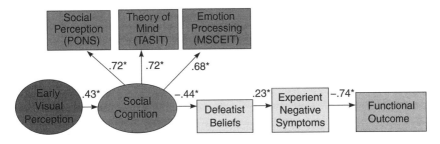

All paths marked with * are significant p < .05

FIGURE 7.1. Multivariate models of how social cognition interacts with other known determinants of poor community functioning in schizophrenia were evaluated with structural equation modeling. Social cognition mediates a relationship between early visual deficits and functioning in schizophrenia. Further, defeatist belief and negative symptoms are part of a single path in which impaired social cognition reduces motivation, which in turn induces negative symptoms and affects poor functioning (adapted from Green et al., 2012b).

Future Directions

Research on social cognition in schizophrenia has expanded rapidly over the past decade. It is now well established that individuals with schizophrenia show impairments across the domains of emotion processing, mental state attribution, and social perception and that these impairments are strongly related to poor community functioning. There has also been some progress in identifying neural regions that may contribute to these impairments. Guided by exciting advances in social cognitive and affective neuroscience, schizophrenia researchers are now beginning to look beyond these areas to achieve a better understanding of the determinants of poor functional outcome. We described recent work on empathy as an example of such efforts and examined emerging evidence of impairments in component processes of empathy in individuals with schizophrenia. Research on social cognition in schizophrenia is a rich and vibrant area, and many issues remain to be addressed in future studies. We will highlight a few of these issues.

First, a basic issue concerns the interrelationships among social cognitive domains. Social cognitive research in schizophrenia has mainly focused on individual domains separately, and little is known about the overarching structure of social cognitive domains in schizophrenia. Further, there appears to be considerable overlap among social cognitive domains, such as the relationship between empathy and other social cognitive domains as we described above. This issue in part reflects our limited understanding of neurobiological mechanisms of social cognitive impairments in schizophrenia. Previous studies have identified neural regions associated with social cognitive impairments in individuals with schizophrenia compared to healthy controls, focusing on key areas (e.g., amygdala for impaired affect recognition; temporoparietal junction for impaired mental state attribution) (also see Hooker, Chapter 5, in this volume). However, these studies tend to examine each social cognitive construct separately, and they are limited in determining how distinct each construct is from each other. Thus, it will be critical to determine the optimal structure and organization of social cognition in schizophrenia using both behavioral and functional neuroimaging methodologies (Mancuso et al., 2011; Green & Lee, 2012) in future studies.

On a related note, there is an increasing understanding that neural circuits involving coordinated activity among multiple key regions (i.e., connectivity) are likely more critical for determining the relationship between brain and social behaviors. The connection between the amygdala and the ventromedial prefrontal cortex has been suggested as a key mechanism of effective emotional regulation (Ochsner et al., 2009). Similarly, functional connectivity of the medial prefrontal cortex and the anterior temporal pole has been proposed to be important for social interactions (Olson et al., 2007; Krueger et al., 2009). Efforts to move beyond investigation of isolated neural regions to connectivity within well-defined neural circuitry and to elucidate neurochemical underpinnings (Holt et al., 2011; Averbeck et al., 2012; Morris et al., 2012) can also provide a more complete picture of social cognition in schizophrenia.

Second, further studies are necessary to determine the full scope of social cognitive impairment in schizophrenia. In addition to the five social cognitive domains reviewed in this chapter, research in this field has already begun to benefit from the rapid growth of social cognitive and affective neuroscience to explore other potential domains such as self-referential processing, social stress, and neuroeconomics that are likely to be relevant to schizophrenia. For example, self-referential processing refers to an ability to attribute traits and dispositions to oneself and others (Macrae et al., 2004) and is regarded as a key component of self versus other processing. Self-referential processing could be relevant to schizophrenia such that certain psychotic symptoms of schizophrenia involve a blurry distinction between self versus other-related processing. Healthy individuals are better at processing traits and dispositions related to themselves (i.e., self-referential bias), but individuals with schizophrenia have failed to show this bias (Harvey et al., 2011). Further, there may be some social cognitive areas in which individuals with schizophrenia are intact. For instance, individuals with schizophrenia were similar to controls when recognizing emotional expressions of faces in the presence of a situational context (Lee et al., 2013; Chung & Barch, 2011), suggesting that individuals with schizophrenia may benefit from social context as much as controls do.

Third, relatively little is known about the course of social cognitive impairments in schizophrenia. In this chapter, we have focused on studies evaluating social cognitive impairment in the chronic phase of schizophrenia. Although these studies are valuable for characterizing social cognitive impairment in schizophrenia, they are limited in determining whether social cognitive impairment in schizophrenia can be a vulnerability marker (i.e., trait-like) or is more likely to be a symptom indicator (i.e., state-like). Social cognitive impairments have been demonstrated among individuals at risk for schizophrenia (Lavoie et al., 2013) and individuals with recent-onset schizophrenia (Green et al., 2012a; Kucharska-Pietura et al., 2005; Pinkham et al., 2007). Further, the level of impairment has been found to be comparable across the phase of illnesses (Green et al., 2012a). Most of these studies utilized cross-sectional designs and provide indirect evidence for social cognitive impairment as a potential vulnerability maker. However, it is critical to examine the level of social cognitive impairment longitudinally to draw a firm conclusion. A few longitudinal studies using individuals with recent-onset schizophrenia have shown the stability of social cognitive impairment over a twelve-month period (Horan et al., 2012; Addington et al., 2006). More studies on individuals at risk for schizophrenia or individuals with first-episode schizophrenia over a longer period will help us determine whether social cognitive impairment in schizophrenia is a stable vulnerability marker.

Fourth, considering the key role of social cognition for social functioning, it is not surprising that social cognition has been examined in other mental disorders characterized by dysfunctional social behavior. For instance, individuals with autism have shown impaired social cognition, but studies have been more focused on certain social cognitive domains than others (e.g., mental state attribution, facial recognition) (Iacoboni & Dapretto, 2006; Weigelt et al., 2012). Social cognitive impairment has been also implicated in depression and bipolar disorder (Cusi et al., 2012; Hoertnagl & Hofer, 2014). However, most of the studies in these disorders (as well as schizophrenia) have focused on characterizing social cognitive impairment among affected individuals compared to psychiatrically healthy individuals, and little is known about the specificity and sensitivity of social cognitive impairment across multiple psychiatric disorders. Further studies using a transdiagnostic approach will help us understand the extent and degree of social cognitive impairment across disorders.

Finally, the strong relationship between social cognition and poor functioning in schizophrenia has generated considerable excitement about the possibility of improving functional outcome through interventions that target social cognition. Emerging evidence indicates that social cognition is amenable to training interventions in schizophrenia (Horan et al., 2011; Combs et al., 2007). In addition, the modulation of social cognition by the neuropeptides oxytocin and vasopressin (Meyer-Lindenberg et al., 2011; Bartz et al., 2011) has also encouraged several efforts to enhance social cognitive impairments in schizophrenia using these neuropeptides (Carter et al., 2009; Pedersen et al., 2011; Davis et al., 2013; Davis et al., 2014). Further, noninvasive brain stimulation such as transcranial direct stimulation (tDCS) has been shown to improve social cognition in healthy individuals (Santiesteban et al., 2012), suggesting that noninvasive brain "current" stimulation could be beneficial for improving social cognitive impairments in individuals with schizophrenia. Further research on social cognitive impairment in schizophrenia in combination with psychopharmacological, psychosocial, and other novel intervention studies (e.g., neurostimulation) may hold the greatest promise for recovery from this disorder.

References

Addington, J., Saeedi, H., & Addington, D. (2006). Influence of social perception and social knowledge on cognitive and social functioning in early psychosis. *British Journal of Psychiatry, 189*, 373–378.

Adolphs, R. (2001). The neurobiology of social cognition. *Current Opinion in Neurobiology, 11*, 231–239.

An, S. K., Kang, J. I., Park, J. Y., Kim, K. R., Lee, S. Y., & Lee, E. (2010). Attribution bias in ultra-high risk for psychosis and first-episode schizophrenia. *Schizophrenia Research, 118*, 54–61.

Anticevic, A., Van Snellenberg, J. X., Cohen, R. E., Repovs, G., Dowd, E. C., & Barch, D. M. (2012). Amygdala recruitment in schizophrenia in response to aversive emotional material: A meta-analysis of neuroimaging studies. *Schizophrenia Bulletin, 38*, 608–621.

Arnstein, D., Cui, F., Keysers, C., Maurits, N. M., & Gazzola, V. (2011). Mu-suppression during action observation and execution correlates with BOLD in dorsal premotor, inferior parietal, and SI cortices. *Journal of Neuroscience, 31*, 14243–14249.

Averbeck, B. B., Bobin, T., Evans, S., & Shergill, S. S. (2012). Emotion recognition and oxytocin in patients with schizophrenia. *Psychological Medicine, 42*(2), 259–266.

Badcock, J. C., Paulik, G., & Maybery, M. T. (2011). The role of emotion regulation in auditory hallucinations. *Psychiatry Research, 185*, 303–308.

Baron-Cohen, S., Wheelwright, S., Hill, J., Raste, Y., & Plumb, I. (2001). The "Reading the mind in the eyes" test revised version: A study with normal adults, and adults with Asperger syndrome or high-functioning autism. *Journal of Child Psychology and Psychiatry and Allied Disciplines, 42*, 241–251.

Bartz, J. A., Zaki, J., Bolger, N., & Ochsner, K. N. (2011). Social effects of oxytocin in humans: Context and person matter. *Trends in Cognitive Science, 15*, 301–309.

Beck, A. T., Rector, N. A., Stolar, N., & Grant, P. M. (2009). *Schizophrenia: Cognitive theory, research and therapy.* New York: Guilford.

Benedetti, F., Bernasconi, A., Bosia, M., Cavallaro, R., Dallaspezia, S., Falini, A., Poletti, S., Radaelli, D., Riccaboni, R., Scotti, G., & Smeraldi, E. (2009). Functional and structural brain correlates of theory of mind and empathy deficits in schizophrenia. *Schizophrenia Research, 114*, 154–160.

Bentall, R. P., Corcoran, R., Howard, R., Blackwood, N., & Kinderman, P. (2001). Persecutory delusions: A review and theoretical integration. *Clinical Psychology Review, 21*, 1143–1192.

Blanchard, J. J., Kring, A. M., Horan, W. P., & Gur, R. (2011). Toward the next generation of negative symptom assessments: The collaboration to advance negative symptom assessment in schizophrenia. *Schizophrenia Bulletin, 37*, 291–299.

Bora, E., Gokcen, S., & Veznedaroglu, B. (2008). Empathic abilities in people with schizophrenia. *Psychiatry Research, 160*, 23–29.

Bora, E., Yucel, M., & Pantelis, C. (2009). Theory of mind impairment in schizophrenia: Meta-analysis. *Schizophrenia Research, 109*, 1–9.

Bowie, C. R., Leung, W. W., Reichenberg, A., McClure, M. M., Patterson, T. L., Heaton, R. K., & Harvey, P. D. (2008). Predicting schizophrenia patients' real-world behavior with specific neuropsychological and functional capacity measures. *Biological Psychiatry, 63*, 505–511.

Bowie, C. R., Reichenberg, A., Patterson, T. L., Heaton, R. K., & Harvey, P. D. (2006). Determinants of real-world functional performance in schizophrenia subjects: Correlations with cognition, functional capacity, and symptoms. *American Journal of Psychiatry, 163*, 418–425.

Brekke, J. S., Kay, D. D., Kee, K. S., & Green, M. F. (2005). Biosocial pathways to functional outcome in schizophrenia. *Schizophrenia Research, 80*, 213–225.

Brune, M. (2003). Social cognition and behavior in schizophrenia. In M. Brune, H. Ribbert, & W. Schiefenhövel (Eds.), *The social brain: Evolution and pathology* (pp. 277–314). Chichester, UK: John Wiley & Sons.

Brune, M., Ozgurdal, S., Ansorge, N., von Reventlow, H. G., Peters, S., Nicolas, V., Tegenthoff, M., Juckel, G., & Lissek, S. (2011). An fMRI study of "theory of mind" in at-risk states of psychosis: Comparison with manifest schizophrenia and healthy controls. *Neuroimage, 55*, 329–337.

Carter, C. S., Barch, D. M., Gur, R., Pinkham, A., & Ochsner, K. (2009). CNTRICS final task selection: Social cognitive and affective neuroscience-based measures. *Schizophrenia Bulletin, 35*, 153–162.

Chung, Y. S., & Barch, D. M. (2011). The effect of emotional context on facial emotion ratings in schizophrenia. *Schizophrenia Research*, 131, 235–241.

Chung, Y. S., Mathews, J. R., & Barch, D. M. (2011). The effect of context processing on different aspects of social cognition in schizophrenia. *Schizophrenia Bulletin*, 37, 1048–1056.

Cohen, A. S., & Minor, K. S. (2010). Emotional experience in patients with schizophrenia revisited: Meta-analysis of laboratory studies. *Schizophrenia Bulletin*, 36, 143–150.

Combs, D. R., Adams, S. D., Penn, D. L., Roberts, D., Tiegreen, J., & Stem, P. (2007). Social Cognition and Interaction Training (SCIT) for inpatients with schizophrenia spectrum disorders: Preliminary findings. *Schizophrenia Research*, 91, 112–116.

Combs, D. R., Penn, D. L., Michael, C. O., Basso, M. R., Wiedeman, R., Siebenmorgan, M., Tiegreen, J., & Chapman, D. (2009). Perceptions of hostility by persons with and without persecutory delusions. *Cognitive Neuropsychiatry*, 14, 30–52.

Corcoran, R., Mercer, G., & Frith, C. D. (1995). Schizophrenia, symptomatology and social inference: investigating "theory of mind" in people with schizophrenia. *Schizophrenia Research*, 17, 5–13.

Corrigan, P. W., & Green, M. F. (1993). Schizophrenic patients' sensitivity to social cues: The role of abstraction. *American Journal of Psychiatry*, 150, 589–594.

Corrigan, P. W., Wallace, C. J., & Green, M. F. (1992). Deficits in social schemata in schizophrenia. *Schizophrenia Research*, 8, 129–135.

Cusi, A. M., Nazarov, A., Holshausen, K., Macqueen, G. M., & McKinnon, M. C. (2012). Systematic review of the neural basis of social cognition in patients with mood disorders. *Journal of Psychiatry & Neuroscience*, 37, 154–169.

Das, P., Lagopoulos, J., Coulston, C. M., Henderson, A. F., & Malhi, G. S. (2012). Mentalizing impairment in schizophrenia: A functional MRI study. *Schizophrenia Research*, 134, 158–164.

Davis, M. (1983). Measuring individual differences in empathy: Evidence for multidimensional approach. *Journal of Personality and Social Psychology*, 44, 113–126.

Davis, M. C., Green, M. F., Lee, J., Horan, W. P., Senturk, D., Clarke, A. D., & Marder, S. R. (2014). Oxytocin-augmented social cognitive skills training in schizophrenia. *Neuropsychopharmacology*, 39(9), 2070–2077.

Davis, M. C., Lee, J., Horan, W. P., Clarke, A. D., McGee, M. R., Green, M. F., & Marder, S. R. (2013). Effects of single dose intranasal oxytocin on social cognition in schizophrenia. *Schizophrenia Research*, 147, 393–397.

Decety, J., & Jackson, P. L. (2004). The functional architecture of human empathy. *Behavioral and Cognitive Neuroscience Review*, 3, 71–100.

Decety, J., & Meyer, M. (2008). From emotion resonance to empathic understanding: A social developmental neuroscience account. *Development and Psychopathology*, 20, 1053–1080.

Derntl, B., Finkelmeyer, A., Toygar, T. K., Hulsmann, A., Schneider, F., Falkenberg, D. I., & Habel, U. (2009). Generalized deficit in all core components of empathy in schizophrenia. *Schizophrenia Research*, 108, 197–206.

Derntl, B., Finkelmeyer, A., Voss, B., Eickhoff, S. B., Kellermann, T., Schneider, F., & Habel, U. (2012). Neural correlates of the core facets of empathy in schizophrenia. *Schizophrenia Research, 136*, 70–81.

Dowd, E. C., & Barch, D. M. (2010). Anhedonia and emotional experience in schizophrenia: Neural and behavioral indicators. *Biological Psychiatry, 67*, 902–911.

Edwards, J., Pattison, P. E., Jackson, H. J., & Wales, R. J. (2001). Facial affect and affective prosody recognition in first-episode schizophrenia. *Schizophrenia Research, 48*, 235–253.

Eisenberg, N., & Miller, P. A. (1987). The relation of empathy to prosocial and related behaviors. *Psychological Bulletin, 101*, 91–119.

Fan, Y., Duncan, N. W., de Greck, M., & Northoff, G. (2011). Is there a core neural network in empathy? An fMRI based quantitative meta-analysis. *Neuroscience and Biobehavioral Reviews, 35*, 903–911.

Fett, A. K., Viechtbauer, W., Dominguez, M. D., Penn, D. L., van Os, J., & Krabbendam, L. (2011). The relationship between neurocognition and social cognition with functional outcomes in schizophrenia: a meta-analysis. *Neuroscience and Biobehavioral Reviews, 35*, 573–588.

Flury, J. M., Ickes, W., & Schweinle, W. (2009). The borderline empathy effect: do high BPD individuals have greater empathic ability? Or are they just more difficult to "read"? *Journal of Research in Personality, 42*, 312–332.

Frith, C. D. (1992). *The cognitive neuropsychology of schizophrenia*. Hove, UK: Lawrence Erlbaum.

Frith, C. D., & Corcoran, R. (1996). Exploring 'theory of mind' in people with schizophrenia. *Psychological Medicine, 26*, 521–530.

Gard, D. E., Kring, A. M., Gard, M. G., Horan, W. P., & Green, M. F. (2007). Anhedonia in schizophrenia: Distinctions between anticipatory and consummatory pleasure. *Schizophrenia Research, 93*, 253–260.

Garety, P. A., & Freeman, D. (1999). Cognitive approaches to delusions: A critical review of theories and evidence. *British Journal of Clinical Psychology, 38*, 113–154.

Gold, R., Butler, P., Revheim, N., Leitman, D. I., Hansen, J. A., Gur, R. C., Kantrowitz, J. T., Laukka, P., Juslin, P. N., Silipo, G. S., & Javitt, D. C. (2012). Auditory emotion recognition impairments in schizophrenia: Relationship to acoustic features and cognition. *American Journal of Psychiatry, 169*, 424–432.

Grant, P. M., & Beck, A. T. (2009). Defeatist beliefs as a mediator of cognitive impairment, negative symptoms, and functioning in schizophrenia. *Schizophrenia Bulletin, 35*, 798–806.

Green, M. F., Bearden, C. E., Cannon, T. D., Fiske, A. P., Hellemann, G. S., Horan, W. P., Kee, K., Kern, R. S., Lee, J., Sergi, M. J., Subotnik, K. L., Sugar, C. A., Ventura, J., Yee, C. M., & Nuechterlein, K. H. (2012a). Social cognition in schizophrenia, Part 1: Performance across phase of illness. *Schizophrenia Bulletin, 38*, 854–864.

Green, M. F., Hellemann, G., Horan, W. P., Lee, J., & Wynn, J. K. (2012b). From perception to functional outcome in schizophrenia: Modeling the role of ability and motivation. *Archives of General Psychiatry, 69*, 1216–1224.

Green, M. F., & Lee, J. (2012). Neural bases of emotional experience versus perception in schizophrenia. *Biological Psychiatry, 71*, 96–97.

Green, M. F., Lee, J., Wynn, J. K., & Mathis, K. I. (2011). Visual masking in schizophrenia: Overview and implications for theories of aberrant visual processing. *Schizophrenia Bulletin, 37*, 700–708.

Green, M. F., Olivier, B., Crawley, J. N., Penn, D. L., & Silverstein, S. (2005). Social cognition in schizophrenia: Recommendations from the MATRICS New Approaches Conference. *Schizophrenia Bulletin, 31*, 882–887.

Green, M. F., Penn, D. L., Bentall, R., Carpenter, W. T., Gaebel, W., Gur, R. C., Kring, A. M., Park, S., Silverstein, S. M., & Heinssen, R. (2008). Social cognition in schizophrenia: an NIMH workshop on definitions, assessment, and research opportunities. *Schizophrenia Bulletin, 34*, 1211–1220.

Gross, J. J. (1998). The emerging field of emotion regulation: An integrative review. *Review of General Psychology, 2*, 271–299.

Haker, H., & Rossler, W. (2009). Empathy in schizophrenia: Impaired resonance. *European Archives of Psychiatry and Clinical Neuroscience, 259*, 352–361.

Happe, F. (1994). An advanced test of theory of mind: Understanding of story characters' thoughts and feelings by able austics, mentally handicapped and normal children and adults. *Journal of Autism and Developmental Disorders, 24*, 129–154.

Harvey, P. O., Lee, J., Horan, W. P., Ochsner, K., & Green, M. F. (2011). Do patients with schizophrenia benefit from a self-referential memory bias? *Schizophrenia Research, 127*, 171–177.

Harvey, P. O., Zaki, J., Lee, J., Ochsner, K., & Green, M. F. (2012). Neural substrates of empathic accuracy in people with schizophrenia. *Schizophrenia Bulletin, 39*, 617–628.

Henry, J. D., Rendell, P. G., Green, M. J., McDonald, S., & O'Donnell, M. (2008). Emotion regulation in schizophrenia: Affective, social, and clinical correlates of suppression and reappraisal. *Journal of Abnormal Psychology, 117*, 473–478.

Herbener, E. S. (2008). Emotional memory in schizophrenia. *Schizophrenia Bulletin, 34*, 875–887.

Hoekert, M., Kahn, R. S., Pijnenborg, M., & Aleman, A. (2007). Impaired recognition and expression of emotional prosody in schizophrenia: Review and meta-analysis. *Schizophrenia Research, 96*, 135–145.

Hoertnagl, C. M., & Hofer, A. (2014). Social cognition in serious mental illness. *Current Opinion in Psychiatry, 27*, 197–202.

Hofelich, A. J., & Preston, S. D. (2012). The meaning in empathy: Distinguishing conceptual encoding from facial mimicry, trait empathy, and attention to emotion. *Cognition & Emotion, 26*, 119–128.

Holt, D. J., Cassidy, B. S., Andrews-Hanna, J. R., Lee, S. M., Coombs, G., Goff, D. C., Gabrieli, J. D., & Moran, J. M. (2011). An anterior-to-posterior shift in midline cortical activity in schizophrenia during self-reflection. *Biological Psychiatry, 69*, 415–423.

Horan, W. P., Green, M. F., DeGroot, M., Fiske, A., Hellemann, G., Kee, K., Kern, R. S., Lee, J., Sergi, M. J., Subotnik, K. L., Sugar, C. A., Ventura, J., & Nuechterlein, K. H. (2012). Social cognition in schizophrenia, Part 2: 12-month stability and prediction of functional outcome in first-episode patients. *Schizophrenia Bulletin, 38,* 865–872.

Horan, W. P., Hajcak, G., Wynn, J. K., & Green, M. F. (2013). Impaired emotion regulation in schizophrenia: Evidence from event-related potentials. *Psychological Medicine, 43,* 2377–2391.

Horan, W. P., Iacoboni, M., Cross, K. A., Korb, A., Lee, J., Nori, P., Quintana, J., Wynn, J. K., & Green, M. F. (2014a). Self-reported empathy and neural activity during action imitation and observation in schizophrenia. *NeuroImage Clinical, 5,* 100–108.

Horan, W. P., Kern, R. S., Tripp, C., Hellemann, G., Wynn, J. K., Bell, M., Marder, S. R. & Green, M. F. (2011). Efficacy and specificity of social cognitive skills training for outpatients with psychotic disorders. *Journal of Psychiatric Research, 45,* 1113–1122.

Horan, W. P., Kring, A. M., & Blanchard, J. J. (2006). Anhedonia in schizophrenia: A review of assessment strategies. *Schizophrenia Bulletin, 32,* 259–273.

Horan, W. P., Nuechterlein, K. H., Wynn, J. K., Lee, J., Castelli, F., & Green, M. F. (2009). Disturbances in the spontaneous attribution of social meaning in schizophrenia. *Psychological Medicine, 39,* 635–643.

Horan, W. P., Pineda, J. A., Wynn, J. K., Iacoboni, M., & Green, M. F. (2014b). Some markers of mirroring appear intact in schizophrenia: Evidence from mu suppression. *Cognitive Affective Behavioral Neuroscience, 14,* 1049–1060.

Horan, W. P., Wynn, J. K., Kring, A. M., Simons, R. F., & Green, M. F. (2010). Electrophysiological correlates of emotional responding in schizophrenia. *Journal of Abnormal Psychology, 119,* 18–30.

Hynes, C. A., Baird, A. A., & Grafton, S. T. (2006). Differential role of the orbital frontal lobe in emotional versus cognitive perspective-taking. *Neuropsychologia, 44,* 374–383.

Iacoboni, M., & Dapretto, M. (2006). The mirror neuron system and the consequences of its dysfunction. *Nature Reviews Neuroscience, 7,* 942–951.

Ickes, W., Stinson, L., Bissonnette, V., & Garcia, S. (1990). Naturalistic social cognition: Empathic accuracy in mixed-sex dyads. *Journal of Personality & Social Psychology, 59,* 730–742.

Janssen, I., Versmissen, D., Campo, J. A., Myin-Germeys, I., van Os, J., & Krabbendam, L. (2006). Attribution style and psychosis: evidence for an externalizing bias in patients but not in individuals at high risk. *Psychological Medicine, 36,* 771–778.

Kee, K. S., Green, M. F., Mintz, J., & Brekke, J. S. (2003). Is emotion processing a predictor of functional outcome in schizophrenia? *Schizophrenia Bulletin, 29,* 487–497.

Kee, K. S., Horan, W. P., Salovey, P., Kern, R. S., Sergi, M. S., Fiske, A. P., Lee, J., Subotnik, K. L., Nuechterlein, K. H., Sugar, C. A., & Green, M. F. (2009). Emotional intelligence in schizophrenia. *Schizophrenia Research, 107,* 61–68.

Kern, R. S., Green, M. F., Fiske, A. P., Kee, K. S., Lee, J., Sergi, M. J., Horan, W. P., Subotnik, K. L., Sugar, C. A., & Nuechterlein, K. H. (2009). Theory of mind deficits for processing counterfactual information in persons with chronic schizophrenia. *Psychological Medicine, 39,* 645–654.

Kettle, J. W., O'Brien-Simpson, L., & Allen, N. B. (2008). Impaired theory of mind in first-episode schizophrenia: Comparison with community, university and depressed controls. *Schizophrenia Research, 99*, 96–102.

Koelkebeck, K., Pedersen, A., Suslow, T., Kueppers, K. A., Arolt, V., & Ohrmann, P. (2010). Theory of Mind in first-episode schizophrenia patients: Correlations with cognition and personality traits. *Schizophrenia Research, 119*, 115–123.

Kohler, C. G., Turner, T. H., Bilker, W. B., Brensinger, C. M., Siegel, S. J., Kanes, S. J., Gur, R. E., & Gur, R. C. (2003). Facial emotion recognition in schizophrenia: intensity effects and error pattern. *American Journal of Psychiatry, 160*, 1768–1774.

Kohler, C. G., Walker, J. B., Martin, E. A., Healey, K. M., & Moberg, P. J. (2010). Facial emotion perception in schizophrenia: A meta-analytic review. *Schizophrenia Bulletin, 36*, 1009–1019.

Krueger, F., Barbey, A. K., & Grafman, J. (2009). The medial prefrontal cortex mediates social event knowledge. *Trends in Cognitive Science, 13*, 103–109.

Kucharska-Pietura, K., David, A. S., Masiak, M., & Phillips, M. L. (2005). Perception of facial and vocal affect by people with schizophrenia in early and late stages of illness. *British Journal of Psychiatry, 187*, 523–528.

Langdon, R., Michie, P. T., Ward, P. B., McConaghy, N., Catts, S., & Coltheart, M. (1997). Defective self and/or other mentalising in schizophrenia: A cognitive neuropsychological approach. *Cognitive Neuropsychiatry, 2*, 167–193.

Lavoie, M. A., Plana, I., Bedard Lacroix, J., Godmaire-Duhaime, F., Jackson, P. L., & Achim, A. M. (2013). Social cognition in first-degree relatives of people with schizophrenia: A meta-analysis. *Psychiatry Research, 209*, 129–135.

Lee, J., Kern, R. S., Harvey, P. O., Horan, W. P., Kee, K. S., Ochsner, K., Penn, D. L., & Green, M. F. (2013). An intact social cognitive process in schizophrenia: situational context effects on perception of facial affect. *Schizophrenia Bulletin, 39*, 640–647.

Lee, J., Quintana, J., Nori, P., & Green, M. F. (2011a). Theory of mind in schizophrenia: Exploring neural mechanisms of belief attribution. *Social Neuroscience, 6*, 569–581.

Lee, J., Zaki, J., Harvey, P. O., Ochsner, K., & Green, M. F. (2011b). Schizophrenia patients are impaired in empathic accuracy. *Psychological Medicine, 41*, 2297–2304.

Lee, S. J., Kang, D. H., Kim, C. W., Gu, B. M., Park, J. Y., Choi, C. H., Shin, N. Y., Lee, J. M., & Kwon, J. S. (2010). Multi-level comparison of empathy in schizophrenia: An fMRI study of a cartoon task. *Psychiatry Research: Neuroimaging, 181*, 121–129.

Leitman, D. I., Hoptman, M. J., Foxe, J. J., Saccente, E., Wylie, G. R., Nierenberg, J., Jalbrzikowski, M., Lim, K. O., & Javitt, D. C. (2007). The neural substrates of impaired prosodic detection in schizophrenia and its sensorial antecedents. *American Journal of Psychiatry, 164*, 474–482.

Leitman, D. I., Wolf, D. H., Laukka, P., Ragland, J. D., Valdez, J. N., Turetsky, B. I., Gur, R. E., & Gur, R. C. (2011). Not pitch perfect: Sensory contributions to affective communication impairment in schizophrenia. *Biological Psychiatry, 70*, 611–618.

Levenson, R. W., & Ruef, A. M. (1992). Empathy: A physiological substrate. *Journal of Personality and Social Psychology, 63*, 234–246.

Li, H., Chan, R. C., McAlonan, G. M., & Gong, Q. Y. (2010). Facial emotion processing in schizophrenia: A meta-analysis of functional neuroimaging data. *Schizophrenia Bulletin, 36*, 1029–1039.

Lieberman, M. D. (2007). Social cognitive neuroscience: A review of core processes. *Annual Review of Psychology, 58*, 259–289.

Livingstone, K., Harper, S., & Gillanders, D. (2009). An exploration of emotion regulation in psychosis. *Clinical Psychology and Psychotherapy, 16*, 418–430.

Macrae, C. N., Moran, J. M., Heatherton, T. F., Banfield, J. F., & Kelley, W. M. (2004). Medial prefrontal activity predicts memory for self. *Cerebral Cortex, 14*, 647–654.

Mancuso, F., Horan, W. P., Kern, R. S., & Green, M. F. (2011). Social cognition in psychosis: Multidimensional structure, clinical correlates, and relationship with functional outcome. *Schizophrenia Research, 125*, 143–151.

McCormick, L. M., Brumm, M. C., Beadle, J. N., Paradiso, S., Yamada, T., & Andreasen, N. (2012). Mirror neuron function, psychosis, and empathy in schizophrenia. *Psychiatry Research, 201*, 233–239.

Meyer-Lindenberg, A., Domes, G., Kirsch, P., & Heinrichs, M. (2011). Oxytocin and vasopressin in the human brain: Social neuropeptides for translational medicine. *Nature Reviews Neuroscience, 12*, 524–538.

Mizrahi, R., Addington, J., Remington, G., & Kapur, S. (2008). Attribution style as a factor in psychosis and symptom resolution. *Schizophrenia Research, 104*, 220–227.

Molenberghs, P., Cunnington, R., & Mattingley, J. B. (2009). Is the mirror neuron system involved in imitation? A short review and meta-analysis. *Neuroscience and Biobehavioral Reviews, 33*, 975–980.

Montag, C., Heinz, A., Kunz, D., & Gallinat, J. (2007). Self-reported empathic abilities in schizophrenia. *Schizophrenia Research, 92*, 85–89.

Morris, R. W., Sparks, A., Mitchell, P. B., Weickert, C. S., & Green, M. J. (2012). Lack of cortico-limbic coupling in bipolar disorder and schizophrenia during emotion regulation. *Translational Psychiatry, 2*, e90.

Oberman, L. M., Pineda, J. A., & Ramachandran, V. S. (2007). The human mirror neuron system: A link between action observation and social skills. *Social Cognitive and Affective Neuroscience, 2*, 62–66.

Ochsner, K. N. (2008). The social-emotional processing stream: Five core constructs and their translational potential for schizophrenia and beyond. *Biological Psychiatry, 64*, 48–61.

Ochsner, K. N., Ray, R. R., Hughes, B., McRae, K., Cooper, J. C., Weber, J., Gabrieli, J. D., & Gross, J. J. (2009). Bottom-up and top-down processes in emotion generation: Common and distinct neural mechanisms. *Psychological Science, 20*, 1322–1331.

O'Connell, G., Christakou, A., Haffey, A. T., & Chakrabarti, B. (2013). The role of empathy in choosing rewards from another's perspective. *Frontiers in Human Neuroscience, 7*, 174.

Olson, I. R., Plotzker, A., & Ezzyat, Y. (2007). The enigmatic temporal pole: A review of findings on social and emotional processing. *Brain, 130*, 1718–1731.

Pedersen, A., Koelkebeck, K., Brandt, M., Wee, M., Kueppers, K. A., Kugel, H., Kohl, W., Bauer, J., & Ohrmann, P. (2012). Theory of mind in patients with schizophrenia: Is mentalizing delayed? *Schizophrenia Research, 137*, 224–229.

Pedersen, C. A., Gibson, C. M., Rau, S. W., Salimi, K., Smedley, K. L., Casey, R. L., Leserman, J., Jarskog, L. F., & Penn, D. L. (2011). Intranasal oxytocin reduces psychotic symptoms and improves Theory of Mind and social perception in schizophrenia. *Schizophrenia Research, 132*, 50–53.

Perry, Y., Henry, J. D., & Grisham, J. R. (2011). The habitual use of emotion regulation strategies in schizophrenia. *British Journal of Clinical Psychology, 50*, 217–222.

Pfeifer, J. H., Iacoboni, M., Mazziotta, J. C., & Dapretto, M. (2008). Mirroring others' emotions relates to empathy and interpersonal competence in children. *Neuroimage, 39*, 2076–2085.

Pinkham, A. E., Penn, D. L., Perkins, D. O., Graham, K. A., & Siegel, M. (2007). Emotion perception and social skill over the course of psychosis: a comparison of individuals "at-risk" for psychosis and individuals with early and chronic schizophrenia spectrum illness. *Cognitive Neuropsychiatry, 12*, 198–212.

Poole, J. H., Tobias, F. C., & Vinogradov, S. (2000). The functional relevance of affect recognition errors in schizophrenia. *Journal of the International Neuropsychological Society, 6*, 649–658.

Roncone, R., Falloon, I. R., Mazza, M., De Risio, A., Pollice, R., Necozione, S., Morosini, P., & Casacchia, M. (2002). Is theory of mind in schizophrenia more strongly associated with clinical and social functioning than with neurocognitive deficits? *Psychopathology, 35*, 280–288.

Rosenthal, R., Hall, J. A., DiMatteo, M. R., Rogers, P. L., & Archer, D. (1979). *Sensitivity to nonverbal communication: The PONS test.* Baltimore: Johns Hopkins University Press.

Santiesteban, I., Banissy, M. J., Catmur, C., & Bird, G. (2012). Enhancing social ability by stimulating right temporoparietal junction. *Current Biology, 22*, 2274–2277.

Savla, G. N., Vella, L., Armstrong, C. C., Penn, D. L., & Twamley, E. W. (2012). Deficits in domains of social cognition in schizophrenia: A meta-analysis of the empirical evidence. *Schizophrenia Bulletin, 39*(5), 979–992.

Schmidt, S. J., Mueller, D. R., & Roder, V. (2011). Social cognition as a mediator variable between neurocognition and functional outcome in schizophrenia: Empirical review and new results by structural equation modeling. *Schizophrenia Bulletin, 37*(Suppl. 2), S41–S54.

Schnell, K., Bluschke, S., Konradt, B., & Walter, H. (2011). Functional relations of empathy and mentalizing: An fMRI study on the neural basis of cognitive empathy. *Neuroimage, 54*, 1743–1754.

Sergi, M. J., Fiske, A. P., Horan, W. P., Kern, R. S., Kee, K. S., Subotnik, K. L., Nuechterlein, K. H., & Green, M. F. (2009). Development of a measure of relationship perception in schizophrenia. *Psychiatry Research, 166*, 54–62.

Sergi, M. J., Rassovsky, Y., Nuechterlein, K. H., & Green, M. F. (2006). Social perception as a mediator of the influence of early visual processing on functional status in schizophrenia. *American Journal of Psychiatry,* 163, 448–454.

Shamay-Tsoory, S. G. (2011). The neural bases for empathy. *The Neuroscientist,* 17, 18–24.

Shamay-Tsoory, S. G., Shur, S., Harari, H., & Levkovitz, Y. (2007). Neurocognitive basis of impaired empathy in schizophrenia. *Neuropsychology,* 21, 431–438.

Silver, H., Bilker, W., & Goodman, C. (2009). Impaired recognition of happy, sad and neutral expressions in schizophrenia is emotion, but not valence, specific and context dependent. *Psychiatry Research,* 169, 101–106.

Singer, T., & Lamm, C. (2009). The social neuroscience of empathy. *Annals of the New York Academy of Sciences,* 1156, 81–96.

Smith, M. J., Horan, W. P., Karpouzian, T. M., Abram, S. V., Cobia, D. J., & Csernansky, J. G. (2012). Self-reported empathy deficits are uniquely associated with poor functioning in schizophrenia. *Schizophrenia Research,* 137, 196–202.

Smith, M. J., Horan, W. P., Cobia, D. J., Karpouzian, T. M., Fox, J. M., Reilly, J. L., & Breiter, H. C. (2014). Performance-based empathy mediates the influence of working memory on social competence in schizophrenia. *Schizophrenia Bulletin,* 40, 824–834.

Snodgrass, S. E., Hecht, M. A., & Ploutz-Snyder, R. (1998). Interpersonal sensitivity: Expressivity or perceptivity? *Journal of Personality and Social Psychology,* 74, 238–249.

Sparks, A., McDonald, S., Lino, B., O'Donnell, M., & Green, M. J. (2010). Social cognition, empathy and functional outcome in schizophrenia. *Schizophrenia Research,* 122, 172–178.

Sprong, M., Schothorst, P., Vos, E., Hox, J., & van Engeland, H. (2007). Theory of mind in schizophrenia: meta-analysis. *British Journal of Psychiatry,* 191, 5–13.

Taylor, S. F., Kang, J., Brege, I. S., Tso, I. F., Hosanagar, A., & Johnson, T. D. (2012). Meta-analysis of functional neuroimaging studies of emotion perception and experience in schizophrenia. *Biological Psychiatry,* 71, 136–145.

Thakkar, K. N., Peterman, J. S., & Park, S. (2014). Altered brain activation during action imitation and observation in schizophrenia: A translational approach to investigating social dysfunction in schizophrenia. *American Journal of Psychiatry,* 171, 539–548.

Ursu, S., Kring, A. M., Gard, M. G., Minzenberg, M. J., Yoon, J. H., Ragland, J. D., Solomon, M., & Carter, C. S. (2011). Prefrontal cortical deficits and impaired cognition-emotion interactions in schizophrenia. *American Journal of Psychiatry,* 168, 276–285.

van den Brink, D., Van Berkum, J. J., Bastiaansen, M. C., Tesink, C. M., Kos, M., Buitelaar, J. K., & Hagoort, P. (2012). Empathy matters: ERP evidence for inter-individual differences in social language processing. *Social Cognitive and Affective Neuroscience,* 7, 173–183.

van der Meer, L., van'tWout, M., & Aleman, A. (2009). Emotion regulation strategies in patients with schizophrenia. *Psychiatry Research,* 170, 108–113.

Varcin, K. J., Bailey, P. E., & Henry, J. D. (2010). Empathic deficits in schizophrenia: The potential role of rapid facial mimicry. *Journal of the International Neuropsychological Society, 16*, 621–629.

Vistoli, D., Brunet-Gouet, E., Lemoalle, A., Hardy-Bayle, M. C., & Passerieux, C (2011). Abnormal temporal and parietal magnetic activations during the early stages of theory of mind in schizophrenic patients. *Social Neuroscience, 6*, 316–326.

Walter, H., Ciaramidaro, A., Adenzato, M., Vasic, N., Ardito, R. B., Erk, S., & Bara, B. G. (2009). Dysfunction of the social brain in schizophrenia is modulated by intention type: An fMRI study. *Social cognitive and affective neuroscience, 4*, 166–176.

Weigelt, S., Koldewyn, K., & Kanwisher, N. (2012). Face identity recognition in autism spectrum disorders: A review of behavioral studies. *Neuroscience and Biobehavioral Reviews, 36*, 1060–1084.

Wynn, J. K., Horan, W. P., Kring, A. M., Simons, R. F., & Green, M. F. (2010a). Impaired anticipatory event-related potentials in schizophrenia. *International Journal of Psychophysiology, 77*, 141–149.

Wynn, J. K., Sugar, C., Horan, W. P., Kern, R., & Green, M. F. (2010b). Mismatch negativity, social cognition, and functioning in schizophrenia patients. *Biological Psychiatry, 67*, 940–947.

Zaki, J., Bolger, N., & Ochsner, K. (2008). It takes two: The interpersonal nature of empathic accuracy. *Psychological Science, 19*, 399–404.

Zaki, J., Weber, J., Bolger, N., & Ochsner, K. (2009). The neural bases of empathic accuracy. *Proceedings of the National Academy of Sciences United States of America, 106*, 11382–11387.

8.

Social Cognition in Those at High Risk of Psychosis

Jean Addington and Mariapaola Barbato

Tʜɪs ᴄʜᴀᴘᴛᴇʀ ꜰᴏᴄᴜsᴇs on social cognition in those who are considered to be at high risk of developing psychosis. It is well established that those with schizophrenia have deficits in social cognition that have implications for social functioning (see Lee, Horan, & Green, Chapter 7, this volume). We will first define the population who are considered at risk of developing psychosis. Then we will present current data on deficits in social cognition that have been observed in these young "at-risk" individuals. The implications of these impairments for psychosis will be discussed as well as the relationship of impaired social cognition to social functioning.

Interest and research in social cognition has had a tremendous growth in the past five to ten years. It has been well established that the performance on a range of social cognitive tasks in persons with schizophrenia is reliably below that of healthy volunteers and even other diagnostic groups. Furthermore, poor social cognition correlates with poorer functional outcomes (Fett et al., 2011). A number of reviews and meta-analytic studies have suggested significant impairment in schizophrenia for several social cognitive domains such as theory of mind (ToM) (Bora & Pantelis, 2013; Bora, Yucel, & Pantelis, 2009; Brüne, 2005; Sprong, Schothorst, Vos, Hox, & Van Engeland, 2007), social perception and social knowledge (Piskulic, Addington, & Maruff, 2010), attributional style (Fiske & Taylor, 1991), and affect recognition, including both facial affect (Kohler, Walker, Martin, Healey, & Moberg, 2010) and emotional prosody (i.e., vocal emotion

perception or the evaluation of emotional nonlexical cues in speech)
(Hoekert, Kahn, Pijnenborg, & Aleman, 2007).

The vast majority of these studies, however, have been based on patients
in the more chronic stage of schizophrenia. It has been unclear if the degree of impairment is different in earlier stages of the illness, such as the
recent onset or first episode of psychosis (FE). As will be demonstrated
below, there does seem to be consistent evidence demonstrating that a significant impairment in the majority of the domains of social cognition is
observed at the first episode of psychosis as well as in more chronic stages
of illness. There is the general sense that these individuals experiencing a
psychotic illness for the first time have deficits in most domains; however,
relatively few studies simultaneously addressed more than one domain of
social cognition and typically used one test per domain. In addition, there
is increasing evidence that these impairments in social cognition are stable
over time (Horan et al., 2012; Penn, Addington, & Pinkham, 2006), although it has to be noted that to date, only a small number of studies have
investigated temporal stability of impaired social cognition.

What is less clear is when these impairments begin. Are they present at
the start of the psychotic illness or do they increase as the illness develops?
Perhaps they begin even before there is evidence of full-blown psychosis.
To examine whether a deficit may occur prior to the onset of illness, research typically focused on young people who were considered at risk of
schizophrenia because of a family history of schizophrenia usually in a first-
degree relative. These individuals are considered at familial high risk for
psychosis. However, researchers are now considering another group of
youth who may be at risk for schizophrenia or other psychotic disorders
based on the presentation of early clinical signs. These young people are
considered to be potentially prodromal for psychosis.

Familial High Risk for Psychosis

Given the strong evidence for the role of genetic factors in the development
of psychotic disorders, there have been a number of studies that examined
social cognitive deficits as potential markers of vulnerability to psychosis.
This approach involves investigating whether deficits identified in individuals with psychosis also occur in their unaffected biological first-degree relatives, that is, those who are at familial high risk for psychosis (FHR). Such
an approach is particularly useful as it avoids many confounding factors
that are typically associated with patient samples, such as medication side
effects, prominent neurocognitive deficits, and relationships to clinical

symptoms of the illness (Kee, Horan, Mintz, & Green, 2004). If social cognitive deficits are indeed enduring vulnerability indicators of psychosis, they would be expected to occur with exceptionally high frequency in individuals at increased risk for schizophrenia (Nuechterlein et al., 1992).

Early Detection of Psychosis

Over the past fifteen years, there has been a major emphasis that could be described as a worldwide movement on the early detection and intervention in schizophrenia and other psychotic disorders. The first goal of this movement was to detect and treat major psychotic illnesses early in the development of the illness so that individuals could receive appropriate treatment at the earliest stage possible and have the best opportunity for recovery (Addington, 2007). This work focused on identifying young people as soon as possible after the onset of the psychotic illness in order to minimize the duration of untreated psychosis. However, more recently, the focus has moved to an even earlier stage of the illness, the prodrome, since there is evidence that subclinical symptoms are present during the prepsychotic period (Fusar-Poli et al., 2013).

In schizophrenia, the prodromal phase of the illness refers to the "subclinical" signs and symptoms that a person experiences prior to the onset of a full-blown syndrome (Yung, Phillips, Yuen, & McGorry, 2004). Recent developments in research have led to the development of reliable criteria to identify individuals who may be at risk of developing psychosis and thus potentially experiencing a prodrome for psychosis (McGlashan, Walsh, & Woods, 2010). The criteria for what can be thought of as a putative prodrome for psychosis was first introduced by Alison Yung and colleagues in Melbourne, Australia (Yung & McGorry, 1996), and incorporated into the Comprehensive Assessment of At-Risk Mental States (CAARMS). These criteria were modified by McGlashan and colleagues to form the Criteria of Psychosis-risk Syndromes (COPS). The COPS are evaluated using the Structured Interview for Prodromal Syndromes (SIPS) and the Scale of Prodromal Symptoms (SOPS) (McGlashan et al., 2010).

Both the Melbourne classification approach and the COPS have three possible criteria. These are brief intermittent psychotic symptoms (BIPS), attenuated positive symptoms (APS), and/or genetic risk and deterioration (GRD). The BIPS state requires the presence of any one or more threshold positive psychotic symptoms that are too brief to meet diagnostic criteria for psychosis. The APS requires the presence of at least one particular positive psychotic symptom of insufficient severity to meet diagnostic criteria for a psychotic disorder. The GRD requires having a combination of both functional decline and genetic risk; genetic risk refers to having either schizotypal personality disorder or a first-degree relative with a schizophrenia-spectrum disorder (McGlashan et al., 2010).

By identifying young people in what could be the prodrome of schizophrenia, researchers have the potential to prospectively follow the course of the illness with the goal of being able to distinguish early on differences for those who go on to develop schizophrenia or other psychotic disorders from those who do not. Current evidence indicates that approximately 25 percent of these at-risk individuals will go on to develop a full-blown illness within one year and 35 percent in two years (Cannon et al., 2008; Fusar-Poli et al., 2013). Several terms have been used to distinguish this population from other high-risk groups such as those with a family history risk or those with schizotypy. These individuals are considered at enhanced high risk, and thus the Melbourne group used the term *ultra-high risk* (UHR). Since the risk is often based on the presence of clinical symptoms, these individuals have also been described as being at clinical high risk (CHR) of developing psychosis. In this chapter, the term *CHR* will be used to describe such samples.

Affect Recognition

Affect recognition is the most studied of the domains of social cognition. It refers to the capacity to recognize and be aware of emotional expressions in oneself and others. It includes identifying emotions, either by observing body language or nonlexical cues in speech. Studies assessing affect recognition typically use a task where faces expressing an emotion are presented and participants have to indicate which emotion the face is showing or else use a measure of affective prosody where participants listen to a recording of spoken sentences that reveal particular emotions. For these tasks, participants have to indicate which emotion they hear. In addition to many studies with individuals experiencing a chronic course of schizophrenia, there is evidence suggesting that even at the first episode of psychosis, individuals perform more poorly than do controls on tests of affect recognition (Addington, Saeedi, & Addington, 2006a; Edwards, Pattison, Jackson, & Wales, 2001), affective acuity (Herbener, Hill, Marvin, & Sweeney, 2005), and affect discrimination (Addington et al., 2006a). Furthermore, these deficits seem to be stable over time (Addington et al., 2006a) and continue to be observed even when patients are in remission (Yalcin-Siedentopf et al., 2014).

Eight studies have investigated affect recognition impairments in those at FHR of psychosis. The results of these studies, however, have been somewhat varied (Alfimova et al., 2009; Bôlte & Poustka, 2003; Eack, Greeno, et al., 2010; Kee et al., 2004; Koelkebeck et al., 2010; Leppänen et al., 2006; Loughland, Williams, & Gordon, 2002). In all of these studies except Davalos et al. (2004), the unaffected relatives performed significantly better on tasks of affect recognition compared to their relatives who had a psychotic illness. However, four studies reported significant trends of reduced performance accuracy in unaffected relatives compared to healthy volunteers (Alfimova et al., 2009; Eack, Greeno, et al., 2010; Kee et al., 2004; Leppänen et al., 2006). Specifically, Kee and colleagues (2004) and Alfimova et al. (2009) reported poorer overall performance on tests of facial affect recognition in nonpsychotic relatives compared to healthy controls. Leppanen et al. (2006) and Eack, Greeno, et al. (2010) reported only specific group deficits in relation to negative emotions and neutral faces, respectively. The other two studies conversely reported no significant difference in the accuracy on facial affect recognition tasks between unaffected relatives and healthy volunteers (Bôlte & Poustka, 2003; Loughland et al., 2002). In a comparison of FHR children to healthy age-matched controls, no differences between groups in accuracy of identifying faces as happy, sad, angry, or fearful (Davalos et al., 2004) were observed.

Several studies have examined affect recognition in those at CHR for psychosis, again with mixed results. Addington and colleagues (Addington, Penn, Woods, Addington, & Perkins, 2008) examined facial affect recognition and facial affect discrimination in a sample of eighty-six young people at CHR based on the COPS criteria and compared their performance to individuals with a chronic course of schizophrenia, individuals experiencing their first episode, and healthy controls. Results demonstrated that on the identification task, the healthy controls performed significantly better than did the CHR and patient groups. On the discrimination task, patient groups performed significantly more poorly than did the normal controls, and the performance of the CHR group fell between that of the patient and control groups without significantly differing from either. Supporting these results, Wölwer et al. (2012) reported poor performance in recognition of facial expression for individuals at CHR compared to healthy controls. These results are in contrast to an early small study ($n = 19$) by Pinkham, Penn, Perkins, Graham, and Siegel (2007), who did not find any differences between a CHR group and healthy controls using a similar task, and to Gee et al. (2012), who used emotion labeling and emotion matching computerized tasks.

A recently published study by Amminger and colleagues (Amminger et al., 2012) compared individuals at CHR based on the CAARMS with a first-episode psychosis group and a healthy control group. This Austrian study used a facial affect task and a measure of affective prosody designed by Edwards (Edwards et al., 2001). Findings were that there were deficits in the recognition of fear and sadness across both face and voice modalities for both the CHR and the FE group compared to the healthy controls. Furthermore, in comparison to the healthy controls, both clinical groups had a significant deficit for fear and sadness recognition in faces and for anger recognition in voices. In reviewing their results, these authors suggest this may be a trait deficit and hypothesized how the amygdala, a key brain structure subserving emotion (see Hooker, Chapter 5, this volume), may be involved. The results of this study were in part confirmed by Comparelli and colleagues (2013), who developed their own task to assess facial emotion naming and recognition in individuals at CHR, as well as first-episode and chronic patients, and observed deficits in the recognition of sadness and disgust in the CHR group and all negative emotions in the patient group.

Only one study to date has examined affect processing longitudinally in CHR individuals to determine if affect processing predicted later conversion to psychosis (Addington et al., 2012). In this study, 172 CHR and 100 help-seeking individuals (HS) were followed for up to twenty-four months. Affect recognition was assessed using two facial affect recognition tasks and a measure of affective prosody. In comparison to previously published data from nonpsychiatric controls, both CHR and HS groups demonstrated deficits on affect recognition. By two years, twenty-five CHR participants converted to psychosis. Interestingly, there were no differences between converters and nonconverters on any affect recognition tasks. This is one of the first studies to longitudinally examine affect processing and its relationship to later conversion to psychosis in individuals at risk for psychosis. While poorer affect recognition may be associated with vulnerability for psychosis, the current results suggest that it may not be a marker of developing a psychotic illness.

Theory of Mind

Theory of mind, also referred to as "mentalizing" or mental state attribution, typically involves the ability to infer the intentions, dispositions, and beliefs of others (Frith & Corcoran, 1996; Green, Olivier, Crawley, Penn, & Silverstein, 2005). Essentially, this is the ability to attribute mental states such as beliefs, intents, desires, pretending, or knowledge to oneself and others and also to understand that others have beliefs, desires, and intentions that are different from one's own. Based on the current research from first-episode studies, which almost exclusively comes from cross-sectional research, there is evidence that first-episode patients have impairments relative to controls and similar to those with a more chronic course of illness.

Theory-of-mind deficits have been well documented in individuals with psychotic illness (Bora et al., 2009; Sprong et al., 2007; Thompson et al., 2012), but the extent to which these deficits occur in unaffected first-degree relatives has not been determined. Impaired theory of mind has been reported for first-degree relatives in several studies (Anselmetti et al., 2009; de Achával et al., 2010; Janssen, Krabbendam, Jolles, & van Os, 2003; Wykes, Hamid, & Wagstaff, 2001), at a nonsignificant trend in some (Irani et al., 2006; Marjoram et al., 2006), and no association in one study (Gibson, Penn, Prinstein, Perkins, & Belger, 2010). Some studies have addressed correlates of theory-of-mind impairments in unaffected relatives of individuals with schizophrenia. Irani et al. (2006) found that relatives with schizotypal personality traits performed significantly more poorly than relatives without such traits. In addition, Keleman and colleagues (Kelemen et al., 2005) and Marjoram et al. (2006) similarly noted poorer theory-of-mind performance in relatives with past or present transient psychotic-like symptoms compared to symptom-free relatives.

Several studies have examined theory of mind in young people who are at CHR for psychosis. A Korean group, Chung and colleagues (Chung, Hyung, Shin, Yoo, & Kwon, 2008), compared the performance of a small CHR group ($n = 33$) on the False Belief task (Perner & Wimmer, 1985), the Strange Story task (Happe, 1994), and a visual cartoon task (Oh et al., 2005) to that of a healthy control group. There were significant differences on both the Strange Story task and the False Belief task, with the CHR group performing more poorly, but no differences were observed on the visual cartoon task. These results were replicated by Hur and colleagues (2013). However, using False Beliefs stories and picture sequencing tasks, two other studies did not show specific deficits for CHR individuals (Brune et al., 2011; Stanford et al., 2011). Brune and colleagues (2011), using a False Beliefs picture sequencing task, compared the performance of CHR individuals with that of schizophrenia patients and controls and observed for the CHR group an altered pattern of activation of the ToM neural network, which comprises the prefrontal cortex, posterior cingulate cortex, and temporoparietal cortex, but no behavioral differences on the task. Schizophrenia patients also activated the ToM neural network differently than did controls. Stanford and colleagues (2011) used the False Beliefs cartoon task, the Strange Stories task, and the Reading the Mind in the Eyes task (Baron-Cohen, Wheelwright, Hill, Raste, & Plumb, 2001) with individuals at CHR, schizophrenia patients, and healthy controls. Results of this study did not show differences in ToM between groups. Thompson and colleagues (2012) used the hinting task and the visual jokes and reported that CHR persons performed more poorly than did controls but not significantly different from FE patients. In another study, Couture and colleagues (Couture, Penn, Addington, Woods, & Perkins, 2008) used the Eyes task. In this study with eighty-six CHR participants, there were no differences between the CHR group and healthy controls. Interestingly, in a later study using the same task with a larger sample, it was demonstrated that baseline performance significantly predicted later conversion to psychosis even when controlling for IQ scores (Healey, Penn, Perkins, Woods, & Addington, 2012). The Eyes task was considered by the authors to be a task of theory of mind, although there is some debate as to whether this is typically a task used in this domain.

Finally, a recent meta-analysis that included twenty-one studies examining ToM in schizophrenia concluded that FE and chronic patients had similar deficits in ToM, and those at FHR and CHR performance fell between that of FE patients and of healthy controls (Bora & Pantelis, 2013).

Social Perception and Social Knowledge

Social perception is the awareness of cues that typically occur in social situations. Social knowledge is the awareness of what is socially expected in different situations in order to guide social interactions (Green et al., 2005). Since the identification of social cues generally requires knowledge of what is expected and acceptable in social situations (Green et al., 2005), social perception and social knowledge are often considered together under the domain of social perception. In schizophrenia research, the concept of social perception and knowledge has not been as extensively researched as other domains. Results of the few studies in this field demonstrated that first-episode individuals were as impaired as chronic schizophrenia patients in their understanding of social relationships (Green et al., 2012) and in their ability to appraise social roles and context, as well as their awareness of rules, goals, and roles that characterize social situations (Addington, Saeedi, & Addington, 2006b).

Only two studies to date have investigated social perception and social knowledge in populations at FHR of psychosis. Toomey and colleagues (Toomey, Seidman, Lyons, Faraone, & Tsuang, 1999), who investigated social perception of nonverbal cues using the Profile of Nonverbal Sensitivity (PONS) test, reported that unaffected relatives of people with schizophrenia demonstrated poorer test performance compared to healthy volunteers. In the second study, Baas et al. (Baas, van't Wout, Aleman, & Kahn, 2008) assessed trustworthiness evaluations about unfamiliar faces with neutral expressions in siblings of individuals with schizophrenia. Healthy siblings displayed similar, although attenuated, bias to affected siblings in judging trustworthiness, whereby they judged faces to be more trustworthy compared to healthy volunteers.

To our knowledge, no studies have examined this domain in the CHR population, although one study by Couture et al. (2008) used the Abbreviated Trustworthiness Task to assess complex social judgments (Adolphs, Tranel, & Damasio, 1998) that could potentially be considered a measure of social perception. In this task, participants were shown forty-two faces of unfamiliar people and were asked to imagine they had to trust the pictured person with their money or with their life. They rated how much they would trust the person on a 7-point scale, ranging from −3 (very untrustworthy) to +3 (very trustworthy). In the study by Couture et al. (2008), there was no difference between the CHR participants and healthy controls in terms of rating the trustworthy faces, but the CHR group rated the untrustworthy faces as more positive significantly more often than the healthy controls did. In a later study with the same task and a larger sample, Healey et al. (2012) reported that relative to help-seeking controls, CHR individuals tended to judge faces to be more approachable relative to a control group. This finding for increasing approachability ratings over time may seem counterintuitive, as CHR status is often associated with paranoia. However, complex social judgments demand higher-level social cognitive processes through the interpretation of more nuanced, subtle social cues. This finding in CHR individuals is consistent with prior research indicating a positive bias in patients with nonparanoid schizophrenia (Baas et al., 2008) and in first-degree family members (Couture et al., 2010).

Attributional Style

Attributional style refers to the causal explanations that individuals attribute to their own behavior and the behavior of others (Fiske & Taylor, 1991). This domain of social cognition is generally assessed in reference to patients who experience hallucinations and delusions, especially persecutory delusions, and their explanation of positive and negative life events. A tendency to internally attribute more positive than negative events to self is referred to as self-serving bias. Most of what is now known about attributional style in psychosis comes from research in chronic schizophrenia, while the stability of attributional style in first-episode psychosis remains unclear. A recent study used the Internal, Personal and Situational Attributions Questionnaire (IPSAQ; Kinderman & Bentall, 1996) to assess attributional bias in first-episode patients and gender-matched healthy controls and did not find any difference between groups (Langdon et al., 2013).

There are few studies addressing this in CHR individuals. An et al. (2010) used a recently developed task, the Ambiguous Intentions Hostility Questionnaire (AIHQ) (Combs, Penn, Wicher, & Waldheter, 2007), which is a self-report questionnaire about negative outcomes that vary intentionally or accidentally or with ambiguous intentions. Using this task, the attributions of twenty-four CHR participants were compared to those of healthy controls ($n = 39$) and FE patients ($n = 20$). Both the FE and CHR participants demonstrated a perceived hostility bias. In the FE group, this was related to persecutory symptoms. Similarly, in the CHR group, their attribution bias for perceiving hostility was linked to a paranoid process (An et al., 2010). Devylder et al. (2013) used the IPSAQ to compare individuals at CHR to age-matched healthy controls and found no differences in attributional bias, although this was a small sample. Thompson and colleagues (Thompson et al., 2013), using the Adult Nowicki Strickland Internal External scale (ANSIE; Nowicki & Duke, 1974a, 1974b), demonstrated that the CHR group had a significantly more externalized locus of control than did controls, and this difference remained statistically significant after adjusting for age, gender, and IQ.

Examining Multiple Domains of Social Cognition

One of the issues about the studies examining individuals at FHR or in CHR of psychosis is that they tended to use a single control group. A potentially more direct test of whether there is increasing deficits from the CHR or potentially prodromal phase to the illness phase would include separate comparison groups that demographically matched each of the clinical groups (Green et al., 2012). In this study, the tasks selected reflected three domains: the Relationships Across Domains (RAD; Sergi et al., 2009) to assess models or rules for interactions, the Awareness of Social Inference Test (Part III) (TASIT) to assess capacities to understand other minds, and the Mayer-Salovey-Caruso Emotional Intelligence Test 2.0 (MSCEIT; Mayer, Salovey, Caruso, & Sitarenios, 2003) to assess emotional communication. Three samples each with their own carefully matched control group were examined: a group of patients with a more chronic course of schizophrenia, an FE group, and a CHR group. Results of this study demonstrated impairment in social cognition across each of the different phases of the illness. However, one of the more interesting observations in this study was a lack of evidence of progression or improvement over the three phases of the illness (i.e., from the period of high risk, to the first episode, and then to the more chronic phase of schizophrenia). This study offers support for the idea that impairment in social cognition begins in the early phases of a psychotic illness and remains stable. Although it was limited to three domains, results were consistent across all three domains.

Thomson and colleagues (2012) compared individuals at CHR, FE individuals, and healthy controls. Tasks used included the adult version of the Diagnostic Analysis of Nonverbal Accuracy–2 (DANVA-2; Nowicki & Carton, 1993; Nowicki & Duke, 1994) for facial and voice affect recognition, as well as the hinting task and the visual jokes task for ToM, and social perception was assessed using the MSCEIT. CHR individuals performed more poorly than did controls only on the ToM task, while FE patients performed more poorly than did controls on all three tasks.

Social Cognition, Neurocognition, and Functioning

Current findings regarding clinical, neurocognitive, and real-life functioning correlates of social cognition in first-episode psychosis are mixed. First, results from cross-sectional studies suggest both the presence and the absence of association between psychopathology and performance on tests across different domains of social cognition. The same is true for longitudinal studies that reported both small reduction (Behere, Venkatasubramanian, Arasappa, Reddy, & Gangadhar, 2009; Frith & Corcoran, 1996; Green et al., 2012) and no change (Addington et al., 2006a, 2006b; Herbener et al., 2005) in social cognitive deficits following improvement in psychopathology. Although social cognition is considered psychometrically distinguishable from neurocognition (Addington & Piskulic, 2013; Mehta et al., 2013; Sergi et al., 2007), evidence from first-episode research suggests that a significant association between the two constructs does exist (Addington et al., 2006a, 2006b; Koelkebeck et al., 2010; Krstev, Jackson, & Maude, 1999). Despite the association, however, social cognitive deficits reportedly persisted even after neurocognitive performance was controlled for (Bertrand, Sutton, Achim, Malla, & Lepage, 2007; Koelkebeck et al., 2010). Finally, there is evidence to suggest that social cognition has a unique association with functional outcome in the early course of psychosis as it was reported as a significant predictor of real-life functioning (Horan et al., 2012) and a mediator of the relationship between neurocognition and poor functional outcome (Addington, Girard, Christensen, & Addington, 2010; Schmidt et al., 2011).

With respect to those at FHR of psychosis, two studies that investigated the association between neurocognitive performance and affect perception in unaffected relatives reported it to be nonsignificant (Alfimova et al., 2009; Eack, Mermon, et al., 2010). Some FHR studies found an association between impairments in cognition and theory of mind in unaffected relatives (Janssen et al., 2003), and others did not (Anselmetti et al., 2009; de Achával et al., 2010; Wykes, 1994).

These relationships have been explored in CHR samples as well (Barbato et al., 2013; Yong et al., 2014). Yong and colleagues (2014) examined the associations between a wide range of neurocognitive tasks and social cognition. Their results showed that poor theory of mind correlated with low ratings on a wide range of neurocognitive tasks, while facial affect was more often associated with low ratings on spatial working memory and attention. Barbato and colleagues (2013) examined the relationship between social cognition, neurocognition, and functioning in individuals at CHR, and although significant associations between social cognition and neurocognition and between neurocognition and functional outcome were observed, social cognition did not mediate the pathway from neurocognition to functioning. It is worth noting that in this study, functional outcome was only assessed with a measure of social attainment.

What Have We Learned?

One important aspect of the study of social cognition is the effort to identify endophenotypes of psychotic disorders. Identifying possible vulnerability markers of psychosis among samples of individuals at either FHR or CHR could have implications for an improved understanding of schizophrenia. To date, methodological issues may prevent sound conclusions being drawn with respect to the "at-risk" samples. Although the number of studies are increasing for the majority of studies, samples are small, and only limited social cognitive domains are assessed. However, from the data available, it appears as if those at CHR of psychosis are already demonstrating impairments in facial affect recognition that is often equivalent to that observed in individuals at their first episode of psychosis or even those with a more chronic course of schizophrenia, and there is some evidence of impairment in tasks assessing theory of mind in those at CHR. Studies examining social perception and social knowledge are rare, and thus limited conclusions can be drawn. Results from the one study on attribution fits with observations from patient populations that deficits are typically linked to paranoid or persecutory symptoms. Thus, at this stage, there is support for the idea that deficits in social cognition are already present in the pre-psychotic period. Clearly, more data are required to make such conclusions more solid. It is possible that those at FHR appear to be less impaired compared to CHR individuals and more impaired compared to healthy individuals without a family risk of psychosis. Therefore, it may be that worsening of social cognitive deficits in FHR is contingent on the emergence of subpsychotic symptoms or even worsening in functioning, both of which are observed in CHR. In fact, in those at FHR who did report psychotic-like experiences or having schizotypy (Eack, Mermon, et al., 2010; Marjoram et al., 2006), there was an increase in social cognitive deficits. Thus, impaired social cognition may be on a continuum parallel to that of subthreshold and full-blown psychotic symptoms.

However, little is known about the extent to which these attenuated deficits are associated with the transition to psychosis in individuals at FHR (Eack, Mermon, et al., 2010). Equally, in examining the role of social cognition in predicting psychosis in those at CHR, studies are few. To date, one study has demonstrated that a combination of neurocognitive tasks and social cognition assessed by a theory-of-mind task was related to conversion (Kim et al., 2011). This result has not been replicated yet, and future studies should further explore this relationship. One study suggested that poor performance on a potential theory-of-mind task may predict transition and another that facial affect deficits were not related to transition (Addington et al., 2012). However, there are clear limitations to the research at this time. Longitudinal studies are rare, and there is no evidence about the longitudinal nature of these social cognitive impairments in these young people. Further work needs to be done in examining the role of such deficits in conversion from the CHR stage to that of full-blown psychosis.

What Are the Implications of Studying Social Cognition in the Early Course of the Illness?

Several studies have demonstrated that impairments in social cognition are present early in the course of a psychotic illness and that such impairments appear to be of a stable magnitude from the period of high risk until the more acute and then chronic phase of illness. Although all of the domains have not been examined in one study, there is evidence of impairment in the key domains of emotion perception, theory of mind, social perception and social knowledge, and attributional style. It is possible that this is early evidence of a vulnerability measure of illness rather than an indicator of either the severity of the illness or of chronicity. For social cognition to be a vulnerability or trait marker, the impairments need to be manifest at all stages of the disorder, including both acute and remitted periods for those who have a diagnosed psychotic illness. In addition, there needs to be evidence of the impairment in high-risk groups such as those at family high risk, those at clinical high risk, and those with schizotypy. Thus, impaired social cognition can be seen as a vulnerability marker in psychosis and possibly somewhat independent of impairment in neurocognition and social functioning. In terms of the social brain, we are seeing evidence of impairment through all phases of the disorder with an increase in impairment that parallels the severity of the phase of the disorder. Future research will have to address the role of social cognition in neurocognition and social functioning in the prepsychotic period. Of course, a greater understanding of the neural underpinnings of social cognition, particularly in this period of risk, which could lead to greater understanding of the illness, would be very relevant for future work. There is an increased interest in the role of social risk factors in the development and early phases of psychosis (van Os, Rutten, & Poulton, 2008); therefore, in future studies, it may be important to review these early social cognitive impairments in the context of other social and early childhood adversities (Addington et al., in press), particularly with the CHR group.

Finally, there are implications for treatment. Treatment effectiveness studies of those at CHR are in the early stages. Since there is support for social cognitive deficits as potential vulnerability markers, improvement of underlying vulnerability may in itself help reduce the risk for later psychosis and limit later functional disability (Cornblatt et al., 2003). Thus, investigating how vulnerability markers can be used as treatment targets is critical to developing early intervention efforts.

References

Addington, J. (2007). The promise of early intervention. *Journal of Early Intervention, 1*, 294–307.

Addington, J., Saeedi, H., & Addington, D. (2006a). Facial affect recognition: A mediator between cognitive and social functioning in psychosis? *Schizophrenia Research, 85*, 142–150.

———. (2006b). Influence of social perception and social knowledge on cognitive and social functioning in early psychosis. *British Journal of Psychiatry,* 189, 373–378.

Addington, J., Penn, D., Woods, S. W., Addington, D., & Perkins, D. O. (2008). Social functioning in individuals at clinical high risk for psychosis. *Schizophrenia Research,* 99, 119–124.

Addington, J., Girard, T. A., Christensen, B. K., & Addington, D. (2010). Social cognition mediates illness-related and cognitive influences on social function in patients with schizophrenia-spectrum disorders. *Journal of Psychiatry and Neuroscience,* 35, 49–54.

Addington, J., Piskulic, D., Perkins, D., Woods, S. W., Liu, L., & Penn, D. L. (2012). Affect recognition in people at clinical high risk of psychosis. *Schizophrenia Research,* 140, 87–92.

Addington, J., & Piskulic, D. (2013). Social cognition early in the course of the illness. In D. Roberts & D. Penn (Eds.), *Social cognition in schizophrenia.* New York: Oxford University Press.

Addington, J., Stowkowy, J., Cadenhead, K., Cornblatt, B., McGlashan, T., Perkins, D., et al. (in press). Early traumatic experiences in those at clinical high risk for psychosis. *Early Intervention in Psychiatry,* 7, 300–305.

Adolphs, R., Tranel, D., & Damasio, A. R. (1998). The human amygdala in social judgment. *Nature,* 393, 470–474.

Alfimova, M. V., Abramova, L. I., Barhatova, A. I., Yumatova, P. E., Lyachenko, G. L., & Golimbet, V. E. (2009). Facial affect recognition deficit as a marker of genetic vulnerability to schizophrenia. *Spanish Journal of Psychology,* 12, 46–55.

Amminger, G. P., Schäfer, M. R., Papageorgiou, K., Klier, C. M., Schlögelhofer, M., Mossaheb, N., et al. (2012). Emotion recognition in individuals at clinical high-risk for schizophrenia. *Schizophrenia Bulletin,* 38, 1030–1039.

An, S. K., Kang, J. I., Park, J. Y., Kim, K. R., Lee, S. Y., & Lee, E. (2010). Attribution bias in ultra-high risk for psychosis and first-episode schizophrenia. *Schizophrenia Research,* 118, 54–61.

Anselmetti, S., Bechi, M., Bosia, M., Quarticelli, C., Ermoli, E., Smeraldi, E., et al. (2009). 'Theory' of mind impairment in patients affected by schizophrenia and in their parents. *Schizophrenia Research,* 115, 278–285.

Baas, D., van't Wout, M., Aleman, A., & Kahn, R. S. (2008). Social judgement in clinically stable patients with schizophrenia and healthy relatives: Behavioural evidence of social brain dysfunction. *Psychological Medicine,* 38, 747–754.

Barbato, M., Liu, L., Penn, D. L., Keefe, R. S., Perkins, D. O., Woods, S. W., et al. (2013). Social cognition as a mediator between neurocognition and functional outcome in individuals at clinical high risk for psychosis. *Schizophrenia Research,* 150, 542–546.

Baron-Cohen, S., Wheelwright, S., Hill, J., Raste, Y., & Plumb, I. (2001). The "Reading the Mind in the Eyes" test revised version: A study with normal adults, and adults with Asperger syndrome or high-functioning autism. *Journal of Child Psychology and Psychiatry,* 42, 241–251.

Behere, R. V., Venkatasubramanian, G., Arasappa, R., Reddy, N., & Gangadhar, B. N. (2009). Effect of risperidone on emotion recognition deficits in antipsychotic-naïve schizophrenia: A short-term follow-up study. *Schizophrenia Research, 113, 72–76.*

Bertrand, M. C., Sutton, H., Achim, A. l. M., Malla, A. K., & Lepage, M. (2007). Social cognitive impairments in first episode psychosis. *Schizophrenia Research, 95, 124–133.*

Bôlte, S., & Poustka, F. (2003). The recognition of facial affect in autistic and schizophrenic subjects and their first-degree relatives. *Psychological Medicine, 33, 907–915.*

Bora, E., & Pantelis, C. (2013). Theory of mind impairments in first-episode psychosis, individuals at ultra-high risk for psychosis and in first-degree relatives of schizophrenia: Systematic review and meta-analysis. *Schizophrenia Research, 144, 31–36.*

Bora, E., Yucel, M., & Pantelis, C. (2009). Theory of mind impairment in schizophrenia: Meta-analysis. *Schizophrenia Research, 109, 1–9.*

Brüne, M. (2005). "Theory of Mind" in schizophrenia: A review of the literature. *Schizophrenia Bulletin, 31, 21–42.*

Brune, M., Ozgurdal, S., Ansorge, N., von Reventlow, H. G., Peters, S., Nicolas, V., et al. (2011). An fMRI study of "theory of mind" in at-risk states of psychosis: comparison with manifest schizophrenia and healthy controls. *NeuroImage, 55, 329–337.*

Cannon, T. D., Cadenhead, K., Cornblatt, B., Woods, S. W., Addington, J., Walker, E., et al. (2008). Prediction of psychosis in youth at high clinical risk: A multisite longitudinal study in North America. *Archives of General Psychiatry, 65, 28–37.*

Chung, Y. S., Hyung, K. D., Shin, N. Y., Yoo, S. Y., & Kwon, J. S. (2008). Deficit of theory of mind in individuals at ultra-high-risk for schizophrenia. *Schizophrenia Research, 99, 111–118.*

Combs, D. R., Penn, D. L., Wicher, M., & Waldheter, E. (2007). The Ambiguous Intentions Hostility Questionnaire (AIHQ): A new measure for evaluating hostile social-cognitive biases in paranoia. *Cognitive Neuropsychiatry, 12, 128–143.*

Comparelli, A., Corigliano, V., De Carolis, A., Mancinelli, I., Trovini, G., Ottavi, G., et al. (2013). Emotion recognition impairment is present early and is stable throughout the course of schizophrenia. *Schizophrenia Research, 143, 65–69.*

Cornblatt, B., Lencz, T., Smith, C. W., Correll, C. U., Auther, A. M., & Nakayama, E. (2003). The schizophrenia prodrome revisited: a neurodevelopmental perspective. *Schizophrenia Bulletin, 29, 633–665.*

Couture, S. M., Penn, D. L., Addington, J., Woods, S. W., & Perkins, D. O. (2008). Assessment of social judgments and complex mental states in the early phases of psychosis. *Schizophrenia Research, 100, 237–241.*

Couture, S. M., Penn, D. L., Losh, M., Adolphs, R., Hurley, R., & Piven, J. (2010). Comparison of social cognitive functioning in schizophrenia and high functioning autism: More convergence than divergence. *Psychological Medicine, 40, 569–579.*

Davalos, D. B., Compagnon, N., Heinlein, S., & Ross, R. G. (2004). Neuropsychological deficits in children associated with increased familial risk for schizophrenia. *Schizophrenia Research, 67, 123–130.*

de Achával, D., Costanzo, E. Y., Villarreal, M., Jáuregui, I. O., Chiodi, A., Castro, M. N., et al. (2010). Emotion processing and theory of mind in schizophrenia patients and their unaffected first-degree relatives. *Neuropsychologia,* 48, 1209–1215.

Devylder, J. E., Ben-David, S., Kimhy, D., & Corcoran, C. M. (2013). Attributional style among youth at clinical risk for psychosis. *Early Intervention in Psychiatry,* 7, 84–88.

Eack, S. M., Greeno, C. G., Pogue-Geile, M. F., Newhill, C. E., Hogarty, G. E., & Keshavan, M. S. (2010). Assessing social-cognitive deficits in schizophrenia with the Mayer-Salovey-Caruso Emotional Intelligence Test. *Schizophrenia Bulletin,* 36, 370–380.

Eack, S. M., Mermon, D. E., Montrose, D. M., Miewald, J., Gur, R. E., Gur, R. C., et al. (2010). Social cognition deficits among individuals at familial high risk for schizophrenia. *Schizophrenia Bulletin,* 36, 1081–1088.

Edwards, J., Pattison, P. E., Jackson, H. J., & Wales, R. J. (2001). Facial affect and affective prosody recognition in first-episode schizophrenia. *Schizophrenia Research,* 48, 235–253.

Fett, A. K., Viechtbauer, W., Dominguez, M. M. G., Penn, D. L., van Os, J., & Krabbendam, L. (2011). The relationship between neurocognition and social cognition with functional outcomes in schizophrenia: A meta-analysis. *Neuroscience & Biobehavioral Reviews,* 35, 573–588.

Fiske, S. T., & Taylor, S. E. (1991). *Social cognition.* New York: McGraw-Hill.

Frith, C. D., & Corcoran, R. (1996). Exploring 'theory of mind' in people with schizophrenia. *Psychological Medicine,* 26, 521–530.

Fusar-Poli, P., Borgwardt, S., Bechdolf, A., Addington, J., Riecher-Rössler, A., Schultze-Lutter, F., et al. (2013). The psychosis high-risk state: A comprehensive state-of-the-art review. *Archives of General Psychiatry,* 70, 120–31.

Gee, D. G., Karlsgodt, K. H., van Erp, T. G., Bearden, C. E., Lieberman, M. D., Belger, A., et al. (2012). Altered age-related trajectories of amygdala-prefrontal circuitry in adolescents at clinical high risk for psychosis: a preliminary study. *Schizophrenia Research,* 134, 1–9.

Gibson, C. M., Penn, D. L., Prinstein, M. J., Perkins, D. O., & Belger, A. (2010). Social skill and social cognition in adolescents at genetic risk for psychosis. *Schizophrenia Research,* 122, 179–184.

Green, M. F., Bearden, C. E., Cannon, T. D., Fiske, A. P., Hellemann, G. S., Horan, W. P., et al. (2012). Social cognition in schizophrenia, Part 1: Performance across phase of illness. *Schizophrenia Bulletin,* 38, 854–864.

Green, M. F., Olivier, B., Crawley, J. N., Penn, D. L., & Silverstein, S. (2005). Social cognition in schizophrenia: Recommendations from the measurement and treatment research to improve cognition in schizophrenia new approaches conference. *Schizophrenia Bulletin,* 31, 882–887.

Happe, F. G. (1994). An advanced test of theory of mind: Understanding by story characters' thoughts and feelings by able autistic, mentally handicapped, and normal children and adults. *Journal of Autism & Developmental Disorders,* 24, 129–154.

Healey, K. M., Penn, D. L., Perkins, D., Woods, S. W., & Addington, J. (2012). *Theory of Mind and complex social judgements in people at clinical high risk of psychosis. Schizophrenia Research,* 150, 498–504.

Herbener, E. S., Hill, S. K., Marvin, R. W., & Sweeney, J. A. (2005). Effects of antipsychotic treatment on emotion perception deficits in first-episode schizophrenia. *American Journal of Psychiatry,* 162, 1746–1748.

Hoekert, M., Kahn, R. S., Pijnenborg, M., & Aleman, A. (2007). Impaired recognition and expression of emotional prosody in schizophrenia: Review and meta-analysis. *Schizophrenia Research,* 96, 135–145.

Horan, W. P., Green, M. F., DeGroot, M., Fiske, A., Hellemann, G., Kee, K., et al. (2012). Social cognition in schizophrenia, Part 2: 12-month stability and prediction of functional outcome in first-episode patients. *Schizophrenia Bulletin,* 38, 865–872.

Hur, J. W., Byun, M. S., Shin, N. Y., Shin, Y. S., Kim, S. N., Jang, J. H., et al. (2013). General intellectual functioning as a buffer against theory-of-mind deficits in individuals at ultra-high risk for psychosis. *Schizophrenia Research,* 149, 83–87.

Irani, F., Platek, S. M., Panyavin, I. S., Calkins, M. E., Kohler, C., Siegel, S. J., et al. (2006). Self-face recognition and theory of mind in patients with schizophrenia and first-degree relatives. *Schizophrenia Research,* 88, 151–160.

Janssen, I., Krabbendam, L., Jolles, J., & van Os, J. (2003). Alterations in theory of mind in patients with schizophrenia and non-psychotic relatives. *Acta Psychiatrica Scandinavica,* 108, 110–117.

Kee, K. S., Horan, W. P., Mintz, J., & Green, M. F. (2004). Do the siblings of schizophrenia patients demonstrate affect perception deficits? *Schizophrenia Research,* 67, 87–94.

Kelemen, O., Erdélyi, R., Pataki, I., Benedek, G., Janka, Z., & Kéri, S. (2005). Theory of Mind and motion perception in schizophrenia. *Neuropsychology,* 19, 494–500.

Kim, H. S., Shin, N. Y., Jang, J. H., Kim, E., Shim, G., Park, H. Y., Hong, K. S., & Kwon, J. S. (2011). Social cognition and neurocognition as predictors of conversion to psychosis in individuals at ultra-high risk. *Schizophrenia Research,* 130, 170–175.

Kinderman, P., & Bentall, R. P. (1996). A new measure of causal locus: The internal, personal and situational attributions questionnaire. *Personality and Individual Differences,* 20, 261–264.

Koelkebeck, K., Pedersen, A., Suslow, T., Kueppers, K. A., Arolt, V., & Ohrmann, P. (2010). Theory of Mind in first-episode schizophrenia patients: Correlations with cognition and personality traits. *Schizophrenia Research,* 119, 115–123.

Kohler, C. G., Walker, J. B., Martin, E. A., Healey, K. M., & Moberg, P. J. (2010). Facial emotion perception in schizophrenia: A meta-analytic review. *Schizophrenia Bulletin,* 36, 1009–1019.

Krstev, H., Jackson, H., & Maude, D. (1999). An investigation of attributional style in first-episode psychosis. *British Journal of Clinical Psychology,* 38, 181–194.

Langdon, R., Still, M., Connors, M. H., Ward, P. B., & Catts, S. V. (2013). Attributional biases, paranoia, and depression in early psychosis. *British Journal of Clinical Psychology,* 52, 408–423.

Leppänen, J. M., Niehaus, D. J. H., Koen, L., Du Toit, E., Schoeman, R., & Emsley, R. (2006). Emotional face processing deficit in schizophrenia: A replication study in a South African Xhosa population. *Schizophrenia Research, 84*, 323–330.

Loughland, C. M., Williams, L. M., & Gordon, E. (2002). Visual scanpaths to positive and negative facial emotions in an outpatient schizophrenia sample. *Schizophrenia Research, 55*, 159–170.

Marjoram, D., Job, D. E., Whalley, H. C., Gountouna, V. E., McIntosh, A. M., Simonotto, E., et al. (2006). A visual joke fMRI investigation into Theory of Mind and enhanced risk of schizophrenia. *NeuroImage, 31*, 1850–1858.

Mayer, J. D., Salovey, P., Caruso, D. R., & Sitarenios, G. (2003). Measuring emotional intelligence with the MSCEIT V2.0. *Emotion, 3*, 97–105.

McGlashan, T., Walsh, B. C., & Woods, S. W. (2010). *The psychosis-risk syndrome: Handbook for diagnosis and follow-up.* New York: Oxford University Press.

Mehta, U. M., Thirthalli, J., Subbakrishna, D. K., Gangadhar, B. N., Eack, S. M., & Keshavan, M. S. (2013). Social and neuro-cognition as distinct cognitive factors in schizophrenia: A systematic review. *Schizophrenia Research, 148*, 3–11.

Nowicki, S., & Carton, J. (1993). The measurement of emotional intensity from facial expressions. *Journal of Social Psychology, 133*, 749–750.

Nowicki, S., & Duke, M. P. (1974a). Adult Nowicki–Strickland internal external control scale. In P. R. Robinson, L. S. Shaver, & L. S. Wrightsman (Eds.), *Measures of personality and social psychological attitudes.* San Diego: Academic Press.

Nowicki, S., & Duke, M. P. (1974b). Locus of control scale for non-college as well as college adults. *Journal of Personality Assessment, 38*, 136–137.

———. (1994). Individual differences in the nonverbal communication of affect: The diagnostic analysis of nonverbal accuracy scale. *Journal of Nonverbal Behaviour, 18*, 9–35.

Nuechterlein, K. H., Dawson, M. E., Gitlin, M., Ventura, J., Goldstein, M. J., Snyder, K. S., et al. (1992). Developmental processes in schizophrenic disorders: Longitudinal studies of vulnerability and stress. *Schizophrenia Bulletin, 18*, 387–425.

Oh, J. E., Na, M. H., Ha, T. H., Shin, Y. W., Roh, K. S., Hong, S. B., et al. (2005). Social cognition deficits of schizophrenia in cartoon task. *Journal of Korean Neuropsychiatric Association, 44*, 295–302.

Penn, D. L., Addington, J., & Pinkham, A. (2006). Social cognitive impairments. In J. A. Lieberman, T. S. Stroup, & D. O. Perkins (Eds.), *A textbook of schizophrenia.* Washington, DC: American Psychiatry Press.

Perner, J., & Wimmer, H. (1985). "John *thinks* that Mary *thinks* that. . . ." attribution of second-order beliefs by 5- to 10-year-old children. *Journal of Experimental Child Psychology, 39*, 437–471.

Pinkham, A. E., Penn, D. L., Perkins, D. O., Graham, K. A., & Siegel, M. (2007). Emotion perception and social skill over the course of psychosis: A comparison of individuals "at-risk" for psychosis and individuals with early and chronic schizophrenia spectrum illness. *Cognitive Neuropsychiatry, 12*, 198–212.

Piskulic, D., Addington, J., & Maruff, P. (2010). Social cognition in schizophrenia: A quantitative review of the literature. *Schizophrenia Research, 117,* 413.

Schmidt, S. J., Mueller, D. R., & Roder, V. (2011). Social cognition as a mediator variable between neurocognition and functional outcome in schizophrenia: Empirical review and new results by structural equation modeling. *Schizophrenia Bulletin, 37,* S41–S54.

Sergi, M. J., Fiske, A. P., Horan, W. P., Kern, R. S., Kee, K. S., Subotnik, K. L., et al. (2009). Development of a measure of relationship perception in schizophrenia. *Psychiatry Research, 166,* 54–62.

Sergi, M. J., Rassovsky, Y., Widmark, C., Reist, C., Erhart, S., Braff, D. L., et al. (2007). Social cognition in schizophrenia: Relationships with neurocognition and negative symptoms. *Schizophrenia Research, 90,* 316–324.

Sprong, M., Schothorst, P., Vos, E., Hox, J., & Van Engeland, H. (2007). Theory of mind in schizophrenia. *British Journal of Psychiatry, 191,* 5–13.

Stanford, A. D., Messinger, J., Malaspina, D., & Corcoran, C. M. (2011). Theory of mind in patients at clinical high risk for psychosis. *Schizophrenia Research, 131,* 11–17.

Thompson, A., Papas, A., Bartholomeusz, C., Allott, K., Amminger, G. P., Nelson, B., et al. (2012). Social cognition in clinical "at risk" for psychosis and first episode psychosis populations. *Schizophrenia Research, 141,* 204–209.

Thompson, A., Papas, A., Bartholomeusz, C., Nelson, B., & Yung, A. (2013). Externalized attributional bias in the ultra high risk (UHR) for psychosis population. *Psychiatry Research, 206,* 200–205.

Toomey, R., Seidman, L. J., Lyons, M. J., Faraone, S. V., & Tsuang, M. T. (1999). Poor perception of nonverbal social-emotional cues in relatives of schizophrenic patients. *Schizophrenia Research, 40,* 121–130.

van Os, J., Rutten, B. P., & Poulton, R. (2008). Gene-environment interactions in schizophrenia: Review of epidemiological findings and future directions. *Schizophrenia Bulletin, 34,* 1066–1082.

Wölwer, W., Brinkmeyer, J., Stroth, S., Streit, M., Bechdolf, A., Ruhrmann, S., et al. (2012). Neurophysiological correlates of impaired facial affect recognition in individuals at risk for schizophrenia. *Schizophrenia Bulletin, 38,* 1021–1029.

Wykes, T. (1994). Predicting symptomatic and behavioural outcomes of community care. *British Journal of Psychiatry, 165,* 486–492.

Wykes, T., Hamid, S., & Wagstaff, K. (2001). Theory of mind and executive functions in the non-psychotic siblings of patients with schizophrenia. *Schizophrenia Research, 49*(Suppl. 1), 148.

Yalcin-Siedentopf, N., Hoertnagl, C. M., Biedermann, F., Baumgartner, S., Deisenhammer, E. A., Hausmann, A., et al. (2014). Facial affect recognition in symptomatically remitted patients with schizophrenia and bipolar disorder. *Schizophrenia Research, 152,* 440–445.

Yong, E., Barbato, M., Penn, D. L., Keefe, R. S., Woods, S. W., Perkins, D. O., et al. (2014). Exploratory analysis of social cognition and neurocognition in individuals at clinical high risk for psychosis. *Psychiatry Research, 218,* 39–43.

Yung, A. R., & McGorry, P. D. (1996). The prodromal phase of first-episode psychosis: Past and current conceptualizations. *Schizophrenia Bulletin, 22,* 353–370.

Yung, A. R., Phillips, L. J., Yuen, H. P., & McGorry, P. D. (2004). Risk factors for psychosis in an ultra high-risk group: Psychopathology and clinical features. *Schizophrenia Research, 67,* 131–142.

9.

Criticism and the Course
of Mental Disorders

Jill M. Hooley

CRITICISM IS a common and inevitable consequence of living in a social world. It provides a signal that our behavior is disliked or disapproved of by others. As such, it can be considered to represent a mild form of social threat. For animals that live in groups, being able to detect threat from the social environment is essential for species survival. It therefore makes sense that, over the course of evolutionary history, criticism has become a highly salient social cue that is stressful to experience and desirable to avoid.

But criticism cannot be avoided. Everyone who lives in the social world experiences criticism from time to time. The familiar children's rhyme tells us that, although sticks and stones may break our bones, words will never hurt us. But is that really so? Rather than threatening our immediate survival, criticism most typically threatens our self-esteem. But to what extent does this constitute a problem? In this chapter, I discuss the role that criticism from close family members plays in the clinical course of psychopathological disorders such as schizophrenia and depression. Having established the link between criticism and poor clinical outcome across a range of disorders, I then consider the biological consequences of criticism, focusing most specifically on how our social brains process this most common and ubiquitous form of social threat.

The Social Environment and Schizophrenia

In the late 1950s, a British sociologist named George Brown made a rather unexpected observation. What Brown and his colleagues noted was that male patients with chronic schizophrenia fared much better if they were discharged from the hospital to live in lodgings or with their brothers or sisters. In contrast, those who returned to live with their wives or with their parents did much less well clinically (Brown, Carstairs, & Topping, 1958). The finding that patients who did not return to live with their families did better than those who lived in ostensibly less supportive social settings was most unexpected. In the British psychiatric literature of the time, there was little to lead anyone to believe that the social environment to which a schizophrenia patient was discharged might make any difference to the course of the disorder. Intrigued by this unusual finding, Brown and his collaborators began a program of research designed to explore the potential role that family relationships might play with respect to clinical outcome in schizophrenia.

One of Brown's most important insights was that it was the more commonplace aspects of family relationships that were likely to be important. This stood in contrast to the approach taken by clinical investigators in the United States who were focusing on extreme aspects of relationships that were more pathological in nature (e.g., Fromm-Reichmann, 1948/1959). Instead, working with Michael Rutter, Brown sought to characterize the emotional climate that existed in otherwise ordinary families (Brown & Rutter, 1966; Rutter & Brown, 1966). Their goal was to describe all forms of emotional expression that members of the research team encountered in the families that they met. The result of this work was the development of the expressed emotion (EE) construct (Brown, Birley, & Wing, 1972).

Expressed Emotion

Expressed emotion is not an especially well-named construct. It does not refer to how willing a person is to show emotions. Rather, EE reflects the extent to which the key relative of a psychiatric patient speaks about that patient in a critical, hostile, or emotionally overinvolved way during the course of a private interview with a researcher. The preferred way of measuring EE is via an interview called the Camberwell Family Interview (CFI) (Hooley & Parker, 2006). Named after the district in London where Brown and his colleagues conducted their seminal research, the CFI is a semistructured interview that is conducted in the absence of the patient. It takes about one to two hours to complete. The CFI contains specific questions that ask about particular symptoms or about the development of the patient's psychiatric difficulties. Most important, however, the CFI is designed to create an opportunity for the relative to talk and tell his or her story. For example, there is a focus on how the relative deals with challenging situations involving the patient. Other questions address the relationship the relative has with the patient more specifically and concern how they get along on a day-to-day basis (Leff & Vaughn, 1985).

Of the three key elements that are used in the rating of EE, criticism is the most important. This was noted by Brown and his colleagues in 1972 and has been confirmed repeatedly by researchers since then. To count as a critical remark, the relative has to say something that indicates obvious dislike or disapproval of some aspect of the patient's behavior (e.g., "I hate the way she loads the dishwasher. Nothing is organized properly."). Critical remarks are rated as such either because they contain critical content (as in the example above) or because the relative uses a negative voice tone when speaking about the patient. Because ratings of EE are derived not only from what the family member says during the CFI but also from the tone of voice that the relative uses when speaking about the patient, the CFI is always recorded for later coding. One problem is that learning to rate EE is time-consuming (two or more weeks of training), and training can be difficult to obtain. It also takes between two and four hours to code each recorded interview. Nevertheless, although some shortcuts to EE assessment do exist (see Hooley & Parker, 2006), the CFI still remains the gold standard form of assessment.

As noted earlier, the most important element of the EE index is criticism. However, for the purposes of coding EE, raters also listen for the presence of hostility. As with criticism, hostile remarks reflect dislike or disapproval. The difference is that the degree of the negativity that is expressed is much more extreme. Some hostile remarks suggest dislike of who the patient is as a person (e.g., "All she cares about is herself. She's very selfish and self-involved. It's always all about her!"). In other cases, the hostility takes the form of rejection ("If he walks into the room, I leave. I don't like being around him anymore.").

These highly negative attitudes are in sharp contrast to the third element of EE. Emotional overinvolvement (EOI) reflects dramatic, exaggerated, overprotective, or devoted attitudes or behaviors toward the patient by the relative (e.g., "We can't be apart. It would kill me. You might as well cut my heart out."). Compared to criticism and hostility, EOI attitudes and behaviors are much less common. EOI tends to be found more often in parents (especially mothers) than in other types of relatives (Goldstein, Miklowitz, & Richards, 2002).

Most relatives are classified as being high EE on the basis of making an above threshold number of critical remarks during the CFI. Absent this, the presence of hostility or a high score (3 or more) on a 0 to 5 scale of EOI will also lead to a high EE rating. The threshold scores that are used for criticism vary according to the diagnosis of the patient. For relatives of patients with schizophrenia, making six or more critical remarks during the CFI will result in a classification of high EE. In contrast, a lower cutting score (two or three critical remarks) is used for relatives of patients with unipolar depression. In cases where patients live with more than one relative (e.g., two parents), the family is classified as high in EE if at least one of the relatives is rated as high EE. Although the rules determining a high versus low EE classification may seem somewhat arbitrary, they were developed based on the variables and scores that provided the best separation between relapsing and nonrelapsing patients and have been well validated in subsequent empirical work (see Hooley, 2007, for more discussion of this issue).

EE and Clinical Outcome

EE is an important construct for one simple reason. Decades of research have established that EE is a highly reliable psychosocial predictor of symptom relapse in psychiatric patients. When patients with schizophrenia or mood disorders live in family environments that are characterized by criticism, hostility, or high levels of EOI, they are at significantly increased risk of early relapse compared to patients who do not live in such family environments. In a meta-analysis, Butzlaff and Hooley (1998) examined twenty-seven prospective outcome studies and reported a weighted mean effect size of $r=.31$ for the association between EE and relapse in schizophrenia. They also noted that, even though EE is a risk factor for relapse in patients with recent-onset schizophrenia, patients with more chronic and long-standing illnesses are at even greater risk of relapse when they live in high EE home environments.

Early work with the EE construct focused only on schizophrenia. However, a now-classic study by Vaughn and Leff (1976) soon established that EE also had predictive validity with respect to clinical outcome in unipolar depressed patients. This finding was later replicated (Hooley, Orley, & Teasdale, 1986) and further extended to patients diagnosed with bipolar mood disorder (Miklowitz et al., 1988). Although one well-conducted study has reported no association between EE and relapse in depression (Hayhurst et al., 1997), even with this study, meta-analysis reveals a highly significant association between EE and relapse in depression (weighted mean effect size, $r = .38$; see Hooley & Gotlib, 2000).

Although beyond the scope of this brief review, it is also important to note that EE has predictive validity for an even broader range of psychopathologies than schizophrenia and mood disorders. As summarized elsewhere, high family levels of EE have been demonstrated to predict worse clinical outcomes for patients with anxiety disorders, eating disorders, and substance abuse problems (Hooley, 2007). What makes EE interesting, then, is that it is a robust predictor of patients doing poorly across a wide range of diagnoses and disorders.

The Experience of Criticism

Why is EE predictive of relapse? Right from the very beginning, it was assumed that high levels of EE might provide a social environment that was too stressful for vulnerable patients with schizophrenia (Brown et al., 1972). In the intervening years, research has tended to support this perspective. The idea that EE constitutes a psychosocial stressor is still very central to current models (Hooley & Gotlib, 2000).

At the level of self-report, patients with schizophrenia who have high EE relatives report feeling more stressed by interactions with those relatives than patients with low EE relatives do (Cutting et al., 2006). Patients with critical caretakers also report higher levels of anxiety (Kuipers et al., 2006). One reason for this may be because high EE relatives are more critical during face-to-face interactions (Hooley, 1986; Miklowitz, Goldstein, Falloon, & Doane, 1984). They are also more behaviorally controlling in their interactions with patients than low EE relatives are (Hooley & Campbell, 2002). The finding that relatives' controlling behaviors also predict relapse in patients with schizophrenia adds further support to the idea that there is something in the interaction styles of high EE relatives that may provide too much stress for vulnerable patients.

Psychophysiological data are also consistent with this perspective. In one study, skin conductance and blood pressure were measured in schizophrenia patients who were in remission and who were tested in their own homes (Tarrier et al., 1979). Recordings were taken for fifteen minutes. During this time, the patient was alone with the experimenter. Then the patient's relative was asked to enter the room and data were collected for an additional fifteen minutes. Patients with high or low EE relatives did not differ in their arousal levels prior to the entry of their relatives. However, after the high EE relative came into the room, the diastolic blood pressure of the patients increased. For patients with low EE relatives, in contrast, there was a decrease in electrodermal arousal (measured as reduced spontaneous fluctuations in skin conductance) after the relative entered. Comparable findings have also been obtained using similar experimental designs with acutely ill patients (Tarrier et al., 1988; Sturgeon et al., 1981). Overall, what tends to be found is that the arrival of a low EE relative seems to facilitate habituation to a novel testing situation in both ill and remitted patients. In contrast, the presence of a high EE relative is associated with continued arousal. Electrodermal reactivity to the presence of a high EE relative has also been linked to an increased likelihood of later relapse (Sturgeon et al., 1984). More recent work further suggests that patients who have higher baseline levels of electrodermal arousal and who live in a high EE family environment are more likely to have worse symptoms at follow-up than patients who do not (Subotnik et al., 2012). In other words, and consistent with a diathesis-stress perspective, it is the interaction between electrodermal activity and psychosocial stress that is most important.

Methodological Issues

Within EE research, relapse is typically assessed on the basis of the symptoms that patients have during a specific follow-up period (usually nine to twelve months after hospital discharge). These symptoms are assessed by independent raters using structured clinical interviews. Importantly, rehospitalization is *not* used to determine relapse. This is because rehospitalization could potentially be confounded with EE. It is reasonable to suggest that families who are high in EE might be less tolerant of having a sick patient at home and so make efforts to get the patient hospitalized at lower symptom levels than might be the case for a low EE family. For this reason, the assessment of relapse is always based on an independent clinical evaluation.

Even with the potential confound between EE and rehospitalization removed, the demonstration of a reliable association between high EE in relatives and poorer clinical outcomes in patients does not mean that we can conclude that EE is playing a causal role in symptom relapse. One way that a significant correlation between EE and relapse could be obtained is if some of the illness characteristics of relapse-prone patients (such as greater severity of illness) cause family members to be more critical. This is highly plausible. It would also lead to a situation where EE and relapse were correlated, but the association between them was driven by a third variable that was correlated with both.

From the very beginning, this possibility was a source of concern to researchers. For example, Brown et al. (1972) noted that patients who had more impaired behavior or more problematic work functioning were at higher risk of relapse than patients who were less impaired or better able to function adequately at work. It was also the patients with more of these difficulties who were more likely to have high EE relatives. Importantly, however, EE still remained a significant predictor of relapse even after these patient variables were statistically controlled. Since that time, other empirical studies that have controlled for potentially important patient variables have further confirmed the independent contribution that is made to relapse by EE (e.g., Nuechterlein et al., 1992).

Does EE Play a Causal Role?

The demonstration of an association between EE and relapse does not necessarily mean that EE plays a causal role in the relapse process. In order to establish causality, true experimental designs must be used. Levels of EE must be modified and the effects of this on resulting relapse rates then examined. One way that this can be done is through treatment studies that are designed to reduce levels of EE. Even then, however, the question of directionality cannot be fully resolved. This is because ethical constraints make it impossible to test whether increasing levels of EE also increases rates of relapse in patients.

With this limitation in mind, the findings of treatment studies are generally consistent with the idea that EE plays a causal role in the relapse process. Of course, we must remember that families may benefit from family-based treatments in a variety of different ways and that decreases in relatives' EE are not always essential to patients' clinical improvement (Miklowitz, 2004). Nonetheless, when families receive interventions designed to reduce or modify aspects of high EE behavior, patient relapse rates decrease relative to controls whose families do not receive the family-based treatments (Leff et al., 1982; Hogarty et al., 1991). Important components of these interventions include providing relatives with education about the illness as well as efforts to help family members improve their communication and problem-solving skills. Studies suggest that, when families of patients with schizophrenia receive interventions of this kind, patient relapse rates over the next six to twelve months decline (Miklowitz & Tompson, 2003). Patient relapse rates in families receiving family-based interventions are approximately 12.5 percent (range, 0–33 percent). In contrast, for families who do not receive these interventions, patient relapse rates average around 42 percent (range, 17–61 percent). There is also evidence that family-based interventions improve clinical outcomes for patients with mood disorders and eating disorders (Eisler et al., 2000; Leff et al., 2000; Miklowitz et al., 2003).

Considered together, the success of family-based interventions in reducing patients' relapse rates supports the idea that EE may play a causal role in the relapse process. However, it is important to avoid an overly simplistic and unidirectional view of EE. EE is not a construct that should be used to assign blame to families. Living with a person with psychopathology presents many challenges. It is also important to know that high levels of EE are quite normative in industrialized countries. In other words, it is the low EE relatives who are unusual in their abilities to cope with the difficulties that severe psychopathology in a loved one can create. We should also keep in mind that high levels of EE do not occur in a vacuum. In short, there is now widespread agreement that EE is a bidirectional construct (Hooley, Rosen, & Richters, 1995; Hooley & Gotlib, 2000) that is most appropriately regarded as "a measure of a set of *patient-relative relationship problems* that are important for the relapse process" (Hooley, Miklowitz, & Beach, 2006).

What Does Criticism Do to the Brain?

The link between EE and relapse as well as the data from family-based intervention studies is consistent with the idea that EE likely plays a causal role in the course of clinical disorders. There is also reason to believe that patients may be at increased risk of relapse because of the stress associated with exposure to a high EE environment. But how, exactly, does EE function as a form of psychosocial stress? More specifically, what happens to people when they experience criticism, and how might this eventually culminate in a relapse of symptoms in a vulnerable patient?

The Effects of Actual Criticism

In an effort to address these issues, Hooley and colleagues have used functional magnetic resonance imaging (fMRI) to examine what happens in the brain when healthy people and people who are vulnerable to depression are exposed to criticism from their own mothers. After the research team

TABLE 9.1. Examples of Critical, Praising, and Neutral Comments

Criticism:
"Melissa, one thing that bothers me about you is your tendency to save every-thing. I really don't care for the fact that you never get rid of anything. You still have T-shirts from high school, and at some point it pays to get rid of things. Maybe they don't clutter your life, but they do take up space in our home. And what is the reason for keeping them? You don't use them. It's time for you really to simplify your life so that you can get on with things, instead of just leaving everything behind in our home."

Praise:
"One thing that I love about you, Melissa, is your artistic ability. Every time I see your artwork in our home I think that you have a special talent. Everything has your unique touch and vision and it speaks to me as I look at what you have done. I love it when you make gifts and cards because it's sometimes something that you have invested your time and talent to create. To know that it is inexpen-sive is just an added bonus. It also reminds me of your desire for simple things and I love it that you are not tied up into material wealth."

Neutral:
"Melissa, let me tell you a little bit about the work on the high school. Uh, you probably wouldn't recognize it. The front lawn is completely torn up and truly looks like a construction zone. They are working double shifts during the summer to speed the process up and hope to have several areas done so there are places for teachers and students to go in the fall. The hallway where the offices are is completely gone, including all those classrooms. They are moving the hallway between the classrooms so that there are no classrooms back to back."

had received permission from the participants, the mothers of these par-ticipants were contacted and asked to make specific comments about their adult child. These comments were required to be critical, praising, or neu-tral in nature (for more details, see Hooley et al., 2005; Hooley et al., 2009). Each comment lasted thirty seconds and always began with the mother addressing the offspring by name. All comments were recorded during a telephone conversation, and mothers were free to choose the content of the praising and criticizing remarks based on their own personal feelings. Importantly, the critical comments were not required to be especially harsh or negative. Rather, they were much better characterized as everyday nag-ging complaints. For the neutral remarks, we asked mothers to describe topics such as the recent weather or other local events that they believed their children would have little interest in. Table 9.1 provides examples of the types of remarks mothers made.

These comments were later played to study participants while they were lying in a MRI scanner. One group of participants contained healthy controls, selected because they had no history of psychopathology. The other group of participants had experienced one or more episodes of clinical depression in the past but were currently fully well and symptom free. Importantly, participants in the control and recovered depressed groups were comparable with regard to their self-reported current levels of depression and negative mood. In other words, there were no mood state differences between the two groups at the time of testing. Where the groups did differ, however, was in their known vulnerability to depression.

The findings revealed that these vulnerability differences were associated with different responses to criticism. In the first study of this type, Hooley and colleagues (2005) reported that, whereas healthy participants showed increased activation in the dorsolateral prefrontal cortex (DLPFC) during criticism, there was a decrease in activation in this brain area in the formerly depressed participants. In a subsequent study involving only females, Hooley et al. (2009) again found that, compared to never-depressed controls, the formerly depressed participants showed significantly reduced activation of DLPFC during criticism. In addition, participants who had been depressed in the past also showed significantly less activation in the anterior cingulate cortex (ACC) and significantly increased activation in the amygdala.

These findings are important because they suggest that criticism is processed differently by people who are vulnerable to depression, even after full clinical recovery. Moreover, the design of this study allows us to rule out the possibility that the findings can be explained by differences in current mood state of participants because the formerly depressed participants were just like the never-depressed controls with respect to their current mood. Of course, we cannot know whether the differences that are revealed by this study might have existed before the onset of depression or whether they are the result of changes that occur in the brain as a result of being depressed. Nonetheless, they tell us that the never-depressed brain handles criticism in a different way than the brain that is vulnerable to depression.

The finding that criticism activates the amygdala in people who are vulnerable to depression is relevant because this limbic region plays a primary role in initiating response to threat, including social threat (see Green & Phillips, 2004). Increased amygdala activity also plays a central role in current models of depression (Davidson et al., 2002; De Raedt & Koster, 2010; Hamilton & Gotlib, 2008). Studies using positron emission tomography (PET) have demonstrated that baseline amygdala activity is elevated in people who are depressed and that this elevation is associated with depression severity (Drevets, Bogers, & Raichle, 2002). Compared to healthy controls, unmedicated depressed patients also show increased and more sustained amygdala activity to negative versus neutral words (Siegle et al., 2007). Moreover, when sad mood was experimentally induced in people who had remitted from an episode of depression, those who showed increased amygdala activation during encoding of negative self-reference words were better able to recall those negative words later on (Ramel et al., 2007). This is relevant because other studies had suggested that amygdala activity normalized following successful treatment for depression (Schaefer et al., 2006). However, challenges such as a sad mood induction, or exposure to criticism, may be able to reinstate it. The fact that criticism is associated with increased amygdala activation may therefore be one route through which high levels of EE may be linked to relapse.

There are also reciprocal connections between the amygdala and prefrontal cortex, with one function of the prefrontal cortex being to inhibit amygdala response following an appraisal of the significance of the threat (Davidson, 2000). A number of researchers have observed that depressed individuals have lower resting state activity in the DLPFC compared to healthy controls (Mayberg et al., 2005). The activity and modulatory role of the PFC also appear to be decreased in depressed individuals during laboratory tasks (Siegle et al., 2007). The lack of prefrontal activation to criticism in people who are vulnerable to depression may therefore mean that limbic reactivity goes unchecked, perhaps leading to other (negative) consequences elsewhere. For example, the DLPFC plays a major role in cognitive control (Fales et al., 2008; Holmes & Pizzagalli, 2008). Decreased activation in the DLPFC is also thought to cause problems when people are required to inhibit negative material. Failure to fully activate the DLPFC during emotionally challenging tasks may lead to a reduced ability to engage in emotion regulation (Joormann, 2010) or stop negative elaborative processes such as rumination (De Raedt & Koster, 2010). In contrast, the pattern of activation in healthy participants may indicate that the DLPFC is actively engaged in the processing of criticism. This may lead to better regulation in limbic regions, reduced risk of rumination, and less potential for the exacerbation of negative mood.

Also highly relevant here is the concept of neuroticism. Neuroticism is a trait that reflects the tendency to experience negative affect. People who score high on neuroticism tend to be highly sensitive to criticism. Moreover, when they are criticized, people who score higher on neuroticism show enhanced functional coupling in brain regions that are involved in cognitive control of negative emotions (Servaas et al., 2013). One way to interpret this is that their brains may have to work harder to regain emotional control when challenged by criticism. It is also the case that, in people who are more neurotic, other connections that regulate negative emotions appear to be relatively weak. The increased functional connectivity in frontal brain areas that is found in more neurotic individuals may therefore be a form of compensation that helps them cope more effectively with emotional challenges.

Studies that have examined the processing of criticism in people with schizophrenia (or with schizophrenia-related traits) are limited in number. They are also inconsistent with regard to their findings. Using an approach similar to that first employed by Hooley et al. (2009), Premkumar and colleagues (2013) examined differences in the processing of relatives' criticism in participants who scored high or low on schizotypal traits. Schizotypal traits include magical thinking, unusual perceptions, speech, and behaviors and are thought to reflect low-level positive symptoms of psychosis. In response to hearing critical (vs. neutral) comments from their relatives, all participants showed increased bilateral activation of the posterior cingulate cortex, as well as the left superior and middle frontal gyri. Reduced activation during criticism (relative to the neutral condition) was also seen in the left middle temporal gyrus extending to the left insula and left temporal transverse gyrus, as well as bilateral cerebellum, and right lingual gyrus and cuneus. However, contrary to expectation, no differences in the neural processing of criticism were found between the participants who scored high or low on schizotypy. This may have been because all participants were drawn from a database of healthy volunteers. The small sample size ($n = 12$ in each group) may also have reduced power to detect significant group differences.

In a related study, Rylands and colleagues (2011) recruited a small sample of patients diagnosed with schizophrenia and, again similar to the work described above, sought to examine the neural correlates of expressed emotion. One interesting feature of the research design was that the patients with schizophrenia heard the very same critical comments that their high EE relatives had made during the Camberwell Family Interview. These were extracted from the interview and later played to patients while they were lying in the scanner. Patients also heard an unfamiliar voice making exactly the same critical comments. In addition, neutral comments made by patients' relatives were extracted from the CFI, and these same neutral comments were again also recorded by a stranger.

The results of the study by Rylands and colleagues (2011) are difficult to interpret because no control sample was used. In other words, we cannot know whether the way in which the patients with schizophrenia processed the critical and neutral comments was different from how people without the illness would have processed the same types of comments made by relatives and strangers. Nonetheless, as was the case in the Premkumar et al.

(2013) study, the researchers did identify several brain regions that seemed
to be differentially activated or deactivated during relatives' criticism. These
brain areas included regions thought to be involved in the processing of
aversive social information (e.g., temporal pole, inferior frontal gyrus, anterior cingulate cortex, medial prefrontal cortex), as well as language areas
such as the precentral gyrus.

In contrast to the findings described earlier for depression, Rylands and
colleagues (2011) did not find evidence of increased amygdala activation
during relatives' criticism. Consistent with the findings of Hooley et al.
(2009), however, they did report deactivation of the anterior cingulate
cortex when patients heard critical comments from their relatives. Hooley
and colleagues have speculated that people who are vulnerable to depression may have an ACC that is relatively more "turned off" and that this
could be a protective strategy to reduce the risk of being challenged by emotional material. Premkumar and colleagues (2012) have provided additional support for this idea. More specifically, they have shown that healthy
individuals with higher levels of schizotypal personality traits show deactivation of the dorsal ACC when viewing scenes of social rejection. In contrast, healthy individuals who scored low on schizotypal traits showed bilateral activation of this brain region when exposed to socially rejecting
images. Although much more research is needed, it is possible that a healthy
response to social rejection requires the activation of brain areas like ACC
that are involved in conflict detection and decision making and that have
connections with other brain areas involved in executive functioning. In
contrast, deactivation of the ACC in the face of social or emotional challenges may be much more characteristic of a less resilient or more vulnerable
brain. Findings such as these highlight the importance of the interaction
between environmental factors and biological vulnerability.

The Effects of Perceived Criticism

There is little doubt that criticism, measured as part of the expressed emotion construct, is tapping into something ecologically valid and clinically
meaningful. However, the practical utility of the EE construct has always
been somewhat limited because objective assessments of criticism are very
time-consuming and costly to obtain.

In an early effort to address these concerns, Hooley and Teasdale (1989)
sought to obtain a measure of subjective criticism by asking depressed patients to rate how critical they thought their relatives were using a simple
1 to 10 scale. Although this perceived criticism (PC) scale was only mod-

estly correlated with objective criticism assessed using the EE interview, it was, more important, a strong predictor of patients' relapse rates (see Hooley & Richters, 1991). Indeed, in the original study, perceived criticism was an even better predictor of symptom relapse over the course of a nine-month follow up than EE was.

Subsequent research has replicated the link between PC and relapse in depression (Kwon, Lee, Lee, & Bifulco, 2006). It has also demonstrated the predictive validity of PC for other disorders (Renshaw, 2008). PC is a significant predictor of future hospital admissions in patients with bipolar disorder even after current symptoms and medication adherence are statistically controlled (Scott, Colon, Pope, Reinares, & Vieta, 2012). In patients with substance abuse problems, PC predicts overall relapse, as well as time to relapse and days abstinent (Fals-Stewart, O'Farrell, & Hooley, 2001). Moreover, PC ratings obtained from people at high risk for the development of psychosis predict an increase in their positive symptoms over the course of a six-month follow-up (Schlosser et al., 2010).

Given how simple PC is to assess, its ability to identify patients at risk of worse clinical outcomes might seem surprising. However, new research is now suggesting that PC may be associated with differential neural activity while processing criticism. When asked to rate how critical their mother was of them using the PC scale, people who scored above the median on PC did not report more negative mood and were not more upset after being criticized than low PC scorers were. However, their brains responded to criticism in a different way. More specifically, high PC scorers showed greater and more prolonged amygdala activity when they heard their mothers criticize them than low PC scorers did. In addition, high PC scorers showed reduced and less sustained activation in the DLPFC (Hooley, Siegle, & Gruber, 2012).

These differences in neural activity were found only during exposure to criticism and not during exposure to praise. In other words, the effects were criticism specific. They were also found in all participants, regardless of whether they were currently suffering from depression, were fully recovered from a past episode of depression, or were healthy, never-depressed controls. Of particular interest is that the differences between the high and low PC scoring individuals involved some of the same brain areas (e.g., amygdala and DLPFC) that have been implicated in depression as well as other disorders (Disner, Beevers, Haigh, & Beck, 2011). Importantly, activity in these two regions was largely independent. This suggests multiple vulnerabilities.

On the other hand, brain areas such as the anterior cingulate cortex, which is considered to play a crucial role in depression, did not show any differences in reactivity across the high and low PC groups. The lack of moderation of ACC activity by perceived criticism is consistent with the idea that the differences in ACC activation are more specifically related to depression and vulnerability to depression, as is suggested by current models (Price & Drevets, 2012). In contrast, PC may be indexing more general vulnerabilities to the effects of criticism, some of which may be independent from those associated with a specific diagnosis.

In the only other neuroimaging study of PC to date, Premkumar et al. (2013) have reported that, in a sample of healthy community residents, higher levels of perceived criticism were correlated with reduced activation of the left middle temporal gyrus. This is a brain area that is involved in detecting prosody—the elements of speech that do not involve word choice or grammar but instead reflect emphasis, rhythm, or intonation. Whether such a form of desensitization might be helpful or even protective for those living in an actual or perceived criticism environment is an issue that warrants further research.

In our current work, we are now examining the role that PC plays in attentional control and emotion processing more broadly. More specifically, we are testing the hypothesis that PC is associated with differences in performance on cognitive processing tasks in the context of negative stimuli. Results obtained from a community sample suggest that people who feel more highly criticized have more difficulty inhibiting socially relevant negative information (Masland, Hooley, Tully, Dearing, & Gotlib, 2015). In particular, it takes them longer to disengage their attention from negative emotional faces. This is an interesting finding because participants in this study were not selected because they were depressed. Rather, the findings suggest that PC may be linked to problems with automatic emotion regulation even in generally healthy participants. If high PC scorers take longer to return to a normal state after an emotional challenge, this could provide a possible explanation for why PC might be associated with poorer clinical outcomes across a range of disorders.

Summary and Future Directions

Criticism is an aversive social stimulus that, in addition to being unpleasant to experience, has implications for our emotional well-being. Although no one likes criticism, criticism is especially problematic for people who are vulnerable to psychopathology. Conceptualized within a diathesis-stress framework, criticism can be regarded as a psychosocial stressor. It is associated with increased risk for relapse across a variety of disorders, including depression and schizophrenia. This highlights the importance of considering interactions of the environment and biological vulnerability.

Researchers are now exploring the mechanism through which criticism might exert its deleterious effects. There is evidence that, when exposed to personally relevant criticisms, people who are vulnerable to depression show increased activation in emotion-processing areas such as the amygdala as well as reduced activation in prefrontal brain areas implicated in cognitive control. In other words, even in fully recovered patients, criticism seems to perturb some of the neural circuits that are implicated in depression. If the brains of vulnerable people take an emotional "hit" from criticism or have to work harder to cope with it, this could be one mechanism through which criticism could, over time, lead to symptom relapse.

Neural responses to criticism are also associated with how critical participants rate the person who is criticizing them as being on a simple self-report measure of perceived criticism. Importantly, these differences in neural activity were found only during exposure to criticism and not during exposure to praise.

What makes perceived criticism an interesting variable is that it is a trans-diagnostic construct. It predicts adverse clinical outcomes but is not a simple measure of negativity or neuroticism. We also know that PC ratings tend to capture destructive rather than constructive forms of criticism (Smith & Peterson, 2008; Peterson & Smith, 2010). As such, it may thus provide a convenient assessment of psychosocial risk.

Although the PC construct was inspired by the EE literature, PC may in some cases be a better predictor of poor clinical outcome because it provides a measure of "how much criticism is getting through to the patient" regardless of what the objectively assessed "reality" might be (Hooley & Teasdale, 1989). Some people may live in genuinely critical social environments, and their high PC ratings may accurately reflect this. There may be other cases, however, where people feel criticized in the absence of objective criticism and for whom PC is a measure of their "thin-skinned" tendencies. It is also possible that some people who live in objectively critical family environments are subjectively unaware of this fact. To the extent that this is true, we might predict that patients who have more negative symptoms or more difficulties with emotion recognition would actually be afforded some psychological protection in the context of living in a high EE home environment. This may perhaps help explain why the magnitude of the relationship between EE and relapse is less strong for patients with schizophrenia (where negative symptoms and emotion perception deficits are common) than it is for patients with depression. It may also help us understand why, in a sample of healthy controls who were selected on the basis of the presence or relative absence of schizotypal traits, more perceived criticism was correlated with reduced activation in a language area involved in the detection of emotional prosody (Premkumar et al., 2013).

In addition to providing an assessment of risk, PC may also be a measure of vulnerability. It is possible that, in the future, high ratings of perceived criticism might be used to identify people with problems in emotion or cognitive control networks and who are thus more vulnerable to the adverse effects of psychosocial stress. This idea fits well with current models that view the inability to disengage from negative mood states as a central issue for understanding depression (Holtzheimer & Mayberg, 2011; Joormann, 2010). If high ratings of PC can be used to identify behavioral subgroups with high amygdala and low DLPFC reactivity to naturally occurring psychosocial stressors, it is also possible that PC ratings could be used to select those people who might benefit most from cognitively based forms of treatment. Given how easy PC ratings are to obtain, this is an idea with important implications for clinical practice.

References

Brown, G., & Rutter, M. (1966). The measurement of family activities and relationships: A methodological study. *Human Relations, 19,* 241–263.

Brown, G. W., Birley, J. L. T., & Wing, J. K. (1972). Influence of family life on the course of schizophrenic disorders: A replication. *British Journal of Psychiatry, 121,* 241–258.

Brown, G. W., Carstairs, G. M., & Topping, G. (1958). Post hospital adjustment of chronic mental patients. *Lancet,* ii, 685–689.

Butzlaff, R. L., & Hooley, J. M. (1998). Expressed emotion and psychiatric relapse. *Archives of General Psychiatry, 55,* 547–552.

Cutting, L., Aakre, J. M., & Docherty, N. M. (2006). Schizophrenic patients' perceptions of stress, expressed emotion, and sensitivity to criticism. *Schizophrenia Bulletin, 32,* 743–750.

Davidson, R. J. (2000). Affective style, psychopathology, and resilience: Brain mechanisms and plasticity. *American Psychologist, 55,* 1196–1214.

Davidson, R. J., Pizzagalli, D., Nitschke, J. B., & Putnam, K. (2002). Depression: Perspectives from affective neuroscience. *Annual Review of Psychology, 53,* 545–574.

De Raedt, R., & Koster, E. H. (2010). Understanding vulnerability for depression from a cognitive neuroscience perspective: A reappraisal of attentional factors and a new conceptual framework. *Cognitive and Affective Behavioral Neuroscience, 10,* 50–70.

Disner, S. G., Beevers, C. G., Haigh, E. A. P., & Beck, A. T. (2011). Neural mechanisms of the cognitive model of depression. *Nature Reviews Neuroscience, 12,* 467–477.

Drevets, W. C., Bogers, W., & Raichle, M. E. (2002). Functional anatomical correlates of antidepressant drug treatment assessed using PET measures of regional glucose metabolism. *European Neuropsychopharmacology, 12,* 527–544.

Eisler, I., Dare, C., Hodes, M., Russell, G., Dodge, E., & Le Grange, D. (2000). Family therapy for adolescent anorexia nervosa: The results of a controlled comparison of two family interventions. *Journal of Child Psychology and Psychiatry, 6,* 727–736.

Fales, C. L., Barch, D. M., Rundle, M. M., Mintun, M. A., Snyder, A. Z., Cohen, J. D., Matthews, J., & Sheline, Y. I. (2008). Altered emotional interference processing in affective and cognitive-control brain circuitry in major depression. *Biological Psychiatry, 63,* 377–384.

Fals-Stewart, W., O'Farrell, T. J., & Hooley, J. M. (2001). Relapse among married or cohabiting substance-abusing patients: The role of perceived criticism. *Behavior Therapy, 32,* 787–801.

Fromm-Reichmann, F. (1948 [1959]). Notes on the development of treatment of schizophrenics by psychoanalytic psychotherapy. In D. M. Bullard (Ed.), *Psychoanalysis and psychotherapy: Selected papers of Freida Fromm-Reichmann.* Chicago: University of Chicago Press.

Goldstein, T. R., Miklowitz, D. J., & Richards, J. A. (2002). The relationship between expressed emotion attitudes and individual psychopathology among relatives of bipolar patients. *Family Process, 41,* 647–659.

Green, M. J., & Phillips, M. L. (2004). Social threat perception and the evolution of paranoia. *Neuroscience and Biobehavioral Reviews, 28,* 333–342.

Hamilton, J. P., & Gotlib, I. H. (2008). Neural substrates of increased memory sensitivity for negative stimuli in major depression. *Biological Psychiatry, 63,* 1155–1162.

Hayhurst, H., Cooper, Z., Paykel, E. S., Vearnals, S., & Ramana, R. (1997). Expressed emotion and depression. *British Journal of Psychiatry, 171,* 439–443.

Hogarty, G. E., Anderson, C. M., Reiss, D. J., Kornblith, S. J., Greenwald, D. P., Ulrich, R. F., & Carter, M. (1991). Family psychoeducation, social skills training, and maintenance chemotherapy in the aftercare of schizophrenia. *Archives of General Psychiatry, 48,* 340–347.

Holmes, A. J., & Pizzagalli, D. A. (2008). Response conflict and frontocingulate dysfunction in unmedicated participants with major depression. *Neuropsychologica, 46,* 2904–2913.

Holtzheimer, P. E., & Mayberg, H. S. (2011). Stuck in a rut: Rethinking depression and its treatment. *Trends in Neurosciences, 34,* 1–9.

Hooley, J. M. (1986). Expressed emotion and depression: Interactions between patients and high- versus low expressed emotion spouses. *Journal of Abnormal Psychology, 95,* 237–246.

———. (2007). Expressed emotion and relapse of psychopathology *Annual Review of Clinical Psychology, 3,* 329–352.

Hooley, J. M., Orley J., & Teasdale, J. D. (1986). Levels of expressed emotion and relapse in depressed patients. *British Journal of Psychiatry, 148,* 642–647.

Hooley, J. M., & Teasdale, J. D. (1989). Predictors of relapse in unipolar depressives: Expressed emotion, marital quality and perceived criticism. *Journal of Abnormal Psychology, 98,* 229–235.

Hooley, J. M., & Richters, J. E. (1991). Alternative measures of expressed emotion: A methodological and cautionary note. *Journal of Abnormal Psychology,* 100, 94–97.

Hooley, J. M., Rosen, L. R., & Richters, J. E. (1995). Expressed emotion: Toward clarification of a critical construct. In G. Miller (Ed.), *The behavioral high risk paradigm in psychopathology* (pp. 88–120). New York, NY: Springer-Verlag.

Hooley, J. M., & Gotlib, I. H. (2000). A diathesis-stress conceptualization of expressed emotion and clinical outcome. *Journal of Applied and Preventive Psychology,* 9, 135–151.

Hooley, J. M., & Campbell, C. (2002). Control and controllability: An examination of beliefs and behavior in high and low expressed emotion relatives. *Psychological Medicine,* 32, 1091–1099.

Hooley, J. M., Gruber, S. A., Scott, L. A., Hiller, J. B., & Yurgelun-Todd, D. A. (2005). Activation in dorsolateral prefrontal cortex in response to maternal criticism and praise in recovered depressed and healthy control participants. *Biological Psychiatry,* 57, 809–812.

Hooley, J. M., Miklowitz, D. M., & Beach, S. R. H. (2006). Expressed emotion and the *DSM-V.* In S. R. H. Beach, M. Wamboldt, N. Kaslow, R. E. Heyman, M. B. First, L. G. Underwood, & D. Reiss (Eds.), *Relational Processes and* DSM-V. Washington, DC: American Psychological Association.

Hooley, J. M., & Parker, H. A. (2006). Measuring expressed emotion: An evaluation of the shortcuts. *Journal of Family Psychology,* 20, 386–396.

Hooley, J. M., Gruber, S. A., Parker, H., Guillaumot, J., Rogowska, J., & Yurgelun-Todd, D. A. (2009). Cortico-limbic response to personally-challenging emotional stimuli after complete recovery from major depression. *Psychiatry Research: Neuroimaging,* 171, 106–119.

Hooley, J. M., Siegle, G., & Gruber, S. A. (2012). Affective and neural reactivity to criticism in individuals high and low on perceived criticism. *PLoS ONE,* 7(9), e44412.

Joormann, J. (2010). Cognitive inhibition and emotion regulation in depression. *Current Directions in Psychological Science,* 19, 161–166.

Kuipers, E., Bebbington, P., Dunn, G., Fowler, D., Freeman, D., Watson, P., Hardy, A., & Garety, P. (2006). Influence of carer expressed emotion and affect on relapse in non-affective psychosis. *British Journal of Psychiatry,* 188, 173–179.

Kwon, J.-H., Lee, Y., Lee, M.-S., & Bifulco, A. (2006). Perceived criticism, marital interaction and relapse in unipolar depression: Findings from a Korean sample. *Clinical Psychology and Psychotherapy,* 13, 306–312.

Leff, J., Kuipers, L., Berkowitz, R., Eberlein-Vries, R., & Sturgeon, D. (1982). A controlled trial of social intervention in the families of schizophrenic patients. *British Journal of Psychiatry,* 141, 121–134.

Leff, J., & Vaughn, C. (1985). *Expressed emotion in families.* New York, NY: Guilford.

Leff, J., Vearnals, S., Brewin, C. R., Wolff, G., Alexander, B., Ases, E., Dayson, D., Jones, E., Chisholm, D., & Everitt, B. (2000). The London depression intervention trial: Randomised controlled trial of antidepressants v couple therapy in the treatment and maintenance of people with depression living with a critical partner: clinical outcome and costs. *British Journal of Psychiatry, 177*, 85–100.

Masland, S. R., Hooley, J. M., Tully, L. M., Dearing, K., & Gotlib, I. H. (2015). Cognitive processing biases in individuals high on perceived criticism. *Clinical Psychological Science, 3*, 3–14.

Mayberg, H. S., Lozano, A. M., Voon, V., McNeeley, H. E., Seminowicz, D., Hamani, C., Schwalb, J. M., & Kennedy, S. H. (2005). Deep brain stimulation for treatment resistant depression. *Neuron, 45*, 651–660.

Miklowitz, D. J. (2004). The role of family systems in severe and recurrent psychiatric disorders: A developmental psychopathology view. *Development and Psychopathology, 16*, 667–688.

Miklowitz, D. J., George, E. L., Richards, J. A., Simoneau, T. L., & Succath, R. L. (2003). A randomized study of family-focused psychoeducation and pharmacotherapy in the outpatient management of bipolar disorder. *Archives of General Psychiatry, 60*, 904–912.

Miklowitz, D. J., & Tompson, M. C. (2003). Family variables and interventions in schizophrenia. In G. P. Sholevar & L. D. Schwoeri (Eds.), *Textbook of marital and family therapy* (pp. 585–617). Washington, DC: American Psychiatric Publishing.

Miklowitz, D. M., Goldstein, M. J., Falloon, I. R., & Doane, J. A. (1984). Interactional correlates of expressed emotion in the families of schizophrenics. *British Journal of Psychiatry, 144*, 482–487.

Miklowitz, D. M., Goldstein, M. J., Nuechterlein, K. H., Snyder, K. S., & Mintz, J. (1988). Family factors and the course of bipolar disorder. *Archives of General Psychiatry, 45*, 225–231.

Nuechterlein, K. H., Snyder, K. S., & Mintz, J. (1992). Paths to relapse: Possible transactional processes connecting patient illness onset, expressed emotion and psychotic relapse. *British Journal of Psychiatry, 161*(Suppl. 18), 88–96.

Peterson, K., & Smith, D. A. (2010). To what does perceived criticism refer? Constructive, destructive, and general criticism. *Journal of Family Psychology, 24*, 97–100.

Premkumar, P., Ettinger, U., Inchley-Mort, S., Sumich, A., Williams, S. C. R., Kuipers, E., & Kumari, V. (2012). Neural processing of social rejection: The role of schizotypal personality traits. *Human Brain Mapping, 33*, 695–706.

Premkumar, P., Williams, S. C. R., Lythgoe, D., Andrew, C., Kuipers, E., & Kumar, V. (2013). Neural processing of criticism and positive comments from relatives in individuals with schizotypal personality traits. *World Journal of Biological Psychiatry, 14*, 57–70.

Price, J. L., & Drevets, W. C. (2012). Neural circuits underlying the pathophysiology of mood disorders. *Trends in Cognitive Science, 16*, 61–71.

Ramel, W., Goldin, P. R., Eyler, L. T., Brown, G. G., Gotlib, I. H., & McQuaid, J. R. (2007). Amygdala reactivity and mood-congruent memory in individuals at risk for depressive relapse. *Biological Psychiatry, 61*, 231–239.

Renshaw, K. D. (2008). The predictive, convergent, and discriminant validity of perceived criticism: A review. *Clinical Psychology Review, 28*, 521–534.

Rutter, M., & Brown, G. W. (1966). The reliability and validity of measures of family life and relationships in families containing a psychiatric patient. *Social Psychiatry, 1*, 38.

Rylands, A. J., McKie, S., Elliott, R., Deakin, J. F., & Tarrier, N. (2011). A functional magnetic imaging paradigm of expressed emotion in schizophrenia. *Journal of Nervous and Mental Disease, 199*, 25–29.

Schaefer, H. S., Putnam, K. M., Benca, R. M., & Davidson, R. J. (2006). Event related functional magnetic resonance imaging measures of neural activity to positive social stimuli in pre-and post-treatment depression. *Biological Psychiatry, 60*, 974–986.

Schlosser, D., Zinberg, J. L., Loewy, R. L., Casey-Cannon, S., O'Brien, M. P., Bearden, C. E., Vinogradov, S., & Cannon, T. D. (2010). Predicting the longitudinal effects of the family environment on prodromal symptoms and functioning in patients at risk for psychosis. *Schizophrenia Research, 118*, 69–75.

Scott, J., Colom, F., Pope, M., Reinares, M., & Vieta, E. (2012). The prognostic role of perceived criticism, medication adherence and family knowledge in bipolar disorders. *Journal of Affective Disorders, 142*, 72–76.

Servaas, M. N., Riese, H., Renken, R. J., Marsman, J.-B. C., Lambregs, J., Ormel, J., et al. (2013). The effect of criticism on functional brain connectivity and associations with neuroticism. *PLoS ONE, 8*(7), e69606.

Siegle, G. J., Thompson, W., Carter, C. S., Steinhauer, S. R., & Thase, M. E. (2007). Increased amygdala and decreased dorsolateral prefrontal BOLD responses in unipolar depression: Related and independent features. *Biological Psychiatry, 61*, 198–209.

Smith, D. A., & Peterson, K. M. (2008). Overperception of spousal criticism in dysphoria and marital discord. *Behavior Therapy, 39*, 300–312.

Subotnik, K. L., Schell, A. M., Chilingar, M. S., Dawson, M. E., Ventura, J., Kelley, K. A., Hellemann, G. S., & Nuechterlein, K. H. (2012). The interaction of electrodermal activity and expressed emotion in predicting symptoms in recent-onset schizophrenia. *Psychophysiology, 49*, 1035–1038.

Sturgeon, D., Kuipers, L., Berkowitz, R., Turpin, G., & Leff, J. (1981). Psychophysiological responses of schizophrenic patients to high and low expressed emotion relatives. *British Journal of Psychiatry, 138*, 40–45.

Sturgeon, D., Turpin, G., Kuipers, L., Berkowitz, R., & Leff, J. (1984). Psychophysiological responses of schizophrenic patients to high and low expressed emotion relatives: A follow-up study. *British Journal of Psychiatry, 145*, 62–69.

Tarrier, N., Vaughn, C., Lader, M. H., & Leff, J. P. (1979). Bodily reactions to people and events in schizophrenics. *Archives of General Psychiatry, 36*, 311–315.

Tarrier, N., Barrowclough, C., Porceddu, K., & Watts, S. (1988). The assessment of psychophysiological reactivity to the expressed emotion of relatives of schizophrenic patients. *British Journal of Psychiatry, 152*, 618–624.

Vaughn, C., & Leff, J. (1976). The influence of family and social factors on the course of psychiatric illness. *British Journal of Psychiatry, 129*, 125–137.

THE SOCIAL WORLD

10.

The Social Brain in a Social World

Russell K. Schutt

Sociology is at its core the science of social relations. Sociologists describe types of social relations, the effects of these relations on individual behavior and attitudes, and their patterning within and across social institutions. It is because Durkheim, Weber, and other early sociologists found in the biology and psychology of the early 1900s no useful insights about social relations that they turned so sharply away from these disciplines. It is because the biologists and psychologists of that period focused on understanding organisms and people as individuals that they gave little attention to social relations. And it is because sociality has come to play such a central role in the biology and psychology of the twenty-first century that sociologists are beginning to reexamine and reconstruct the foundations of their discipline (cf. Schutt, 2011).

Efforts to incorporate into sociological theorizing biological and psychological insights about sociality have already begun, and some notable successes have been achieved, but progress has been slow and the outcome remains uncertain. While 2001 American Sociological Association president Doug Massey (2002, p. 25) urged sociologists to "end our hostility to the biological sciences and work to incorporate the increasingly well-understood biological foundations of human behavior," he also characterized his discipline as having "allowed the fact that we are social beings to obscure the biological foundations upon which our behavior ultimately rests" (p. 1). Our chapter author and renowned sociological theorist Jonathan Turner describes sociologists as having "an almost primal fear response to efforts seeking to bring biology into sociological explanations, soon followed by an anger response" (Turner, 2007, pp. 11–12). Social psychologist Thomas Scheff (1990, pp. 4–5) described the division Durkheim proposed between sociology and psychology as "frozen into rigid separation, with tragic consequences for both disciplines."

No credible scientific methods or bodies of evidence in the late nineteenth and early twentieth centuries connected the operation of the human brain to human sociality, but this position is no longer tenable; sociologists' disconnection from biology and psychology is therefore no longer productive. The chapters in this book's first two sections have described the consequences of our species' evolution as social beings for our neurobiology and in turn the consequences of this neurobiology for our feelings about and reactions to social experience. These insights provide new explanatory connections for sociologists who study human development, family interaction, group processes, and other forms of social relations. Chapters in this last section focus more directly on how social experience influences mental and neural processes throughout the life course.

In this chapter, I return to the foundation that Durkheim and Weber constructed for sociology at the start of the twentieth century and identify the biological and psychological premises that led them to reject interdisciplinary connections at that time. My review of this classical theory demonstrates that Durkheim's and Weber's arguments reflected an understanding of human evolution and of human psychology that has been called into question, where it has not been completely refuted, by subsequent research. I focus specifically on the transformation made possible by social neuroscience research in our understanding of the dynamics of human evolution, the biology of human sociality, and the psychology of human rationality. It is because Durkheim and Weber understood the importance of human sociality that they rejected the individualist biology and psychology available to them; it is because social neuroscience now makes human sociality a key focus of these disciplines that it is time to chart a new direction for sociology.

In the last part of this chapter, I review several promising theoretical directions in sociology that incorporate the neurobiological foundations of human sociality and the findings of socially oriented psychology. I then introduce the contributions made by our chapter authors in this section to the creation of this new biopsychosocial paradigm for sociology. The representation within these chapters of psychiatrists and psychologists as well as sociologists is itself testament to the synergies that can arise in scholarship informed by this interdisciplinary perspective.

The Classical Divorce of Sociology from Biology and Psychology

Written as his doctoral dissertation and first published in 1893, Durkheim's (2014) *Division of Labor in Society* created the foundation for sociology in the twentieth century, but like his American contemporaries,[1] Durkheim had to explain why he did not follow the social Darwinist approach already popularized for the discipline by Herbert Spencer. After all, in the words of Lester Frank Ward (1894, p. 857), the soon-to-be first president of the American Sociological Society, "the astonishing power that he [Spencer] has become in the thought of the world" reflects "the high degree to which it [his thought] rests on the firm foundations of truth"—except, in Ward's opinion, for Spencer's extension into sociology. Throughout the *Division of Labor,* Durkheim therefore propounds "a radical sociologism" as "the one way of maintaining the autonomy of sociology as an independent discipline" (Merton, 1938/1990, p. 21).

Durkheim (1893/1984, p. 144) characterized Spencer's theory of societal development as beginning with the belief that primitive humanity's "sole passions" were hunger and thirst, with the competition to survive being "a logical consequence of Darwinian principles." Social life, and society itself, developed because individuals found that exchange relationships helped them pursue their own self-interest. According to Durkheim (1893/1984, p. 79), Spencer believed that the development of industrial societies and their use of contracts as "the supreme legal expression of cooperation" would in turn reduce the need for a regulatory apparatus like the state.

In contrast to Spencer, Durkheim (1893/1984, pp. 220–221) argued that "collective life did not arise from individual life; on the contrary, it is the latter that emerged from the former." It was not egoism that was "the point of departure for humanity," but altruism—"everywhere that societies exist" (Durkheim, 1893/1984, p. 145). In fact, Durkheim (1893/1984, p. 173) argued, "Altruism is not destined to become, as Spencer would wish, a kind of pleasant ornament of our social life, but one that will always be its fundamental basis. How indeed could we ever do without it? Men cannot live together without agreeing, and consequently without making mutual sacrifices, joining themselves to one another in a strong and enduring fashion."

Durkheim thus recognized unequivocally the fundamental nature of human sociality, in both primitive and modern societies. It was because Durkheim accepted Spencer's characterization of biological evolution as precluding social impulses that he found no value in a disciplinary connection

with biological science. Similarly, Durkheim linked the "sphere of psychological life" to the individual organism and its states, physical needs, and
sensations; as a result, psychology would also be of no value for sociologists' efforts to analyze the "collective type" of life. It was essential for the
discipline of sociology not to be "established on the psychological consti-
tution of the individual" but on "the only object proper to it" (Durkheim,
1951/1997, pp. 37–38):

> It is not realized that there can be no sociology unless societies exist, and that
> societies cannot exist if there are only individuals.

Durkheim's fundamental methodological postulate thus became that social
phenomena must be a given a social explanation (Alpert, 1939/1990, p. 238).

Like Durkheim, and at about the same time, German sociologist Max
Weber also "sought to advance the scientific study of society as a phenomenon *sui generis*" and rejected the social Darwinist focus on biological determinants (Bendix, 1962, p. 473). In addition, Weber argued that psychology was "no more relevant to sociology than any other science which
dealt with factors conditional to human behavior, like physics, geology, etc."
(Parsons, 1947, p. 25). Unlike Durkheim, Weber emphasized the importance
of understanding the subjective meanings that individuals give to their actions, but he used this as a basis for distinguishing the focus of sociology
from that of psychological phenomena (such as memory, habituation, fatigue) and of biological influences that may create some uniformities that
are "not understandable" in terms of subjective meaning. Sociologists,
Weber (1947, p. 94) argued, must treat such influences as "given data," like
the physiological need for nutrition.

Despite his conclusion that it was not possible to understand the meaning
of the behavior of "primitive men," Weber (1947, p. 106) thought that a
biological analog could help to identify the role of mechanical and instinc-
tive factors in "the early stages of human social differentiation." Psychology
could also be of value in explaining "irrationalities of action," but it could not
contribute to understanding the rational human action that characterizes
modern society (Weber, 1947, pp. 108–109).

In their construction of a framework for understanding human sociality,
both Durkheim and Weber thus concluded they had to reject connections
to biology. The theories of society that they developed on the basis of this
rejection helped to create a veritable "wall within academia" that restricted
for a century "the study of evolution to biology and a few human-related subjects such as human genetics, physical anthropology, and specialized branches
of psychology" (Wilson, 2007, p. 2). Yet the rationale for this disciplinary
divorce vanishes in light of new discoveries about human evolution, about

the neurobiology of human sociality, and about the neuropsychology of human rationality.

Evolution and Sociality

The development of group-level selection theory in evolutionary biology began with the recognition that the ties that bind individual humans to one another are of critical importance for survival (Keysers & Gazzola, 2014). Several characteristics of our species created a unique "human adaptive complex" that made cooperation both possible and necessary within and across families. The long human life span and an extended period of juvenile dependence required multigenerational resource flows and support of reproduction by post-reproductive individuals, male support of reproduction through aiding women and their children, and substantial cooperation between kin and nonkin in food production and sharing (Kaplan, Hooper, & Gurven, 2009).

Although it was overlooked even while he was alive, Darwin had recognized in *The Descent of Man* (1871, p. 166) that the functioning of social groups required members to help each other in ways that might not be directly advantageous for the altruistic individuals. As modern evolutionary biologists David Sloan Wilson and Edward O. Wilson (2007, p. 328) explain, "[s]elfish individuals might out-compete altruists within groups, but internally altruistic groups out-compete selfish groups" (see also Barkow, Cosmides, & Tooby, 1992, p. 161).[2] In this volume (Chapter 3), Jonathan S. Turner highlights the importance of social bonding for the effectiveness and hence survival of early human groups who faced fierce predators on the open African savanna.

The diversity and uncertainty of early human environments also heightened the importance of cooperation and sharing (Kaplan, Hooper, & Gurven, 2009). Since the ability of foragers and hunters to secure sufficient food would vary greatly over time and location, a culture of sharing would smooth out the resource flow and improve survival for the larger group. It was only when environmental conditions provided more concentrated resources, and when large-scale agriculture began to produce surplus resources, that dominance hierarchies became the new normal form of human organization.

Anthropological and archaeological evidence supports the expectations of this group-level selection process. Throughout premodern history, humans lived and survived in small interdependent groups of about 150 to 200 individuals (Gazzaniga, 2012, chap. 5; Van Vugt & Kameda,

2014, p. 336). The dominant pattern, still reflected within the twentieth century in those groups largely isolated from outside influence, was one of enduring supportive relations within groups, long-term nurturance of children by parents, monogamous male-female bonds, and egalitarian distribution of resources (e.g., Diamond, 2012; Thomas, 2006). This cooperative intragroup social pattern did not prevent intergroup conflict; in fact, it seems that intergroup conflict was both ubiquitous and frequently lethal (Diamond, 2012; Pinker, 2011). But what is crucial to understanding the evolution of our social brains is that the environment in which the human species evolved was intensely social; it was adaptation to this environment that determined whether infants could thrive and whether groups of kin and others who lived together would endure.

Group-level selection thus provides a biologically based rationale for rejecting social Darwinism's central tenet of the survival of individuals based solely on competition with other individuals:

> Our ability to function as team players in coordinated groups enabled our species to achieve worldwide dominance, replacing other hominids and many other species along the way. . . . Only when we could trust our social partners to work toward shared goals could we rely upon them to share meaningful cooperation. (Wilson & Wilson, 2007, p. 343)

The importance of sociality for survival in turn required supporting neural structures:

> To play the game the human way, it was necessary for the evolving populations to acquire an ever higher degree of intelligence. They had to feel empathy for others, to measure the emotions of friend and enemy alike, to judge the intentions of all of them, and to plan a strategy for personal social interactions. As a result, the human brain became simultaneously highly intelligent and intensely social. (Wilson, 2012, p. 17)[3]

Human success in replacing the Neanderthals in Eurasia may be one of the indications of the success of this evolved strategy of sociality. Genetic evidence suggests that part of the underlying genetic difference between Neanderthals and modern humans was in two genes that can result in an inability to read social cues and explain some cases of human autism (Kolbert, 2011).

Emotions provide a quick form of communication between group members and others that can improve safety, so the emotional capacities of the human brain and body would have enhanced the species' evolutionary advantage in group effectiveness (Christakis & Fowler, 2009, pp. 32, 36–37; Kahneman, 2011; Turner, Chapter 3, this volume).

The development of emotions in humans, the display of emotions, and the ability to read the emotions of others helped coordinate group activity by three means: facilitating interpersonal bonds, synchronizing behavior, and communicating information. (Christakis & Fowler, 2009, p. 36)

Recognizing the importance of group selection in human evolution also allows a key role for cultural influence, since new behavioral patterns can emerge and spread much more quickly within the culture of a group than would be possible if fitness-enhancing mutations could only occur biologically and be transmitted genetically in the course of reproduction (Richerson & Boyd, 2005). The faster adaptation made possible by the spread of cultural patterns would also have facilitated the adaptation of humans to many different environments (Boyd & Richerson, 2009, p. 3284). Culturally evolved cooperative social environments would also favor selection within groups of individuals disposed to more prosocial motives, thus resulting in genetic transmission of neural structures that support sociality (Boyd & Richerson, 2009, p. 3281; Wilson, 2012, pp. 289–290). Christakis and Fowler (2009, p. 233) estimate the resulting genetic component of human sociality at 47 percent. Simply put, humans are wired to connect.

Neurobiology and Human Social Ties

Émile Durkheim's concern with the bases and functions of social solidarity is the foundation for much of the scholarship that guides this book. His path-breaking research on *Suicide* (Durkheim, 1951/1997) identified the association between variation in suicide rates and indicators of social solidarity and continues to inspire productive research in our disciplines. However, Durkheim (1895/1964, pp. 50–59) also insisted that patterns in social solidarity could be understood by sociologists only as "social facts"— *external* constraints on the individual that were to be analyzed sui generis, without reference to individuals or their bodies (Durkheim, 1895/1964, p. 3; Lukes, 1990, p. 85). Durkheim (1895/1964, pp. 50–59) even proposed that children's development of social feeling and sensitivity was imposed externally through education; there was nothing innate or natural about it.

But there is now abundant evidence of neurobiological mechanisms that promote human sociality during human development and in group interaction throughout the life course. Neuropeptide hormones, particularly oxytocin and arginine vasopressin, encourage sociality (Bales, 2014), while genetic changes allowed greater communication in *Homo sapiens* (Zihlman & Bolter, 2004). Vicarious motor activation within the brain in response to observing others allows humans to experience the world from the standpoint of others and thus interact more effectively (Keysers & Gazzola, 2014). Multiple brain regions, including the amygdala, dorsolateral prefrontal cortex, orbitofrontal cortex, and mirror neurons, are part of the evolved social brain (Burns, 2006, p. 79).

As a result of the operation of our "social brain," the default condition for humans appears to be social proximity and interaction, not being alone (Coan, Brown, & Beckes, 2014, pp. 94–95). Social connections are associated with being "happier, healthier, and better citizens" (Lieberman, 2013, p. 250). From partner hand-holding and secure infant-caregiver attachment to peer bond quality and romantic love, social connection has positive effects at both the biological and affective levels (Acevedo & Aron, 2014; Cassidy, Ehrlich, & Sherman, 2014; Coan, Brown, & Beckes, 2014; Watanabe & Smuts, 2004). By contrast, social loss has adverse hormonal effects that can result in depression (Panksepp et al., 2014), while exposure to violence and trauma can damage the hippocampus and reduce prefrontal cortical gray matter (TenHouten, 2013, pp. 89–90). In the words of psychologist Matthew D. Lieberman (2013, p. 238), "Evolution has bet time and time again on making us more social." Sociality, in other words, is biologically programmed into the human brain.

Neurobiology and Human Rationality

Weber's (1947, p. 92) dualistic vision of the role of reason and emotion presumed that "irrational, affectually determined" influences were deviations from a rational ideal. The anger provoked by problems in interpersonal relations was "derived from irrational motives" and thus clearly distinguishable from action carried out in pursuit of rational goals (Weber, 1947, pp. 95–96). Since modern societies characterized by "legal-rational authority" are legitimated to their citizens by impersonal rules and procedures, they could largely leave emotion behind (Weber, 1947, pp. 328–330). Weber thus translated Enlightenment ideals and Cartesian philosophy into an analysis of societal development and a conception of organizational functioning (Damasio, 1994, pp. 247–250; TenHouten, 2013, pp. 93–102).

Notwithstanding Weber's disinterest in biological connections, human rationality can also be understood in relation to neurobiology. It is the size of the human brain's prefrontal cortex (PFC) that most distinguishes human from primate neurobiology, and it is the PFC that supports the "executive functioning" that underlies rationality (TenHouten, 2013, pp. 221–224). Executive functioning is involved when flexible models of the world are used to control interpersonal competition and goal attainment, when structured information is retrieved from memory, when automatic, involuntary and habitual responses are inhibited and new sequences of behavior are initiated. Through the executive functioning it makes possible, the prefrontal cortex thus largely controls human planning, weighing alternatives, and making decisions. It is the seat of human self-control (Lieberman, 2013, pp. 112–115).

If the enlarged human PFC allowed *Homo sapiens* to operate as rational beings, coolly calculating the means required to reach desirable ends, neurobiology would seem to support Weber's portrayal of reason and emotion as incompatible (TenHouten, 2013, pp. 123–124). But this is neither how the brain operates nor how decisions are made. Emotions are required for the exercise of human reason, in order to restrict the range of options considered and focus attention on critical information (TenHouten, 2013, p. 122). Emotional reactions to events travel through faster circuits in the brain that can then shape the actions taken in response to evaluation of alternatives without any conscious recognition of the influence of emotions. Reason and emotion are therefore by design intended to be synergistic in their influence (Damasio, 1994).

And since social connections have positive value for both surviving and thriving (Coan, Brown, & Beckes, 2014, pp. 94–96), both reason and emotion are attuned to the need to make us "walk the walk" required to maintain social connections (Lieberman, 2013).

> Evolution has wired us with panoptic self-control in which the mere possibility of being judged and evaluated by others dramatically increases our tendency to behave in line with society's values and morals. (Lieberman, 2013, p. 228)

It is thus both natural, and rational, to enhance social connection and avoid the (emotional) pain of social rejection.

Interdisciplinary Directions in Sociology

The development of social capital theory reflects increasing attention by sociologists in recent decades to the importance of social ties as sources of knowledge and other resources and as signals to potential employers and others of these resources (Lin, 2001, pp. 19–20). However, this approach does not yet incorporate an understanding of humans' evolved neurobiological capacities for social interaction or of the resulting psychological need for secure ties. Prior to the development of social neuroscience, social psychologist Thomas Scheff's "microsociology" came closest to an inter-disciplinary understanding of sociality and human society.

Building on the work of sociologist Erving Goffman (1967) and psychol-ogist Helen Block Lewis (1971), Thomas Scheff (1990, p. 4) rejected the effort to explain human motives and actions as comprehensible at the level of individuals. Disputing the continuing preference of sociologists, following Durkheim, to view social order as dependent on "exterior and constraining bonds," Scheff (1990, p. 5) proposed *"maintenance of bonds"* as the most crucial human motive and secure social bonds as the "force that holds a society together." Shame, Scheff (1990, pp. 73, 76) asserted,

> is *the* social emotion, arising as it does out [of] the monitoring of one's own actions by viewing one's self from the standpoint of others. (p. 80)

Social bonds in simpler societies that maximized the use of shame would thus be stronger than those in societies with an advanced division of labor (Sheff, 1990, pp. 23–24, 73).

By anticipating key findings of social neuroscience, Scheff's theory indi-cates how helpful this interdisciplinary approach is for investigating core sociological concerns. As more recent research has demonstrated (Dutra et al., 2008; Talbot, Talbot, & Tu, 2004), and as Scheff's theory would pre-dict, both brain and mind are adversely affected when feelings of shame rather than positive self-regard emerge from social interaction. When se-vere trauma is accompanied by feelings of shame, the likelihood of post-traumatic stress disorder increases sharply (Andrews et al, 2000; Feirig & Taska, 2006; van der Kolk, 2005, 2006).

Chapter author Jonathan H. Turner (1988, p. 3) also anticipated in his theory of social interaction the value of social neuroscience, for he recog-nized that "[t]he basic unit of sociological analysis is not [individual] ac-tion, but *inter*action." Turner (1988) defined interactional processes as in-volving skills in what we have termed in this volume social cognition.

> Interactional processes are what people actually do when they influence each other's behavior. . . . In broad strokes, these capacities involve signaling a course of behavior and interpreting both one's own behavioral signals and those of others. (p. 15)

The emotions arising from interpersonal interaction in turn underlie deci-sion making, including ostensibly rational decisions about instrumental needs, since they attach a valence to alternative choices (Damasio, 1994; Turner, 2007, p. 36). In Chapter 3 of this volume, Turner has identified how he expanded on these prior insights to develop a theory of human emo-tions and an understanding of human evolution.

Bernice Pescosolido focuses her chapter (Chapter 11) on the potential for multilevel analysis of human functioning, rather than on the evolutionary origins of human capacities. Through a careful review of research on suicide and on religious affiliation, drawing on Durkheim's insights about social factors in suicide rather than on his unwillingness to take account of biological factors in his theorizing, Pescosolido is able to demonstrate the ubiquity of cross-level influences from molecules to communities. Her grand synthesis of the biological effects of social factors and of the social effects of biological variation charts a direction for productive new research within a biopsychosocial paradigm.

The chapter by psychiatrists Michael Behen and Harry Chugani (Chapter 12) provides an arresting example of the biological effects of social conditions on children raised in socially isolating conditions in Romanian orphanages. In addition to documenting the profoundly devastating physiological and neurological effects of severe social deprivation, they also show that enriching the social environment can reverse some of these harmful effects. Sociologists Patrick Sharkey and Robert Sampson (Chapter 13) then turn our attention to the impact of the larger social environment by identifying the negative cognitive effects of neighborhood violence on schoolchildren. The resulting discoveries about the neurological effects of what might be termed "normal" variation in the social environment helps establish the need for multilevel analyses connecting social structure to human biology.

Alan Horwitz (Chapter 14) provides further evidence of the negative impact of problems in the social environment in his review of the consequences of bereavement. At the same time, however, Horwitz strikes a cautionary note by distinguishing carefully the effects of the stress of bereavement from those of the more profound and unexpected social deprivations that result in psychiatric disorder and neural damage.

In the final chapter in this section (Chapter 15), social work researcher Shaun Eack and psychiatrist (and coeditor) Matcheri Keshavan focus on the cognitive and neurological benefits of a social environment that is intentionally enriched with cognitive enhancement therapy. Their demonstration that a carefully structured, highly supportive social environment can reverse the neurological deficits in social circuitry of people with schizophrenia is a reminder that neuroplasticity can be both a biological boon as well as a bane in human development and functioning.

The inclusion in this section of chapters by psychiatrists and a psychologically oriented social work researcher indicates the growing awareness of the brain-mind-society link in all three of our disciplines. Taken together, these contributions illustrate how research in psychology and neuroscience can improve understanding of social processes.

Conclusions

It is now clear that the interpenetration of individual and society that both Durkheim and Weber recognized does not occur solely at the level of social norms and behavior, on which they focused; it instead is instantiated in the human brain in a way that influences subsequent behavior and consciousness and thus the way in which individuals interact with the social world. This interpenetration shaped the human species, it is reflected in societal organization, and it guides human development and human action.

The extensive powers of both reason and emotion that are the natural products of human evolution have created a mind that supports enhanced functioning of humans as individuals, but always and necessarily in the context of connections with others. "Naturalizing the human" thus allows multilevel analysis of patterns of human behavior and orientation (Smith & Franks, 1999, pp. 13–14).

If our species evolved and succeeded because of its sociality, if our genes prepare us for living in a social world, and if our development is enabled by social connections, we can only understand our functioning in relation to our interaction with the social world. If chance mutations or environmental insults have altered the neural circuits that support sociality, our ability to function effectively will be challenged. If the social environment hinders our ability to function socially, our neural circuitry may be altered in ways that have enduring harm. By contrast, when we are able to develop and maintain supportive social ties, both our ability to engage in the larger social world and our health and well-being will benefit. Each chapter in this section helps use to understand this bidirectional link.

British sociologist Nikolas Rose concludes his book on neurobiology with Joelle Abi-Rached by acknowledging that social neuroscience now supports

> the core contention of the human sciences, that human societies are not formed by aggregations of such isolates, each bounded by the surfaces of its individual body. (Rose & Abi-Rached, 2013, p. 234)

It is now Spencer's commitment to egoism, not Durkheim's awareness of altruism, that can be rejected as inconsistent with human biology.

Notes

1. A good example of the intellectual turmoil generated in the late nineteenth century by Spencer's approach to sociology is represented in an article about social Darwinism by proponent D. Collin Wells (1907) in an early issue of the *Amer-*

ican Journal of Sociology (volume 12, number 5) and the comments in response to it in that same issue.

2. The bases for and nature of group selection are strenuously debated among evolutionary biologists (e.g., West et al., 2008; Wilson & Wilson, 2007), including the role of true group selection compared to kin selection (Clutton-Brock et al., 2009, p. 3130; Wilson, 2014). Many but by no means all now accept the existence of some form of multilevel selection process.

3. Wilson (2012, p. 17) notes specifically the importance for social functioning of rapid processing of mental scenarios, good long-term memory, and emotion-controlling centers of the brain like the amygdala and autonomic nervous systems that could motivate decisions about alternative plans of action.

References

Acevedo, B. P., & Aron, A. P. (2014). Romantic love, pair-bonding, and the dopaminergic reward system. In M. Mikulincer & P. R. Shaver (Eds.), *Mechanisms of social connection: From brain to group* (pp. 55–53). Washington, DC: American Psychological Association.

Alpert, H. ([1939] 1990). Explaining the social socially. In P. Hamilton (Ed.), *Emile Durkheim: Critical assessments* (Vol. II, pp. 238–243). New York: Routledge.

Andrews, B., Brewin, C. R., Rose, S., & Kirk, M. (2000). Predicting PTSD symptoms in victims of violent crime: The role of shame, anger, and childhood abuse. *Journal of Abnormal Psychology, 109*(1), 69–73.

Bales, K. L. (2014). Comparative and developmental perspectives on oxytocin and vasopressin. In M. Mikulincer & P. R. Shaver (Eds.), *Mechanisms of social connection: From brain to group* (pp. 15–31). Washington, DC: American Psychological Association.

Barkow, J. H., Cosmides, L., & Tooby, J. (1992). "Cooperation." In J. H. Barkow, L. Cosmides, & J. Tooby (Eds.), *The adapted mind: Evolutionary psychology and the generation of culture* (pp. 161–162). New York: Oxford University Press.

Bendix, R. (1962). *Max Weber: An intellectual portrait.* Garden City, NY: Doubleday Anchor.

Boyd, R., & Richerson, P. J. (2009). Culture and evolution of human cooperation. *Philosophical Transactions of the Royal Society B, 364,* 3281–3288.

Burns, J. (2006). The social brain hypothesis of schizophrenia. *World Psychiatry,* 5, 77–81.

Cassidy, J., Ehrlich, K. B., & Sherman, L. J. (2014). Child-parent attachment and response to threat: A move from the level of representation. In M. Mikulincer & P. R. Shaver (Eds.), *Mechanisms of social connection: From brain to group* (pp. 125–143). Washington, DC: American Psychological Association.

Christakis, N. A., & Fowler, J. H. (2009). *Connected: The surprising power of our social networks and how they shape our lives.* Boston: Little, Brown.

Clutton-Brock, T., West, S., Ratnieks, F., & Foley, R. (2009). Introduction: The evolution of society. *Philosophical Transactions of the Royal Society B, 364,* 3127–3133.

Coan, J. A., Brown, C. L., & Beckes, L. (2014). Our social baseline: The role of social proximity in economy of action. In M. Mikulincer & P. R. Shaver (Eds.), *Mechanisms of social connection: From brain to group* (pp. 89–104). Washington, DC: American Psychological Association.

Damasio, A. (1994). *Descartes' error: Emotion, reason, and the human brain.* New York: Putnam.

Darwin, C. (1871). *The descent of man, and selection in relation to sex.* New York: Appleton.

Diamond, J. (2012). *The world until yesterday: What can we learn from traditional societies?* New York: Viking.

Durkheim, É. ([1893] 1984). *The division of labor in society.* With an introduction by Lewis A. Coser. Translated by W. D. Halls. New York: Free Press.

———. ([1893] 2014). *The division of labor in society.* Edited and with an Introduction by Steven Lukes. Translation by W. D. Halls. New York: Free Press.

———. ([1895] 1964). *The rules of sociological method* (Solovay, Sarah A., & Mueller, John H., Trans.; Catlin, George E., Ed.). New York: Free Press.

———. ([1951] 1997). *Suicide: A study in sociology.* New York: Free Press.

Dutra, L., Callahan, K., Forman, E., Mendelsohn, M., & Herman, J. (2008). Core schemas and suicidality in a chronically traumatized population. *Journal of Nervous and Mental Disease, 196*(1), 71–74.

Feiring, C., & Taska, L. S. (2005). The persistence of shame following sexual abuse: A longitudinal look at risk and recovery. *Child Maltreatment, 10*(4), 337–349.

Gazzaniga, M. S. (2012). *Who's in charge?* New York: HarperCollins.

Goffman, E. (1967). *Interaction ritual.* Garden City, NY: Anchor Doubleday.

Kahneman, D. (2011). *Thinking, fast and slow.* New York: Farrar, Straus and Giroux.

Kaplan, H. S., Hooper, P. L., & Gurven, M. (2009). The evolutionary and ecological roots of human social organization. *Philosophical Transactions of the Royal Society B, 364,* 3289–3299.

Keysers, C., & Gazzola, V. (2014). The vicarious brain. In M. Mikulincer & P. R. Shaver (Eds.), *Mechanisms of social connection: From brain to group* (pp. 71–88). Washington, DC: American Psychological Association.

Kolbert, K. (2011). Sleeping with the enemy. *The New Yorker, 87*(24), 64.

Lewis, H. B. (1971). *Shame and guilt in neurosis.* New York: International Universities Press.

Lieberman, M. D. (2013). *Social: Why our brains are wired to connect.* New York: Crown.

Lin, N. (2001). *Social capital: A theory of social structure and action.* New York: Cambridge University Press.

Lukes, S. (2014). Introduction. In S. Lukes (Ed.), Émile Durkheim, *The division of labor in society.* New York: Free Press.

Massey, D. S. (2002). A brief history of human society: The origin and role of emotion in social life. 2001 Presidential Address, American Sociological Association. *American Sociological Review, 67,* 1–29.

Merton, R. K. ([1938] 1990). Durkheim's *Division of labor in society*. In P. Hamilton (Ed.), *Emile Durkheim: Critical assessments* (Vol. II, pp. 20–27). New York: Routledge.

Panksepp, J., Solms, M., Schläpfer, T. E., & Coenen, V. A. (2014). Primary-process separation-distress (PANIC/GRIEF) and reward eagerness (SEEKING) processes in the ancestral genesis of depressive affect and addictions. In M. Mikulincer & P. R. Shaver (Eds.), *Mechanisms of social connection: From brain to group* (pp. 33–53). Washington, DC: American Psychological Association.

Parsons, T. (1947). Introduction. In T. Parsons (Ed.), *Max Weber: The theory of social and economic organization* (pp. 3–86). New York: Oxford University Press.

Pinker, S. (2011). *The better angels of our nature: Why violence has declined*. New York: Viking.

Richerson, P. J., & Boyd, R. (2005). *Not by genes alone: How culture transformed human evolution*. Chicago: University of Chicago Press.

Rose, N., & Abi-Rached, J. M. (2013). *Neuro: The new brain sciences and the management of the mind*. Princeton, NJ: Princeton University Press.

Scheff, T. J. (1990). *Microsociology: Discourse, emotion, and social structure*. Chicago: University of Chicago Press.

Schutt, R. K. (with Goldfinger, S. M.). (2011). *Homelessness, housing, and mental illness*. Cambridge, MA: Harvard University Press.

Smith, T. S., & Franks, D. D. (1999). Introduction: Summaries and comments. In D. D. Franks (Ed.), *Mind, brain, and society: Toward a neurosociology of emotion in social perspectives on emotion* (Vol. 5, pp. 3–17). Stanford, CA: JAI Press.

Talbot, J. A., Talbot, N. L., & Tu, X. (2004). Shame-proneness as a diathesis for dissociation in women with histories of childhood sexual abuse. *Journal of Traumatic Stress, 17*(5), 445–448.

TenHouten, W. D. (2013). *Emotion and reason: Mind, brain, and the social domains of work and love*. New York: Routledge.

Thomas, E. M. (2006). *The old way: A story of the first people*. New York: Farrar, Straus, Giroux.

Turner, J. H. (1988). *A theory of social interaction*. Stanford, CA: Stanford University Press.

———. (2007). *Human emotions: A sociological theory*. New York: Routledge.

van der Kolk, B. A. (2005). Child abuse and victimization. *Psychiatric Annals, 35*(5), 374–378.

———. (2006). Clinical implications of neuroscience research in PTSD. *Annals of New York Academy of Science, 1071*, 277–293.

Van Vugt, M., & Kameda, T. (2014). Evolution of the social brain: Psychological adaptations for group living. In M. Mikulincer & P. R. Shaver (Eds.), *Mechanisms of social connection: From brain to group* (pp. 335–355). Washington, DC: American Psychological Association.

Ward, L. F. (1894). Spencer-smashing at Washington. *The Popular Science Monthly, 44*, 856–857. http://en.wikisource.org/wiki/Popular_Science_Monthly/Volume_44/April_1894/Popular_Miscellany. Accessed July 5, 2014.

Watanabe, J. M., & Smuts, B. B. (2004). Cooperation, commitment, and communication in the evolution of human sociality. In R. W. Sussman & A. R. Chapman (Eds.), *The origins and nature of sociality* (pp. 288–309). New York: Aldine de Gruyter.

Weber, M. (1947). *Max Weber: The theory of social and economic organization.* Edited and with an introduction by Talcott Parsons. Translated by A. M. Henderson and Talcott Parsons. Glencoe, IL: Free Press.

Wells, D. C. (1907). Social Darwinism. *American Journal of Sociology, 12*(5), 695–716.

West, S. A., El Mouden, C., & Gardner, A. (2008). *Social evolution theory and its application to the evolution of cooperation in humans.* Working paper. http://www.zoo.ox.ac.uk/group/west/social.html

Wilson, D. S. (2007). *Evolution for everyone: How Darwin's theory can change the way we think about our lives.* New York: Delta.

Wilson, D. S., & Wilson, E. O. (2007). Rethinking the theoretical foundation of sociobiology. *The Quarterly Review of Biology, 82*(4), 327–348.

Wilson, E. O. (2012). *The social conquest of Earth.* New York: Liveright.

Wilson, E. O. (2014). *The meaning of human existance.* New York: Liveright.

Zihlman, A., & Bolter, De. R. (2004). Mammalian and primate roots of human sociality. In R. W. Sussman & A. R. Chapman (Eds.), *The origins and nature of sociality* (pp. 23–52). New York: Aldine de Gruyter.

11.

Linking the Social Brain to the Social World through Network Connections

Bernice A. Pescosolido

THE HUMAN GENOME PROJECT (HGP) was expected to change the world of medicine and science. It did. The mapping of human DNA, with a working draft by 2000 (International Human Genome Sequencing Consortium, 2001; Venter et al., 2001) and a complete map by 2003 (International Human Genome Sequencing Consortium, 2004), was achieved in record time with many important discoveries, but at least one stunning conclusion: the nature-nurture debate was now obsolete.

While this was a widely anticipated outcome of the Human Genome Project, the reasons for that conclusion were at least partially unexpected. The result was not conquest but "consilience" (Wilson, 1998). The HGP did not produce the "book of life." The studies that followed in the next decade revealed the limited predictive power of DNA, in and of itself. In response, they brought to the fore the role of RNA and epigenetics, once considered the epiphenomenal "junk of nature." As "the markings on genes that program their function" (Szyf, quoted in Lee, 2009) but do not involve a change in the nucleotide sequence itself, how methylation-demethylation and histones come to be, what they do, and how and whether they are passed from generation to generation pointed increasingly to gene-environment interactions (GxE; see Bird, 2007). The knowledge of the now-separate disciplines would have to come together to arrive at a more holistic understanding of the complicated interactions that produce human behavior, including health and illness.

As E. O. Wilson (1998, p. 8) had predicted, this linking of "facts and fact-based theories across disciplines to create a common groundwork of explanation" became the flashpoint of new directions and the centerpiece of National Institutes of Health's Roadmap (Zerhouni, 2003). The HGP pointed to the environment more directly than anyone, including many social scientists, had supposed. In the first decade of the twenty-first century, some of the best scientists in the United States concluded that "the relations among genes, the brain, and social behavior have complex entanglements across several different time scales," leading to "increasing appreciation that social information can alter gene expression and behavior" (Robinson, 2004, p. 399).

Here, I argue that consilience, more recently expressed as transdisciplinarity,[1] requires (1) three fundamental understandings—biological foundations, biological embedding, and social embeddedness—and (2) a framework linking them. Together, they serve as the platform to facilitate cross-communication across the natural, social, behavioral, physical, medical, and public health sciences that 100 years of development *within* each of these traditions has downplayed. I leave the first fundamental understanding to those who know it, but I describe the latter two and end by suggesting one possible new framework, the Social Symbiome. It draws from a Networks and Complex Systems (N&CS) science approach, which offers enough of a shared perspective and language to deconstruct the "Tower of Babel" that plagues efforts at serious integration of insights across the disciplines (Pescosolido, 2006, 2011; Pescosolido et al., in press).

As the Institute of Medicine (IOM, 2006) noted, one of the basic challenges that faces transdisciplinary integration lies in the scores of factors and forces that the social and behavioral sciences bring to the table regarding human health and development. I argue that networks can serve as a prime organizational vector of transdisciplinary integration that can narrow those possibilities. Finally, though I draw on examples across health problems, I often focus on issues surrounding mental health and substance abuse, targeting suicide as a key research question. The concern with suicide has a long research tradition in both the medical and the social sciences. In fact, understanding how such a private act is patterned by larger social forces such as religion and marriage supplied sociology with its empirical foundation (Durkheim, 1897/1951; Pescosolido, 1994). These issues, clearly connected to the brain, resonate across the sciences and provide a rich set of empirical findings that, together, support the development of an approach linking biology and society. Yet, they also raise challenges in schizophrenia and other mental disorders of adaptation to social context, for example, as to how scientific teams integrate the best of what they bring to the proverbial transdisciplinary table (van Os et al., 2008; van Os et al., 2010).

The Nature of the Social

Powerful support for linking the social brain to the social world through network interaction comes out of the research agenda on mice, stress, and maternal behavior (see Meaney, 2001, for a review). Looking at the psychosocial development of mouse pups, researchers in Canada have documented that the network tie between mother and pup is critical to adult mouse "mental health." Reminiscent of the early Harlow monkey studies on attachment and neurosis, those pups with attentive mothers grew to exhibit behaviors more consistent with a healthy adult mouse. They demonstrated better spatial learning, had less fearful demeanors, and, for both males and females, even went on to demonstrate better parental care themselves (see de Jong et al., 2012, on males). Those without such maternal attention were characterized with "abnormal neural and behavioral development" (D'Amato et al., 1992). In brief, mother mice that groomed and licked their pups raised pups that were more "successful" as adults. The nature of the maternal care bond modified the expression of genes that regulate the behavioral and neuroendocrine responses to stress (i.e., the pups produced less stress hormone). Researchers linked these responses to a chemical change, specifically a group of molecules, a methyl group, which attached itself to the control center of genes regulating stress and, essentially, switched it off. This DNA methylation, a chemical coating of the genes, results from the social behaviors of mothers and alters the epigenome, endophenotypes, and phenotypes while leaving the genome intact.

In fact, according to Meaney and Szyf (2005), the mechanism through which detrimental environments "coat" the DNA structure occurs at a glucocorticoid receptor gene promoter in the hippocampal structure of the brain. Altered histone acetylation and transcription factors associated with nerve growth bind to the promoter. Further, DNA methylation changes glucocorticoid receptor expression because it modifies chromatin structure. Finally, by targeting these processes with drugs, the stress effects on the mice pups could be successfully reversed.

This example illustrates two key links between the social brain and the social world. The most obvious is the role of *biological embedding*—that is, how social factors and processes "get under the skin" to affect health and development. Yet, considering only that link is too simplistic. To move transdisciplinary integration forward, we must also understand and incorporate the complexities of *social embeddedness,* how individuals are connected to layers of environmental structures, providing an understanding of context. Both are addressed below.

Biological Embedding

First coined by Hertzman (2000), this concept was developed to explain the nearly universal social class gradient in health. That is, across a wide spectrum of diseases and disorders, individuals with lower socioeconomic (SES) status have higher rates of morbidity and mortality across the life course. Hertzman hypothesized that, as an "emergent property" of the interaction between individuals' developmental, material experiences and psychosocial conditions, the brain is "sculpted" in childhood. This interaction conditions other immediate and prolonged interactions between defense systems and the brain. Indeed, research has revealed that children exposed to adverse psychosocial experiences, often associated with disadvantaged social position, show elevated disease risk in adulthood (Danese et al., 2011; Shonkoff & Phillips, 2000). From this, Hertzman proposed that theorizing, describing, and hypothesizing the biological mechanisms through which disadvantage translates into risk was critical. In particular, tying biological embedding to sensitive periods in the development of neural circuitry would show how environmental influences on both genetic variation and epigenetic regulation generate "socially partitioned developmental trajectories with impact on health across the life course" (Hertzman & Boyce, 2010, p. 329).

Thus, biological embedding alters biological processes caused by social experiences and circumstances and, in turn, either protects or predisposes individuals to health and disease. Because this "stamping" appears to be stable and long term and can be multiplied over time, individuals who are persistently in lower social class statuses can cumulate adverse effects over their development. This works primarily thorough four neurobiological systems that can create pathways to translate social experiences into biological effects (Hertzman & Boyce, 2010, p. 336). First, the hypothalamic-pituitary-adrenal (HPA) axis is involved in the secretion of cortisol, still considered a good biomarker of the stress response. Second, the autonomic nervous system regulates the production and release of neurotransmitters such as norepinephrine and other chemicals implicated across numerous brain disorders such as anxiety and depression (Higgins & George, 2007). Third, the prefrontal cortex affects memory, attention, and other executive functions implicated in brain disorders from Alzheimer's disease to attention-deficit hyperactivity disorder (ADHD). Finally, the primitive amygdala locus coeruleus and higher-order cerebral connections influence skills central to social affiliation implicated in health problems from autism to schizophrenia (Barr & Kolb, 2007).

Biological embedding results from day-to-day experiences as well as exceptional traumas, producing cumulative advantage, disadvantage, or amelioration over time. In line with other recent views on susceptibility, ideas about biological embedding are nonlinear and nonspecific. That is, even similar environmental experiences can produce different health problems because they are embedded in complex interactions over time. Researchers studying genetic influences on mental illness, for example, no longer limit themselves to disease-specific phenotypes (e.g., parental schizophrenia linked to schizophrenia in offspring) but rather to a wide spectrum of psychiatric disease and disorders (i.e., examining a family pedigree that involves schizophrenia in parents for schizophrenia, bipolar disorder, depression, ADHD in their children, etc.; see Gottesman & Gould, 2005).

Some suggest that at the core of this process lie recurring, network-based interactions. Hertzman and Boyce (2010, p. 332), for example, see health disparities as a function of power differences that produce regular and routine *social interactions* marked by discrimination. In turn, such encounters translate into direct biological effects "at least partially attributable to differences in individuals' sense of identity, respect, and position within societies, small or large, marked by nonegalitarian structures and values."

Social Embeddedness

The last statement reveals why it is not enough to consider biological embedding alone, even as it stands as the necessary link between the biomedical and sociobehavioral sciences. An individual's "position within society," in and of itself, marks an entire range of psychological, social, economic, and cultural forces. "Societies, small or large," references a range of social groupings; in sociological terms, anything from the family and peer group to the nation-state and historical epochs. "Nonegalitarian structures and values" points to both vertical dimensions of social hierarchy and to deep cultural content.

The social environment is intricate, dense, and multifaceted. Elucidating the mechanism of biological embedding requires understanding the nature and range of social influence and the social structures that shape them. To that end, social embeddedness offers one way to conceptualize and break down the connection between the social brain and the social world. As the degree to which social actors are enmeshed in social networks, this concept can be extended to include the overlap of social ties within and between social units. Introduced by sociologist Mark Granovetter (1985), it is derived from a social network perspective with early and deep roots in sociology and anthropology (Freeman, 2004) and with renewed vigor in an emerging "network science" (Barabasi, 2009). Seminal ideas that became the concept of social embeddedness were employed by Granovetter (1974) to describe how men's social networks shaped the process of acquiring jobs with better or worse salaries, benefits, and job satisfaction. The key here was that Granovetter hypothesized and provided empirical evidence that economic outcomes, in his case, were fundamentally influenced by social process and structures that were noneconomic in goals or content. Thus, social systems or levels are fundamentally bound up in one another. Social-network ties can have effects beyond their explicit purpose, and even "weak ties" play an important function, connecting different groups and sectors (Granovetter, 1983). Further, even the social and temporal embeddedness of social institutions themselves can be traced through individuals' personal networks (Cleaver, 2002).

Over time, social embeddedness has come to take on the wider meaning of how social actors, whether individuals (Wellman & Wortley, 1990), organizations (Aldrich, 2007), institutions (Tilly, 1984), or even nations (Beckfield, 2010), are inevitably and fundamentally tied into larger social environments represented by network connections. It is a dynamic process with networks as the mechanisms linking individuals and institutions across levels, time, and place. In health, social networks describe the nature of the community as well as individuals' access to and participation in rich, supportive, advantaged environments or decimated, difficult, and disadvantaged ones known to be associated with well-being or disease risk. A large body of research supports the critical role that human connections play in health, illness, and disease status (Kawachi, 2001; Pescosolido & Levy, 2002). In health care, networks describe the hopeful, compassionate, or distressing sterile climates and bonds formed within offices, hospitals, and systems. Social networks shape pathways to care (Pescosolido, Brooks-Gardner, & Lubell, 1998a; Pescosolido et al., 1998b). They shape the nature of provider communication (West et al., 1999) and influence health system change (Swan, 2009). Considered together, individuals', providers', and systems' health and illness "careers" (Pescosolido, 1991) are facilitated or impeded by the interaction of treatment and community networked systems.

Developing a Shared Framework Linking the
Social Brain to the Social World

All science models, at this point, understand that microprocesses do not operate in a vacuum. The fundamental concepts of biology provide the foundation of behavior, including health and disease. The concept of social embeddedness sets multiple levels of the social world, viewing entire processes constituted and operating through social networks. Biological embedding represents the concept linking the social brain to the social world.

To offer a transdisciplinary framework linking biology, biological embedding, and social embeddedness, several conditions must be met. Such a theoretical scaffolding (1) considers and articulates the full set of contextual levels documented to have an impact in past empirical research; (2) offers a dynamic underlying mechanism or "engine of action" that connects levels, allowing for a way to narrow focal influences; (3) employs a metaphor and analytic language familiar to both social and natural sciences to facilitate synergy; (4) understands the need for and uses the full range of methodological tools from the social and natural sciences (Pescosolido, 2006); and (5) provides a tangible pathway to intervention, whether through medical treatment, legal policy changes, or community-based activism (Pescosolido, 2011).

What individuals know, how they evaluate the potential efficacy and suitability of a range of behavior, and what they eventually do are fundamentally tied to, negotiated in, and given meaning through social interactions. These draw from and are translated back to the individual as social experiences recorded on the genome. Cutting-edge approaches across the physical (Vespignani, 2009), biological (Sporns, 2011), medical (Christakis & Fowler, 2007), public health (Valente, 2010), and social (Liu, King, & Bearman, 2010) sciences support the network perspective as a potential solution.

Network models privilege one explanation—social interaction through and in network ties—providing a fundamentally different starting point and placing different priorities on sets of explanatory factors already found to be useful (Pescosolido, 1992). For example, in health care, the Network Episode Model (NEM; Pescosolido, 1991) took this approach in light of frustrations with the inability of existing individually focused and static models of help seeking to provide basic explanatory power. The NEM began with the premise that responding to illness or prevention is a phenomenon structured and given meaning through a social process managed by individuals' social networks in the community and the treatment system. Since individuals have both agency and habit (i.e., practical consciousness), they improvise and routinize within the possibilities and limits of social network structures in their community, organizations, and historical period. As pragmatists with commonsense knowledge and cultural routines, individuals face changes in their health status by interacting with others who may recognize (or deny) a problem, send them to (or provide) treatment, and support, cajole, or nag them about appointments, medications, or lifestyle. However, as part of a society that includes institutions of social control, they may also encounter the health care system with resistance and under coercive requirements (e.g., required examinations for employment or sports; involuntary commitment for mental health problems; Pescosolido, 1991, 1992).

As the NEM developed, the layers of the network in the community and treatment system were differentiated from personal networks. Pathways to care were described; network influences in interaction with biological and genetic factors were documented; and, over time, the frame of reference was pushed back to illness onset as well as behavior in response to illness (e.g., Carpentier & White, 2002; Lindsey et al., 2010; Pescosolido, 2006; Pescosolido & Boyer, 1999; Pescosolido et al., 1998a; Pescosolido et al., 2010; Pescosolido et al., 1998b; Rogers, Hassell, & Nicolaas, 1999). Most recently transformed in sync with goals and language of the "omics" revolution, the Social Symbiome (Pescosolido, 2011; Pescosolido et al., in press) began to construct an explicit N&CS science base for linking biology, biological embedding, and social embeddedness. The foundations of the framework are described below.

Durkheim's Theory of Suicide as Illustrative, Predictive Network Foundation

Suicide represents one of the foremost problems that historically captured the attention of medicine, public health, and social science. In fact, the last decade of the twentieth century witnessed increased attention to suicide from medical professionals, public health researchers, expert policy makers, and legislators. This focus produced the Surgeon General's *Call to Action* (U.S. Public Health Service, 1999), the Institute of Medicine's *Reducing Suicide: A National Imperative* (Goldsmith et al., 2002), the Centers for Disease Control and Prevention's (CDC's) report on preventing suicide through social connectedness (CDC, 2008), and the Garrett Lee Smith Memorial Act for suicide prevention (2004; see Wray, Colen, & Pescosolido, 2011).

In research, certain factors have demonstrated robust effects at different levels of aggregation (individual to geographical areas within countries to cross-national comparison), across disciplinary frameworks (e.g., suicide tends to increase with age, for men, and in occupations [medical professionals, police]), and across time (see Pritchard & Baldwin, 2000; Stockard & O'Brien, 2002, as recent exceptions). Yet, over the past three decades, scientific research and conceptual thinking have converged to suggest that suicide comes from a combination of social, cultural, physiological/health, developmental, and genetic factors operating through diverse, complex pathways. As a result, both biological embedding and social embeddedness likely play important etiological roles. Suicide may have a basis in depression or substance abuse, yet even these are tied to social factors like the loss of social relations, economic conditions, or political violence.

However, scientific progress on understanding and examining multiple levels and different pathways to suicide has been limited. Contemporary suicide research tends to be bifurcated along clinical/biological/individual and social science/public health/aggregate lines (Blackmore et al., 2008). Biomedical epidemiology tends to draw data from treated populations, individual death certificates, and psychological autopsies, often with matched controls. Social epidemiology tends to use official rates of suicide organized by geographical areas such as county, state, and country or by time periods (e.g., years). Even when social and contextual factors are acknowledged, suicide continues to be framed and understood as a problem faced by individuals. Bringing the basic ideas of the NEM and N&CS science together with classic social science theories of suicide presents the possibility of developing a foundation for a transdisciplinary approach to link the social brain to the social world.

Though not the first empirical investigation at the population level, Durkheim's (1897/1951) theory of suicide resonates with the CDC's (2008) contemporary focus on "connectedness" in suicide research and prevention. And, connectedness ties directly into a network perspective (Bearman, 1991; Brashears, 2010; Pescosolido, 1994; Pescosolido & Georgianna, 1989; Segre, 2004). Focusing on the group level, Durkheim conceptualized two critical dimensions as defining the nature of social groups. Integration refers to the presence of ties that offer love, care, and concern to group members—elements often synonymous with issues of social support, a commonly used and long-standing concept in health, illness, and health care (Berkman, 1985; Cohen & Syme, 1985). Regulation refers to guidance, appraisal, pressure, and even coercion—all factors that establish normative boundaries of social groups. While less often studied, the latter notion has been used to show that certain individuals "prod" others in their network toward health behavior (Reczek & Umberson, 2012). Thus, any group can be described on both dimensions as having "more" or "less" integration and regulation.

In network terms, then, intergroup connectedness is seen as a major way that society affects suicide. For example, differences between Norway and Denmark's suicide rates have been traced to difference in social integration, and in Norway, where the level of integration among young men was in decline, suicide rates increased (Bille-Brahe, 1987; Institute of Medicine, 2002). The doubling of the suicide rate in Ireland from 1945 to the 1990s has also been seen as directly related to lower levels of regulation and integration (Swanwick & Clare, 1997). Using Granovetter's notion of social embeddedness, recent research has found that even the suicide attempts of "weak-tie" network members push at-risk youth toward more suicide/ideation (Baller & Richardson, 2009). In sum, social networks both create and "hold" culture—emotions, stress, values and beliefs, and action scripts.

Figure 11.1 provides a graphical rendering of Durkheim's theory translated into the current language and perspective of social networks (Pescosolido & Levy, 2002). Each dimension of group connectedness runs from dense to sparse in terms of network ties. When these two are considered simultaneously, four poles represent the kinds of network structures that predispose individuals to suicide. Specifically, when individuals exist in social structures with too little integration or regulation, the social net is loose or open, and there is little in the social structure to "catch" individuals when crisis destabilizes their equilibrium. In the face of challenge, social network ties provide an insufficient buffer and individuals "fall" through the net. Thus, the absence of network ties that provide support *or* oversight results in problems—disease, death, inadequate care, lonely neighborhoods, unmethylated stress-related genes, and so on. For Durkheim, location on the spatial network map with too little integration produced a state of egoism in the social structure, a higher egoistic suicide rate (disconnectedness at the aggregate level), or a greater probability of egoistic suicide (isolation at the individual level). For similar topographical reasons, but fundamentally different social reasons, locations characterized by underregulation also put individuals and societies at a similar level of risk. With networks that provide too little regulation, the social structure is in a state of anomie (normlessness), the individual is in a state of anomia (rootlessness), and the probability of suicide is also high. Both locations produce "diseases of the infinite" because they provide no grip in the societal safety net that supports people during times of individual or community crises.

Figure 11.1 also depicts problem locations in societies that are too regulated or too integrated. Here, social networks are overbearing and the safety net closes up. With no "give" to the social net, the domineering nature of social connectivity results in an inflexible, unsupportive social environment. Like the situation of "too little," the situation of "too much" has dire con-

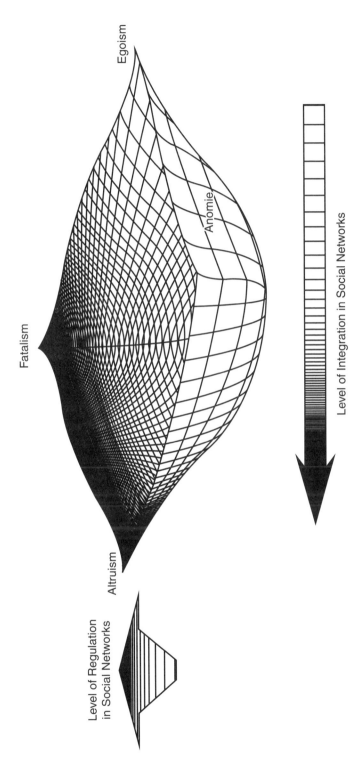

FIGURE 11.1. Theoretical predictive plane for a Network and Complex Systems (N&CS) science framework (adapted from Pescosolido & Levy, 2002; Institute of Medicine, 2002; reprinted with permission).

sequences. Confronting challenges in the context of an overintegrated social structure produces altruistic social structures and correspondingly altruistic suicide (e.g., war heroes, saints), while the overregulated location produces a fatalistic social structure with fatalistic suicides (e.g., mass cult suicides; Pescosolido, 1994). In both cases, the individual becomes fused with the group, losing individual identity and the capacity for independent decision making and self-protection.

The middle (or lowest point) in the social safety net offers the greatest support in the face of biological or social challenges. Here, social networks are optimal (i.e., moderate on both dimensions) and together result in the lowest number or rate of suicides. For example, the intersection of moderate levels of integration and regulation is thought to underlie the fairly consistent finding of lower suicide rates for married men. To use Durkheim's terms, men "profit" in marriage, at least in part, because their wives cajole, coerce, or demand that their husbands engage in healthier behavior, as well as provide the companionship and support more typically ascribed to marriage (Umberson, 1987; Umberson & Greer, 1990). As individuals fall on places on the net that are higher (e.g., more extreme values or amounts of marital regulation, as in domestic abuse), the predictions are more grave for suicide (see Kushner & Sterk, 2005, on an alternate hypothesis; Neeleman, 1998).

From Genes to Global Cultures

What is most crucial to understand about the net is that it does not depict what any one individual "has." Rather, it depicts a fixed theoretical space that describes the possible configurations and consequences of network structures. Biological and social systems have a network structure that predisposes or protects individuals from suicide. Individuals have stronger or weaker connections into those structures. Together, this constructs a personal world of social and biological influence. The IOM (2002) reports the heritability of liability to suicidal behavior to be somewhere between 30 and 50 percent. Both biological embedding and social embeddedness likely play important etiological roles in the remaining 50 to 70 percent.

In network imagery, membership in Durkheim's "societies" or "social groups" translates into sets of networks at different levels of aggregation. He considered country-level differences (e.g., Italy vs. England), organizational or institutional differences (e.g., family structures, religions), and individual differences (e.g., marital status) in integration and regulations. If we then bring to the N&CS science new data on networks at biological levels (e.g., brain networks; Sporns, 2011), we end with six core systems, each with a theoretical prediction plane, modeled in infinite remission (i.e., a fractal structure; Abbott, 2001; Pescosolido, 2011; Pescosolido et al., in press). The community or "place," institutions or "organizations," the support system or "personal networks," the individual or "self," the biology or "body systems," and the molecular system or "genes" and "proteins" all shape pathways to health, morbidity, and mortality, as well as responses to them (see Duberstein et al., 2004, on support for multiple types and levels of social integration). The interconnections among these large, interacting units align directly with the basic definition of complexity theory and the potential of a network perspective to provide direction (Mitchell, 2009).

In sum, Durkheim's notion of the centrality of social interactions in understanding suicide corresponds to the primary starting point for an N&CS science framework linking the social brain to the social world. The nature of social interactions defines the mechanism underlying the impact of social structures and process. Taking it one step further, these mechanisms exist both within levels of the social and biological environment and also connect their influence across levels. Combining the theoretical specification at each level (Figure 11.1) with a consideration of the multiplicity of levels of society and biology that may work to influence health and health care produces the Social Symbiome (Pescosolido, 2011; Pescosolido et al., in press). Fleshing out this frame within and across levels and guidance by a focus on how one social influence—religion—has been implicated in suicide may facilitate understanding of how biological foundations interact with social embeddedness to produce biological embedding.

Key Research Question: How Does Religion Operate as a Prime Vector of Social Environmental Influence?

Religious groups represent one form of many natural "communities" dependent upon factors such as member socialization and participation (Gustafson, 1961; Tilly, 1984). According to social scientists, the potential protective or destructive power of religion depends on the ability of religious networks to provide a source of support and guidance. This is interwoven with the ability of religious groups to draw individuals to their activities and actually participate in a religious network (Collins, 1982; Pescosolido & Georgianna, 1989). For example, what differentiates religious groups in their ability to restrain or facilitate suicidal impulses lies in the degree to which religions provide social and historical communities that provide emotional support and instrumental help. In Durkheim's original hypothesis on the role of religion in the transition to modern industrial society at the end of the nineteenth century, those who stood with Catholicism were seen as having a base of strong and continuing network affiliation located in the church and the wide range of other social institutions (e.g., hospitals and schools) that it controlled. Suicide rates in predominantly Catholic areas were relatively low because of the continued guidance (i.e., regulation) and institutional supports (i.e., integration) the church provided in the modern age. Those who affiliated with the more liberal religions resulting from the Protestant Reformation chose tolerance, free inquiry, and diversity. They traded emotional and institutional support and, in turn, faced greater psychological tensions, ambiguity, and ultimately higher suicide rates. This "one law" dominated much of the debate on religion and suicide over the twentieth century (Bankston, Allen, & Cunningham, 1983; Johnson, 1965). Research generally supported Durkheim's original claim but not without evidence to the contrary.

Reconsidering these ideas through a network translation of the more general proposition (i.e., religions with greater integration produce a lower suicide rate) rather than the specific hypothesis (i.e., Catholicism vs. Protestantism), we argued that three sociohistorical trends (secularization, ecumenicalism in the 1960s, and the post–World War II evangelical revival) had realigned religion in the United States (Pescosolido & Georgianna, 1989). In fact, we found that areas with greater representation of Catholicism and Judaism continued to post lower suicide rates. Further, Protestant religions labeled liberal, mainline, or institutional (e.g., Episcopal, Congregational) appeared to aggravate suicide, as Durkheim saw in Western Europe at the turn of the nineteenth century. However, Protestant religions classified as evangelical or conservative (e.g., Seventh-Day Adventists, Southern Baptists) seemed to have a protective effect on suicide, similar to Catholicism and Judaism.

In sum, the original *hypotheses* in Durkheim did not stand; yet, considered under a network frame, the general theory was supported. Conservative, evangelical Protestants are more likely to participate in religious activities and to name fellow congregation members as best friends than their liberal counterparts (Pescosolido & Georgianna, 1989; Stark & Glock, 1973). These churches are seen as strong, primary groups and "some of the most cohesive non-ethnic communities in the United States" (Roof & McKinney, 1987). To the contrary, mainline or liberal Protestants are seen as "dormant" because their studies document that adherents to these religious "societies" do not attend church frequently, often do not know one another, and participate in hierarchical church structures that translate into a passive role for members (Idler et al., 2003; Kelley, 1972; Quinley, 1974; Seybold & Hill, 2001).

There is an inherent complexity to religious influence that requires a rejection of a reductionist approach. The consideration of a number of components part and partial of the institution of religion represents a part of the self-organizing influence of religion on suicide. Specifically, the influence of religion depends on the context in which religions exist, on the network structure of the religious community, on the religious composition of any individuals' personal networks, and on the strength of the tie that binds the individual to a particular religious community. Religious communities are, in and of themselves, more or less likely to provide an integrative and regulative network of support. But, individuals can forge stronger or weaker ties with these religious communities and choose to participate (or not). For example, beliefs and values that shaped norms of behavior regarding suicide are deeply rooted in social networks that reinforce established ideas about right and wrong, as well as about appropriate ways to solve problems (Colucci & Martin, 2008; Pescosolido & Georgianna, 1989).[2] Thus, in line with Figure 11.2, social embeddedness in religion reflects the basic logic of complexity theory. There are large, interacting levels at which religion operates. Individuals, groups, institutions, and context, *together*, shape the religious landscape and create the social force on individual suicide.

New questions arise. Who in these highly Catholic areas had lower suicide rates? Was it just Catholics, or did the fabric of Catholicism, which had always included educational institutions from kindergarten to college, hospitals and social services, generally protect those who lived among the Catholics? And, were those who did commit suicide, even in these low-rate areas, *only* Protestants, members of other religious groups, those who were atheists, or even Catholics?

Only by considering multiple contextual levels of biology and society can we begin to unravel the etiological complexities of social and biological influences underlying suicide that are shaped by religious community. Table 11.1 provides examples of factors at each level that research has implicated in suicide. However, research attention has not been focused equally across levels, under a network perspective, or in some cases (i.e., molecular networks and religion) not at all. Given the reliance of social science on aggregated suicide rates, more research has been done on the upper levels on the Social Symbiome. Finally, given the focus of medical science on biological systems and disease, little research has brought social factors of any kind to bear across levels.

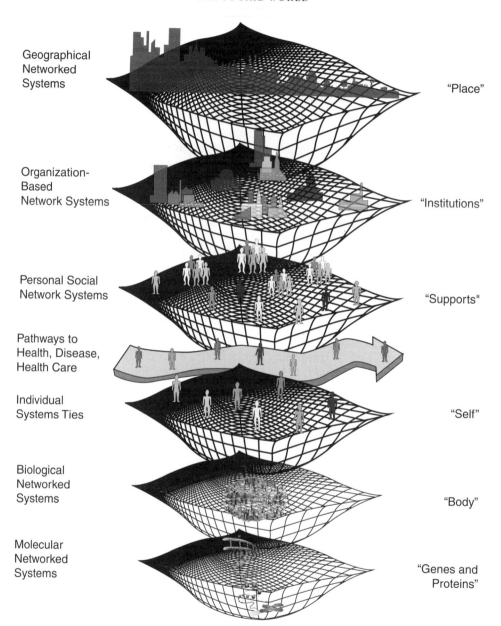

Geographical Networked Systems — "Place"

Organization-Based Network Systems — "Institutions"

Personal Social Network Systems — "Supports"

Pathways to Health, Disease, Health Care

Individual Systems Ties — "Self"

Biological Networked Systems — "Body"

Molecular Networked Systems — "Genes and Proteins"

FIGURE 11.2. The Social Symbiome, based in Network and Complex Systems (N&CS) science, for human health, disease, and health care.

TABLE 11.1. Social and Individual Levels of the Social Symbiome and Examples of Religious Influences on Suicide

Network Levels	Examples of Religion Variables
Community Networked Systems	Presence of religious denominations Location of a religion in a historical hub of strength Religious homo/heterogeneity
Organizational Networked Systems	Integration and regulation in the "home" church, temple, congregation, etc. Religious pressure on medicolegal officials
Personal Networked Systems	Co-religious composition of friends, kin, network ties
Individual Ties w/o Networks	Religious affiliation and participation Religiously anchored meaning systems
Biological Networked Systems	Depression, other psychiatric diagnosis, HPA axis dysregulation
Molecular Networked Systems	No current research on religion
Cross-Level Interactions	Religious presence × divorce rate Catholicism × attendance Religious presence × health care system access Religious tie × depression, anxiety Religious tie × alcohol use Religious tie × divorce status Religious tie × stress Religious tie × HPA dysregulation Religious tie × inflammatory response

In the section that follows, a broad reporting of existing research is addressed, guided by the Social Symbiome. While some levels are sparse, the discussion ends with the rich potential in cross-level interactions suggested by current synergies.

The Community Network

Recent research on the presence of religious communities in an area and its suicide rate continues to demonstrate a clear effect of community-based religious networks. The proportion of conservative religious adherents *in a neighborhood* is negatively associated with individual-level suicide attempts (Maimon & Kuhl, 2008). Similarly, Van Tubergen and colleagues (2005) found that suicide rates in the Netherlands decreased as the proportion of church members within a given *municipality* increased. Indeed, they argue that religious communities have a protective effect for all individuals in an area, whether or not they participate.

However, the larger context has also been implicated, as much by the absence of religion's effects as its presence. In Sweden, for example, Stack (1991) was unable to find an effect of religious affiliation on male or female suicide rates, and only limited support for an influence on youth. He argued that governments providing greater social connections (e.g., the Welfare State in the Nordic countries) may dilute the need for or influence of religion. Further, in the United States, the effects of religious affiliation appear to be more pronounced in *regions* of traditional historical strength for a particular religion. In these places, the opportunity to construct and maintain strong ties comes from the greater likelihood of locating co-religionists and the greater possibility of participating in organizations and institutions formed, supported, or otherwise assisted by religions with a longer and more pronounced presence. For example, while Catholicism's influence on suicide in the United States appears to be both large and consistently protective overall, its effect in the South, a region of relatively few Catholics, is to aggravate suicide. Similarly, in the Northeast, where the presence of Judaism has been historically and numerically strong, its greater presence also decreases suicide, but in all other regions of the country, Judaism is associated with an increase in suicide rates (e.g., in the South; Pescosolido, 1990; Bankston et al., 1983; Kowalski, Faupel, & Starr, 1987).

Finally, technology has created new forms of connected communities that escape geography. As Wellman et al. (1996, p. 213) noted early in the Internet age, "When computer networks link people as well as machines, they become social networks." They are seen as capable of creating and maintaining strong to weak ties; positive to negative ones; and religious, health, and friendship bonds (including ones relevant to suicide, suicide prevention, and suicide support groups; Eysenbach et al., 2004).

As listed in Table 11.1, these studies suggest the potential effect of the sheer presence of a religion, religious homogeneity, and contextual history.

Organizational Network Systems

Societies are made up of sets of organizations or groups that, together, form the basic social institutions—the family, religion, the economy, the educational system, the polity, and, particularly for health and illness, the health care system. While on one level, these help to shape the overall community context, each of these units can be conceptualized, per se, as having an integration/regulation profile. For example, the connectedness within any individual's home church, temple, or mosque might matter, providing even more insight into the context under which religions might protect individuals from suicidal impulses. However, there has been little research at this level on religion. In Turkey (Eskin, 2004), we have a glimpse into the potential protective effects of institutional sectors affiliated with religion. Youth educated in religious versus secular institutions reported lower acceptability of suicide. Further, in the debate over the validity of official suicide rates, stronger ties of medicolegal officials to their communities have been seen as possible sources of bias in suicide rates. In the classic critique (Douglas, 1966), misreporting was directly tied to officials being pressured by religious or other community (e.g., local government) groups to conceal suicide rates. Individual and organizational differences in medicolegal systems have, indeed, been associated with rate reporting, though not always in the directions anticipated (CDC, 2008; Conwell, Duberstein, & Caine, 2002; Pescosolido & Mendelsohn, 1986; Timmermans, 2005; U.S. Public Health Service, 1999).

Other sets of social institutions, and the organizations that comprise them, have been prime research targets in suicide. While they do not implicate the influence of religion, the sheer dedicated research at this level calls for a consideration of the potential interaction of religious and other institutions (see bottom row of Table 11.1). For example, can a strong presence of religion moderate the consistent effects of other institutions? Here, a short description of the most robust influences on suicide rates is listed for such consideration.

The strength or weakness of the family institution in geographical areas has been routinely linked to suicide rates. In general, discord within families has been correlated with suicide, while parental and family connectedness produces the opposite effect, especially among youth (Cicchetti & Toth, 1998; Institute of Medicine, 2002, p. 3). In addition, health care systems can provide different levels of support in treatment centers and can set the connectedness between inpatient (organizational) and outpatient (community-based) services. For example, individuals discharged from mental health facilities, who had their outpatient care reduced at their last session, were documented to be at much greater risk of suicide in the weeks immediately following discharge (Institute of Medicine, 2002).

Personal Social Networks

While the levels above set the conditions for the likelihood that individuals can form particular kinds of network ties, any one person's set of networks results in a unique configuration. Aggregate-level research suggests that the proportion of co-religionists in a person's network likely underlies the protective influence of particular religions (Pescosolido & Georgianna, 1989). At the individual level, involvement in religious activity has been associated with less suicide (Duberstein et al., 2004; Nooney, 2005). In fact, Brashears (2010) documents that an individual's ties with religiously similar others decreases feelings of restlessness and unhappiness. In general, those who enjoy close relationships cope better with various stresses, including bereavement, job loss, and illness, and enjoy better psychological and physical health (Institute of Medicine, 2002, p. 3). Conversely, individuals described as "rootless" or socially withdrawn are more likely than case-controls to complete suicide (Appleby, Shaw, & Amos, 1999; Nor, 2000; Trout, 1980).

The Individual

A long research line suggests that religious involvement works, in part, by shaping beliefs that can influence positive outcomes through "the inner experience of spiritual and religious feelings" (Anglin, Gabriel, & Kaslow, 2005; Colucci & Martin, 2008; Dervic et al., 2011; Greening & Stoppelbein, 2002). Religion also provides some individuals with a sense of meaning and purpose (Werner, 1992, 1996). Since conservative, evangelical denominations, for example, often require more frequent and active participation, individuals' religious commitment and beliefs have been tied together (Gearing & Lizardi, 2009; Stack & Wasserman, 1992).

Historically, however, individual and psychological explanations of suicide have focused squarely on conflicts, whether internal or social (see Jamison, 1999; Maltsberger & Goldblatt, 1996, for overviews). While religious involvement can result in conflict, the role of religion as a buffer of conflict and problems, including health, has been a mainstay of social science research. For example, belief in eternal life has been demonstrated to reduce the negative health effects of discrimination (e.g., Bierman, 2006) or anxiety (Inzlicht, Tullett, & Good, 2011).

Being divorced, separated, or widowed increases suicide, while being a parent, particularly for mothers, decreases suicide risk. Histories of mental illness, childhood maltreatment, and hopelessness have all been implicated in individuals' deaths by suicide (Abramson et al., 2000; Beck et al., 1974; Conwell, Pearson, & DeRenzo, 1996; Gonda et al., 2008; Institute of Medicine, 2002; Joiner et al., 2001; Weishaar & Beck, 1990). Again, these suggest possible interactions with stress across individual levels of the Social Symbiome (see bottom row, Figure 11.2).

Biology

Little research has been focused on the biological embedding of religious ties, participation, or effects (see Modai et al., 2002, on neural networks; Tai & Chiu, 2007). Most discussion on this topic focuses on the historical debates between evolutionary biology and religious teachings (e.g., Grinde, 1998), though some research has addressed biological pathways (e.g., Seeman, Dubin, & Seeman, 2003). For example, religious practices have demonstrated immediate effects on biological measurements such as blood pressure (Williams & Sternthal, 2007).

Further, while systems biology increasingly looks to network perspectives (Kreeger & Lauffenburger, 2010; Weiss, Yang, & Qu, 2006), this fairly new approach has not turned to biological predispositions to suicide. However, dysregulation of the HPA axis, as the primary stress response system, and variation in the functioning of the serotonergic and noradrenic systems have been implicated (Arango & Mann, 1992; Brunner et al., 2001; Goldsmith et al., 2002). The very recent establishment of a scientific journal, *Religion, Brain, and Behavior,* speaks to the growing interest in cross-level interactions that may prove useful in understanding the role of religion in suicide.

Molecular

According to the IOM *Report* (2002), the search for candidate genes for suicidal behavior has thus far been inconclusive. However, family studies (Statham, Heath, & Madden, 1998), particularly studies of adoptees from families with multiple suicides (Wender, Kety, & Rosenthal, 1986) and twin studies (Roy et al., 1991), have documented a sixfold increase among first-degree relatives. New avenues of research, though not directed to suicide, have moved to a network perspective. As Al-Shahrour et al. (2006, p. 472) note, "Genes do not operate alone in the cell, but in a sophisticated network of interactions that we only recently started to envisage." And, if we return to the fundamental concept of biological embedding, the potential impact of religion may lie with its influence on the epigenome.

The Complexity of Cross-Level Influences

Under an N&CS science perspective, a complete sketch of the Social Symbiome requires moving beyond an accounting of level effects. Interactions are evidenced. Targeting complex interactions with religion using a cross-national perspective and examining over 50,000 individuals in fifty-six nations, Stack and Kposowa (2011) find that individuals who live in countries with high levels of religiosity and participate in religious activities report low acceptability of suicide. Actively religious individuals are also much less likely than nonreligious people to abuse drugs and alcohol, or to divorce, both additional risk factors for suicide (Batson, Schoenrade, & Ventis, 1993; Braam et al., 1997a; Braam et al., 1997b; Colasanto & Shriver, 1989; Gorsuch, 1995; Institute of Medicine, 2002; Pressman et al., 1990). Moreover, lower rates of depression are found among religious persons, and depression appears to be a significantly stronger predictor of suicide attempts within secular as opposed to religious neighborhoods (Kendler, Gardner, & Prescott, 1997; Kennedy et al., 1996; Koenig et al., 1992; Koenig et al., 1997; Pressman et al., 1990). Even on the biological level, immune-inflammatory responses were lower in individuals who regularly participated in religious activities, net of depression or negative life events (Institute of Medicine, 2002; Koenig et al., 1997).

Other complex interactions have been implicated in suicide. Among individuals, losing network ties and increasing alcohol use predisposes individuals to suicide (Duberstein, Conwell, & Caine, 1993; Murphy, 1992; Murphy et al., 1979). Similarly, hopelessness appears to arise from the co-occurrence of low self-esteem, interpersonal losses, and low self-efficacy to shape how individuals solve personal problems (Antoni et al., 2001; Bandura, 1982, 1992; Catanzaro, 2000; Cruess et al., 2000; Dieserud et al., 2001; Green & Rodgers, 2001; Institute of Medicine, 2002). Even among suicide bombers, Pedahzur and Perlinger (2006) have found that cohesive networks surround the design of suicide attacks, but, ironically, the bombers themselves often stand in peripheral locations within the network.

A Note on Generalizability

While religion has served as the focal research question here, many other social factors can be similarly considered. The effect of marriage and divorce has always had strong associations with suicide rates at the individual and national levels. But more importantly, the links are complex and suggest similar contextual import. For example, while marriage has been documented to have protective effects, the effect is reversed for young men who "marry too young" (i.e., overregulated in Durkheim's sense) and for women, historically, who lived in societies prohibiting divorce.

Similar theoretical logics can be fleshed out for the social power of education, the economy, and political crises, all which have documented effects on suicide (e.g., see Pridemore et al., 2007).

Conclusion

The job of linking the social brain to the social world, even for the one outcome identified here, suicide, remains. Standing back, two issues are clear. First, research has provided risk and protective factors that are promising targets for understanding self-harm and for configuring new suicide reduction efforts. Second, these factors work in concert to predispose or protect individuals' well-being (Institute of Medicine, 2002).

Theorizing about multiple levels of influence that are at work may produce new research, prevention, and interactive directions. For example, policy and intervention efforts would be quite different if research findings suggest that the overall domestic profile of a community is of greater importance in reducing suicide than an individual's marital and/ or family status. That is, initiatives that target the creation and maintenance of support institutions available to all community members, regardless of family structure, would look quite different than those directed only toward members of families, for example, that have experienced divorce.

Some of the greatest challenges that face contemporary society lie in the puzzle presented by chronic disease and mental health issues and, in particular, their comorbidity. Further, the complications that comorbidities present to individuals with other brain disorders (e.g., traumatic brain injury, Alzheimer's disease, Parkinson's disease) call for paving new roads in research, intervention, and prevention. Adopting N&CS science offers one direction. To define the "core subsystems" is a first step; to lay out illustrative concepts is only a modest beginning; to measure them in a comprehensive research design remains a grand challenge (Ostrom, 2009, p. 420).

Notes

1. Wilson, however, had no vision of transdisciplinarity; rather, he saw the absorption of all that might be useful into the natural sciences (see Pescosolido, 2006, on this issue).
2. Religions can go too far. The 1978 mass suicide at Jonestown provides evidence of an overregulated social structure. Ties outside of the People's Temple were strongly discouraged and bonds of marital or family intimacy, which could provide an opposing source of integration or regulation, were disrupted. Tape-recorded testimonials on discrimination at the hands of "the man" (i.e., primarily the American government) and the purity of a "socialist dream" gave a sense of purpose and belonging to individuals they had not felt, wherever they were from. Thus, what united them was a sense of connectedness. However, as the People's

Temple came under greater scrutiny, frequent suicide drills and other extreme behaviors turned Jonestown into a "greedy group" (Coser & Coser, 1979), demanding total commitment and sliding the religious community to the fatalistic pole and over 900 deaths (see Pescosolido, 1994, for examples and detail).

References

Abbott, A. (2001). *Chaos of disciplines.* Chicago: University of Chicago Press.

Abramson, L. Y., Alloy, L. B., Hogan, M. E., Whitehouse, W. G., Gibb, B. E., & Hanklin, B. L. (2000). The hopelessness theory of suicidality. In T. E. Joiner & M. D. Rudd (Eds.), *Suicide science: Expanding the boundaries* (pp. 17–32). Boston, MA: Kluwer Academic.

Aldrich, H. (2007). *Organizations and environments* (Reprint ed.). Stanford, CA: Stanford Business Books.

Al-Shahrour, F., Minguez, P., Tarraga, J., Montaner, D., Alloza, E., Vaquerizas, J. M., et al. (2006). BABELOMICS: A systems biology perspective in the functional annotation of genome-scale experiments. *Nucleic Acids Research, 34*(Suppl. 2), W472–W476.

Anglin, D. M., Gabriel, K. O. S., & Kaslow, N. J. (2005). Suicide acceptability and religious well-being: A comparative analysis in African American suicide attempters and non-attempters. *Journal of Psychology and Theology, 33*(2), 140–150.

Antoni, M. H., Lehman, J. M., Klibourn, K. M., Boyers, A. E., Culver, J. L., Alferi, S. M., et al. (2001). Cognitive-behavioral stress management intervention decreases the prevalence of depression and enhances benefit finding among women under treatment for early-stage breast cancer. *Health Psychology, 20,* 20–32.

Appleby, L., Shaw, J., & Amos, T. (1999). Suicide within 12 months of contact with mental health services: National clinical survey. *British Medical Journal, 318,* 235–239.

Arango, V., & Mann, J. J. (1992). Relevance of serotonergic postmortem studies to suicidal behavior. *International Review of Psychiatry, 4,* 131.

Baller, R. D., & Richardson, K. K. (2009). The "dark side" of the strength of weak ties: The diffusion of suicidal thoughts. *Journal of Health and Social Behavior, 50,* 261–276.

Bandura, A. (1982). Self-efficacy mechanism in human agency. *American Psychologist, 37,* 122–147.

———. (1992). Self-efficacy mechanism in psychobiologic functioning. In R. Schwarzer (Ed.), *Self-efficacy: Thought control of action* (pp. 355–394). Washington, DC: Hemisphere Publishing.

Bankston, W. B., Allen, H. D., & Cunningham, D. S. (1983). Religion and suicide: A research note on sociology's "One Law." *Social Forces, 62,* 521–529.

Barabasi, A.-L. (2009). Scale-free networks: A decade and beyond. *Science, 325*(412), 412–413.

Barr, R. G., & Kolb, B. (2007). *Proposal for renewal: 'Biological embedding': Moving from metaphor to mechanisms.* Director's Rep. Experience-based Brain Biol. Development Program (EBBD), Canadian Institute of Advanced Research (CIFAR).

Batson, C. D., Schoenrade, P., & Ventis, W. L. (1993). *Religion and the individual: A social-psychological perspective.* New York: Oxford University Press.

Bearman, P. (1991). The social structure of suicide. *Sociological Forum, 6,* 501–524.

Beck, A. T., Weisman, A., Lester, D., & Trexler, L. (1974). The measurement of pessimism: The hopelessness scale. *Journal of Consulting & Clinical Psychology, 42,* 861–865.

Beckfield, J. (2010). The social structure of the world polity. *American Journal of Sociology, 115,* 1018–1068.

Berkman, L. A. (1985). The relationship of social networks and social support to morbidity and mortality. In S. Cohen & S. L. Syme (Eds.), *Social support and health* (pp. 241–262). New York, NY: Academic Press.

Bierman, A. (2006). Does religion buffer the effects of discrimination on mental health? Differing effects by race. *Journal for the Scientific Study of Religion, 45,* 551–565.

Bille-Brahe, U. (1987). The reliability of Scandinavian suicide statistics: Introduction. *Acta Psychiatrica Scandinavica, 76*(Suppl. 336), 9–10.

Bird, A. (2007). Perceptions of epigenetics. *Nature, 447,* 396–398.

Blackmore, E. R., Weller, M. S., Zagorski, B., Stansfeld, S. A., Stewart, D. E., Caine, E. D., & Conwell, Y. (2008). Psychosocial and clinical correlates of suicidal acts: Results from a national population survey. *British Journal of Psychiatry, 192,* 279–284.

Braam, A. W., Beekman, A. T., Deeg, D. J., Smit, J. H., & van Tilburg, W. (1997a). Religiosity as a protective or prognostic factor of depression in later life: Results from a community survey in The Netherlands. *Acta Psychiatrica Scandinavica, 96,* 199–205.

Braam, A. W., Beekman, A. T., van Tilburg, T. G., Deeg, D. J., & Van Tilburg, W. (1997b). Religious involvement and depression in older Dutch citizens. *Social Psychiatry and Psychiatric Epidemiology, 32,* 284–291.

Brashears, M. E. (2010). Anomia and the sacred canopy: Testing a network theory. *Social Networks, 32,* 187–198.

Brunner, J., Stalla, G. K., Stalla, J., Uhr, M., & Grabner, A. (2001). Decreased corticotropin-releasing hormone (CRH) concentrations in the cerebrospinal fluid of eucortisolemic suicide attempters. *Journal of Psychiatric Research, 35,* 1–9.

Carpentier, N., & White, D. (2002). Cohesion of the primary social network and sustained service use before the first psychiatric hospitalization. *Journal of Behavioral Health Services and Research, 29,* 404–418.

Catanzaro, S. J. (2000). Mood regulation and suicidal behavior. In T. E. Joiner & M. D. Rudd (Eds.), *Suicide science: Expanding the boundaries* (pp. 81–103). Norwell, MA: Kluwer Academic.

Centers for Disease Control and Prevention. (2008). Strategic direction for the prevention of suicidal behavior: Promoting individual, family, and community connectedness to prevent suicidal behavior. Atlanta, GA: Centers for Disease Control and Prevention.

Christakis, N. A., & Fowler, J. H. (2007). The spread of obesity in a large social network over 32 years. *New England Journal of Medicine, 357,* 370–379.

Cicchetti, D., & Toth, S. L. (1998). The development of depression in children and adolescents. *American Psychologist, 53,* 221–241.

Cleaver, F. (2002). Reinventing institutions: Bricolage and the social embeddedness of natural resource management. *European Journal of Development Research, 14,* 11–30.

Cohen, S., & Syme, S. L. (1985). *Social support and health.* New York: Academic Press.

Colasanto, D., & Shriver, J. (1989). Mirror of America: Middle-aged face marital crisis. *Gallup Report, 284,* 34–38.

Collins, R. (1982). *Sociological insight.* New York: Oxford University Press.

Colucci, E., & Martin, G. (2008). Religion and spirituality along the suicidal path. *Suicide and Life-Threatening Behavior, 38,* 229–244.

Conwell, Y., Pearson, J., & DeRenzo, E. G. (1996). Indirect self-destructive behavior among elderly patients in nursing homes: A research agenda. *American Journal of Geriatric Psychiatry, 4,* 152–163.

Conwell, Y., Duberstein, P. R., & Caine, E. D. (2002). Risk factors for suicide in later life. *Biological Psychiatry, 52,* 193–204.

Coser, R. L., & Coser, L. A. (1979). Jonestown as perverse utopia. *Dissent, 26,* 158–263.

Cruess, D. G., Antoni, M. H., McGregor, B. A., Kilbourn, K. M., Boyers, A. E., Alferi, S. M., Carver, C. S., & Kumar, M. (2000). Cognitive-behavioral stress management reduces serum cortisol by enhancing benefit finding among women being treated for early stage breast cancer. *Psychosomatic Medicine, 62,* 304–308.

D'Amato, F. R., Cabib, S., Puglisi-Allegra, S., Patacchioli, F. R., Cigliana, G., Maccari, S., & Angelucci, L. (1992). Effects of acute and repeated exposure to stress on the hypothalamo-pituitary-adrenocortical activity in mice during postnatal development. *Hormone Behavior, 26,* 474–485.

Danese, A., Caspi, A., Williams, B., Ambler, A., Sugden, K., Mika, J., et al. (2011). Biological embedding of stress through inflammation processes in childhood. *Molecular Psychiatry, 16,* 244–246.

de Jong, T. R., Korosi, A., Harris, B. N., Perea-Rodriguez, J. P., & Saltzman, W. (2012). Individual variation in paternal responses of virgin male California mice (*Peromyscus californicus*): Behavioral and physiological correlates. *Physiological and Biochemical Zoology, 85*(6), 740–751.

Dervic, K., Carballo, J. J., Baca-Garcia, E., Galfalvy, H. C., Mann, J. J., Brent, D. A., & Oquendo, M. A. (2011). Moral or religious objections to suicide may protect against suicidal behavior in bipolar disorder. *Journal of Clinical Psychiatry, 72,* 1390–1396.

Dieserud, G., Roysamb, E., Ekeberg, O., & Kraft, P. (2001). Toward an integrative model of suicide attempt: A cognitive psychological approach. *Suicide and Life-Threatening Behavior, 31,* 153–168.

Douglas, J. (1966). On suicide: The sociological analysis of social meanings of suicide. *European Journal of Sociology*, 7, 249–275.

Duberstein, P. R., Conwell, Y., & Caine, E. D. (1993). Interpersonal stressors, substance abuse, and suicide. *Journal of Nervous & Mental Disease*, 181, 80–85.

Duberstein, P. R., Conwell, K. R., Conner, S., Eberly, S., Evinger, J. S., & Caine, E. D. (2004). Poor social integration and suicide: Fact or artifact? A case control study. *Psychological Medicine*, 34, 1331–1337.

Durkheim, É. ([1897] 1951). *Suicide*. New York: Free Press.

Eskin, M. (2004). The effects of religious versus secular education on suicide ideation and suicidal attitudes in adolescents in Turkey. *Social Psychiatry and Psychiatric Epidemiology*, 39, 536–542.

Eysenbach, G., Powell, J., Englesakis, M., Rizo, C., & Stern, A. (2004). Health related virtual communities and electronic support groups: Systematic review of the effects of online peer to peer interactions. *British Medical Journal*, 328, 1–6.

Freeman, L. C. (2004). *The development of social network analysis: A study in the sociology of science*. Vancouver, BC: Empirical Press.

Gearing, R. E., & Lizardi, D. (2009). Religion and suicide. *Journal of Religion and Health*, 48, 332–341.

Goldsmith, S., Pellmar, T. C., Kleinman, A., & Bunney Jr., W. E. (2002). *Reducing suicide: A national imperative*. Washington, DC: National Academies Press.

Gonda, X., Fountoulakis, K., Kaprinis, G., & Rihmer, Z. (2008). Prediction and prevention of suicide in patients with unipolar depression and anxiety. *Annals of General Psychiatry*, 7(Suppl. 1), S323.

Gorsuch, R. L. (1995). Religious aspects of substance abuse and recovery. *Journal of Social Issues*, 51, 65–83.

Gottesman, I. I., & Gould, T. D. (2005). The endophenotype concept in psychiatry. In N. Andreasen (Ed.), *Research advances in genetics and genomics: Implications for psychiatry* (pp. 63–84). Washington, DC: American Psychiatric Publishers.

Granovetter, M. (1974). *Getting a job: A study of contacts and careers*. Cambridge, MA: Harvard University Press.

———. (1983). The strength of weak ties: A network theory revisited. *Sociological Theory*, 1, 201–233.

———. (1985). Economic action and social structure: The problem of embeddedness. *American Journal of Sociology*, 91, 481–510.

Green, B. L., & Rodgers, A. (2001). Determinants of social support among low-income mothers: A longitudinal analysis. *American Journal of Community Psychology*, 29, 419–441.

Greening, L., & Stoppelbein, L. (2002). Religiosity, attributional style, and social support as psychosocial buffers for African American and white adolescents' perceived risk for suicide. *Suicide and Life-Threatening Behavior*, 32, 404–417.

Grinde, B. (1998). The biology of religion: A Darwinian gospel. *Journal of Social and Evolutionary Systems*, 21, 19–28.

Gustafson, J. F. (1961). *Treasure in earthen vessels*. New York: Harper & Brothers.

Hertzman, C. (2000). The biological embedding of early experience and its effects on health in adulthood. *Annals of the New York Academy of Sciences, 896*, 85–95.

Hertzman, C., & Boyce, T. (2010). How experience gets under the skin to create gradients in developmental health. *Annual Review of Public Health, 31,* 329–347.

Higgins, E. S., & George, M. S. (2007). *The neuroscience of clinical psychiatry: The pathophysiology of behavior and mental illness.* New York: Lippincott, Williams, & Wilkins.

Idler, E., Ellison, C. G., George, L. K., Krause, N., Ory, M., Pargament, L., Powell, L., Williams, D., & Underwood, L. (2003). Measuring multiple dimensions of religion and spirituality for health research: Conceptual background and findings from the 1998 General Social Survey. *Research on Aging, 25,* 327–365.

Institute of Medicine. (2002). *Reducing suicide: A national imperative.* Washington, DC: National Academies Press.

———. (2006). *Genes, behavior, and the social environment.* Washington, DC: National Academies Press.

International Human Genome Sequencing Consortium. (2001). Initial sequencing and analysis of the human genome. *Nature, 409,* 860–921.

———. (2004). Finishing the euchromatic sequence of the human genome. *Nature, 431,* 931–945.

Inzlicht, M., Tullett, A. M., & Good, M. (2011). The need to believe: A neuroscience account of religion as a motivated process. *Religion, Brain, and Behavior, 1,* 192–251.

Jamison, K. R. (1999). *Night falls fast: Understanding suicide* New York: Knopf.

Johnson, B. (1965). Durkheim's one cause of suicide. *American Sociological Review, 30,* 875–886.

Joiner, T. E., Steer, R. A., Abramson, L. Y., Alloy, L. B., Metalsky, G. I., & Schmidt, N. B. (2001). Hopelessness depression as a distinct dimension of depressive symptoms among clinical and non-clinical samples. *Behaviour Research and Therapy, 39,* 523–536.

Kawachi, I. (2001). Social ties and mental health. *Journal of Urban Health, 78,* 458–467.

Kelley, D. M. (1972). *Why conservative churches are growing: A study in the sociology of religion.* New York: Harper & Row.

Kendler, K. S., Gardner, C. O., & Prescott, C. A. (1997). Religion, psychopathology, and substance use and abuse: A multimeasure, genetic-epidemiologic study. *American Journal of Psychiatry, 154,* 322–329.

Kennedy, G. J., Kelman, H. R., Thomas, C., & Chen, J. (1996). The relation of religious preference and practice to depressive symptoms among 1,855 older adults. *Journals of Gerontology: Series B, 51,* P301–P308.

Koenig, H. G., Cohen, H. J., Blazer, D. G., Pieper, C., Meador, K. G., Shelp, F., Goli, V., & DiPasquale, B. (1992). Religious coping and depression among elderly, hospitalized medically ill men. *American Journal of Psychiatry, 149,* 1693–1700.

Koenig, H. G., Cohen, H. J., George, L. K., Hays, J. C., Larson, D. B., & Blazer, D. G. (1997). Attendance at religious services, interleukin-6, and other biological parameters of immune function in older adults. *International Journal of Psychiatry in Medicine, 27,* 233–250.

Kowalski, G., Faupel, C., & Starr, P. (1987). Urbanism and suicide. *Social Forces, 66,* 85–101.

Kreeger, P. K., & Lauffenburger, D. A. (2010). Cancer systems biology: A network modeling perspective. *Carcinogenesis, 31,* 2–8.

Kushner, H. I., & Sterk, C. E. (2005). The limits of social capital: Durkheim, suicide, and social cohesion. *American Journal of Public Health, 95,* 1139–1143.

Lee, C. (2009). When science and humanities collide. In *McGill Reporter.* Montreal, Quebec, Canada: McGill University. http://publications.mcgill.ca/reporter /2009/04/moshe-szyf-james-mcgill-professor-of-pharmacology-and-therapeutics/.

Lindsey, M. A., Barksdale, C. L., Lambert, S. F., & Ialongo, N. S. (2010). Social network influences on service use among urban, African American youth with mental health problems. *Journal of Adolescent Health, 47,* 367–373.

Liu, K.-Y., King, M., & Bearman, P. S. (2010). Social influence and the autism epidemic. *American Journal of Sociology, 115,* 1387–1434.

Maimon, D., & Kuhl, D. C. (2008). Social control and youth suicidality: Situating Durkheim's ideas in a multilevel framework. *American Sociological Review, 73,* 921–943.

Maltsberger, J. T., & Goldblatt, M. J. (Eds.). (1996). *Essential papers on suicide.* New York: New York University Press.

Meaney, M. J. (2001). Maternal care, gene expression, and the transmission of individual differences in stress reactivity across generations. *Annual Review of Neuroscience, 24,* 1161–1192.

Meaney, M. J., & Szyf, M. (2005). Environmental programming of stress responses through DNA methylation: Life at the interface between a dynamic environment and a fixed genome. *Dialogues in Clinical Neuroscience, 7,* 103–123.

Mitchell, M. (2009). *Complexity: A guided tour.* New York: Oxford University Press.

Modai, I., Kurs, R., Ritsner, M., Oklander, S., Silver, H., Segal, A., Goldberg, I., & Mendel, S. (2002). Neural network identification of high-risk suicide patients. *Informatics for Health and Social Care, 27,* 39–47.

Murphy, G. E. (1992). *Suicide in alcoholism.* New York: Oxford University Press.

Murphy, G. E., Armstrong, J. W., Jr., Hermele, S. L., Fischer, J. R., & Clendenin. W. W. (1979). Suicide and alcoholism: Interpersonal loss confirmed as a predictor. *Archives of General Psychiatry, 36,* 65–69.

Neeleman, J. (1998). Regional suicide rates in the Netherlands: Does religion still play a role? *International Journal of Epidemiology, 27,* 466–472.

Nooney, J. G. (2005). Religion, stress, and mental health in adolescence: Findings from Add Health. *Review of Religious Research, 46,* 341–354.

Nor, Z. Z. (2000). A study of social network of suicide attempters in University Malaya Medical Centre, Kuala Lumpur. *Malaysian Journal of Psychiatry, 8,* 3–10.

Ostrom, E. (2009). A general framework for analyzing sustainability of social-ecological systems. *Science, 325,* 419–422.

Pedahzur, A., & Perlinger, A. (2006). The changing nature of suicide attacks: A social network perspective. *Social Forces, 84*, 1987–2008.

Pescosolido, B. A. (1990). The social context of religious integration and suicide: Pursuing the network explanation. *The Sociological Quarterly, 31*, 337–357.

———. (1991). Illness careers and network ties: A conceptual model of utilization and compliance. In G. L. Albrecht & J. A. Levy (Eds.), *Advances in medical sociology* (pp. 161–84). Greenwich, CT: JAI Press.

———. (1992). Beyond rational choice: The social dynamics of how people seek help. *American Journal of Sociology, 97*, 1096–1138.

———. (1994). Bringing Durkheim into the 21st century: A social network approach to unresolved issues in the study of suicide. In D. Lester (Ed.), *Emile Durkheim: Le Suicide—100 years later* (pp. 264–295). Philadelphia: The Charles Press.

———. (2006). Of pride and prejudice: The role of sociology and social networks in integrating the health sciences. *Journal of Health and Social Behavior, 47*, 189–208.

———. (2011). Organizing the sociological landscape for the next decades of health and health care research: The Network Episode Model III-R as cartographic subfield guide. In B. A. Pescosolido, J. K. Martin, J. D. McLeod, & A. Rogers (Eds.), *The handbook of the sociology of health, illness, and healing: Blueprint for the 21st century* (pp. 39–66). New York: Springer.

———. (2013). The public stigma of mental illness: What do we think; what do we know; what can we prove? *Journal of Health and Social Behavior, 54*, 1–21.

Pescosolido, B. A., & Mendelsohn, R. (1986). Social causation or social construction? An investigation into the social organization of suicide rates. *American Sociological Review, 51*, 80–101.

Pescosolido, B. A., & Georgianna, S. (1989). Durkheim, religion, and suicide: Toward a network theory of suicide. *American Sociological Review, 54*, 33–48.

Pescosolido, B. A., Brooks-Gardner, C., & Lubell, K. M. (1998a). How people get into mental health services: Stories of choice, coercion and 'muddling through' from 'first-timers'. *Social Science and Medicine, 46*, 275–286.

Pescosolido, B. A., Wright, E. R., Alegria, M., & Vera, M. (1998b). Social networks and patterns of use among the poor with mental health problems in Puerto Rico. *Medical Care, 36*, 1057–1072.

Pescosolido, B. A., & Boyer, C. A. (1999). How do people come to use mental health services? Current knowledge and changing perspectives. In A. V. Horwitz & T. L. Scheid (Eds.), *A handbook for the study of mental health: Social contexts, theories, and systems* (pp. 392–411). New York: Cambridge University Press.

Pescosolido, B. A., & Levy, J. A. (2002). The role of social networks in health, illness, disease and healing: The accepting present, the forgotten past, and the dangerous potential for a complacent future. *Social Networks & Health, 8*, 3–25.

Pescosolido, B. A., Martin, J. K., Long, J. S., Medina, T. R., Phelan, J. C., & Link, B. G. (2010). 'A disease like any other? A decade of change in public reactions to schizophrenia, depression and alcohol dependence. *American Journal of Psychiatry,* 167, 1321–1330.

Pescosolido, B. A., Olafsdottir, S., Sporns, O., Perry, B. L., Meslin, E., Grubesic, T. H., Martin, J. K., Koehly, L. M., Pridemore, W., Vespignani, A., Foroud, T., & Shekhar, A. (in press). The social symbiome framework: Linking *genes-to-global* cultures in public health using network science. In Z. Neal, (Ed.), *Handbook of Applied Systems Science.* New York: Routledge.

Pressman, P., Lyons, J. S., Larson, D. B., & Strain, J. J. (1990). Religious belief, depression, and ambulation status in elderly women with broken hips. *American Journal of Psychiatry,* 147, 758–760.

Pridemore, W. A., Chamlin, M. B., & Cochran, J. K. (2007). An interrupted time series analysis of Durkheim's social deregulation thesis: The case of the Russian Federation. *Justice Quarterly,* 24, 271–290.

Pritchard, C., & Baldwin, D. (2000). Effects of age and gender on elderly suicide rates in Catholic and Orthodox countries: An inadvertent neglect? *International Journal of Geriatric Psychiatry,* 15, 904–910.

Quinley, H. E. (1974). *The prophetic clergy.* New York: John Wiley.

Reczek, C., & Umberson, D. A. (2012). Gender, health behavior, and intimate relationships: Lesbian, gay, and straight contexts. *Social Science & Medicine,* 74, 1783–1790.

Robinson, G. E. (2004). Beyond nature and nurture. *Science,* 304, 397–399.

Rogers, A., Hassell, K., & Nicolaas, G. (1999). *Demanding patients? Analysing the use of primary care.* Philadelphia: Open University Press.

Roof, W. C., & McKinney, W. (1987). *American mainline religion.* London: Rutgers University Press.

Roy, A., Segal, N. L., Centerwall, B., & Robinette, D. (1991). Suicide in twins. *Archives of General Psychiatry,* 48, 29–32.

Seeman, T. E., Dubin, L. F., & Seeman, M. (2003). Religiosity/spirituality and health: A critical review of the evidence for biological pathways. *American Psychologist,* 58, 53–63.

Segre, S. (2004). A Durkheimian network theory. *Journal of Classical Sociology,* 4, 215–235.

Seybold, K. S., & Hill, P. C. (2001). The role of religion and spirituality in mental and physical health. *Current Directions in Psychological Science,* 10, 21–24.

Shonkoff, J. P., & Phillips, D. A. (2000). *From neurons to neighborhoods: The science of early childhood development. Institute of Medicine committee report.* Washington, DC: National Academies Press.

Sporns, O. (2011). *Networks of the brain.* Cambridge, MA: MIT Press.

Stack, S. (1991). The effect of religiosity on suicide in Sweden: A time series analysis. *Journal for the Scientific Study of Religion,* 30, 462–468.

Stack, S., & Wasserman, I. (1992). The effect of religion on suicide ideology: An analysis of the networks perspective. *Journal for the Scientific Study of Religion,* 31, 457–466.

Stack, S., & Kposowa, A. J. (2011). Religion and suicide acceptability: A cross-national analysis. *Journal for the Scientific Study of Religion,* 50, 289–306.

Stark, R., & Glock, C. Y. (1973). Are we entering a post-Christian era. In C. Y. Glock (Ed.), *Religion in sociological perspective* (pp. 284–296). Belmont, CA: Wadsworth.

Statham, D. J., Heath, A. C., & Madden, P. A. (1998). Suicidal behaviour: An epidemiological and genetic study. *Psychological Medicine, 28,* 839–855.

Stockard, J., & O'Brien, R. M. (2002). Cohort variations and changes in age-specific suicide rates over time: Explaining variations in youth suicide. *Social Forces, 81,* 605–642.

Swan, M. (2009). Emerging patient-driven health care models: An examination of health social networks, consumer personalized medicine and quantified self-tracking. *International Journal of Environmental Research and Public Health, 6,* 492–525.

Swanwick, G. R., & Clare, A. W. (1997). Suicide in Ireland 1945–1992: Social correlates. *Irish Medical Journal, 90,* 106–108.

Tai, Y.-M., & Chiu, H.-W. (2007). Artificial neural network analysis on suicide and self-harm history of Taiwanese soldiers. In *Second International Conference on Innovative Computing, Information and Control* (p. 363). Kumamoto, Japan: IEEE.

Tilly, C. (1984). *Big structures, large processes, huge comparisons.* New York: Russell Sage.

Timmermans, S. (2005). Suicide determination and the professional authority of medical examiners. *American Sociological Review, 70,* 311–333.

Trout, D. L. (1980). The role of social isolation in suicide. *Suicide and Life-Threatening Behavior, 10,* 10–23.

Umberson, D. A. (1987). Family status and health behavior: Social control as a dimension of social integration. *Journal of Health and Social Behavior, 28,* 306–319.

Umberson, D. A., & Greer, M. (August 1990). *Social relationships and health behavior: The wellness regulation model.* Paper presented at the Annual Meeting of the American Sociological Association, Washington, DC.

U.S. Public Health Service. (1999). *The Surgeon General's call to action to prevent suicide.* Washington, DC: U.S. Public Health Service.

Valente, T. W. (2010). *Social networks and health: Models, methods, and applications.* Oxford, UK: Oxford University Press.

van Os, J., Rutten, B. P. F., & Poulton, R. (2008). Gene-environment interactions in schizophrenia: Review of epidemiological findings and future directions. *Schizophrenia Bulletin, 34*(6), 1066–1082.

van Os, J., Kenis, G., & Rutten, B. P. F. (2010). The environment and schizophrenia. *Nature, 468,* 203–212.

Van Tubergen, F., Grotenhuis, M., & Ultee, W. (2005). Denomination, religious context, and suicide: Neo-Durkheimian multilevel explanations tested with individual and contextual data. *American Journal of Sociology, 111,* 797–823.

Venter, J. C., Adams, M. D., Myers, E. W., Li, P. W., Mural, R. J., Sutton, G. G., et al. (2001). The sequence of the human genome. *Science, 291*(5507), 1304–1351.

Vespignani, A. (2009). Predicting the behavior of techno-social systems. *Science, 325*(5939), 425–428.

Weishaar, M. E., & Beck, A. T. (1990). Cognitive approaches to understanding and treating suicidal behavior. In S. Blumenthal & D. Kupfer (Eds.), *Suicide over the life cycle: Risk factors, assessment, and treatment of suicidal patients* (pp. 469–498). Washington, DC: American Psychiatric Press.

Weiss, J. N., Yang, L., & Qu, Z. (2006). Systems biology approaches to metabolic and cardiovascular disorders: Network perspectives of cardiovascular metabolism. *Journal of Lipid Research, 47,* 2355–2366.

Wellman, B., & Wortley, S. (1990). Different strokes from different folks: Community ties and social support. *American Journal of Sociology, 96,* 558–588.

Wellman, B., Salaff, J., Dimitrova, D., Garton, L., Gulia, M., & Haythornthwaite, C. (1996). Computer networks as social networks: Collaborative work, telework, and virtual community. *Annual Review of Sociology, 22,* 213–238.

Wender, P., Kety, S., & Rosenthal, D. (1986). Psychiatric disorders in the biological and adoptive families of adopted individuals with affective disorders. *Archives of General Psychiatry, 43,* 923–929.

Werner, E. E. (1992). The children of Kauai: Resiliency and recovery in adolescence and adulthood. *Journal of Adolescent Health, 13,* 262–268.

———. (1996). Vulnerable but invincible: High risk children from birth to adulthood. *European Child & Adolescent Psychiatry, 5*(Suppl. 1), 47–51.

West, E., Barron, D. N., Dowsett, J., & Newton, J. N. (1999). Hierarchies and cliques in the social networks of health care professionals: Implications for the design of dissemination strategies. *Social Science & Medicine, 48,* 633–646.

Williams, D. R., & Sternthal, M. (2007). Spirituality, religion and health: Evidence and research directions. *Medical Journal of Australia, 186,* 47–50.

Wilson, E. O. (1998). *Consilience: The unity of knowledge.* New York: Knopf.

Wray, M., Colen, C., & Pescosolido, B. A. (2011). The sociology of suicide. *Annual Review of Sociology, 37,* 505–528.

Zerhouni, E. (2003). The NIH Roadmap. *Science, 302*(5642), 63–72.

12.

Functional and Structural Correlates of Early Severe Social Deprivation

Michael E. Behen and Harry T. Chugani

S TUDIES IN CHILDREN raised from birth in orphanages have demonstrated that institutional rearing is associated with neurocognitive dysfunction and socioemotional difficulties. While it is assumed that such findings are reflective of abnormal neurologic development resulting from early social deprivation (e.g., Schore, 1994), only recently has there been much direct investigation of the impact of early, severe, social deprivation on brain anatomy and function. Animal studies, including those in nonhuman primates, strongly indicate that early postnatal neglect and deprivation may be associated with both short-term and long-term changes in brain function (reviewed in Suomi, 1997; Hofer, 1996; Kaufman et al., 2000); only recently has there been much empirical investigation of the effects of early social deprivation on neural function and structure in humans.

In this chapter, we summarize our work (and that of others) addressing the functional outcomes (i.e., global and specific neurocognitive and behavioral outcomes) and functional and structural neural correlates of early severe social deprivation. First, we outline the demographic and orphanage-specific characteristics of our study sample of children, all of whom have been raised from birth in international orphanages. We then present findings on global and specific neurocognitive and behavioral outcomes in children with histories of orphanage rearing and consider these alongside findings on other samples of children with similar histories. Summaries of the functional and structural neural correlates follow, including findings from functional (positron emission tomography with 2-deoxy-2(18F)fluoro-D-glucose [FDG-PET], functional magnetic resonance imaging [fMRI], electroencephalography [EEG]/event-related potential [ERP]) and structural (volumetric MRI, diffusion tensor imaging) brain imaging studies that have been conducted on children with histories of early deprivation. We then consider predictors of functional and structural outcomes, and conclude with a discussion of the mechanisms for such brain plasticity, including (1) the lack of exposure to adequate domain-specific and experience-expectant stimuli during sensitive period(s) of development and (2) the deleterious effects of chronic unmitigated stress on the developing nervous system.

Sample Characteristics

One hundred fifty-six children, all raised from birth in Eastern Europe (including Romania, Bulgaria, Poland, Armenia, Ukraine, and Slovakia), Northern Asia (Russia, Kazakhstan, and Georgia), South Asia (China and Vietnam), or Central/South America (Guatemala and Mexico) and later adopted in the United States, were included in the study. The study involved several components over two visits: (1) a neurologic screening, (2) neuropsychological evaluation, and (3) FDG-PET or functional and structural MRI studies. On the first visit, all the children enrolled in the study underwent neurologic exam and neuropsychological evaluation to ensure that they met all the criteria for further participation in the study. Scans took place on a separate visit.

All children were recruited through advertisements presented to local and national parent-support groups as well as newsletters for various international adoption groups. All were separated from their biological mothers at birth and placed into orphanages immediately upon release from the hospital nursery. The demographic and orphanage-specific characteristics of the group are presented in Table 12.1. All children in the study were monolingual English speaking and attended school regularly following adoption.

In order to minimize the occurrence of major confounding factors with known neurobiological effects, children with current and/or historical indication of any of the following were excluded from the study: prematurity, pre- or perinatal difficulties, current or historical medical problems, epilepsy, documented suspicion of or known prenatal exposure to alcohol and/or other substances, and/or focal findings on neurologic examination. Alcohol exposure was directly assessed by a neurologist as part of the

TABLE 12.1. Demographic Characteristics of the Sample ($N = 155$)

	Mean	Standard Deviation
Age at testing (in months)	115.6	28.4
Gender	63 males/91 females	
Duration of time in the orphanage	29.4	19.9
Duration of time in the adoptive home	89.5	33.6
Body mass index	17.4	2.8
Head circumference t-score	33.5	19.4
Adopted mother's years of education	16.5	2.1
Adopted father's years of education	16.8	2.5
Region of adoption	55% Eastern Europe	
	22% Northern Asia	
	22% Eastern Asia	

neurological examination using the Miller et al. (2006) criteria. Children with a "high" phenotypic suggestion of alcohol exposure (greater than 12) were not included in the study.

Functional Correlates of Early Deprivation

Global Cognition

It has long been reported that children raised in institutions evidence global developmental delay and/or cognitive impairment (Spitz, 1945). More recently, a number of studies have found that 70 to 90 percent of such children have impaired global cognition and/or multifaceted developmental delays at the time of adoption (Judge, 2003; Rutter, 1998). Longitudinal studies of these children, however, have reported an impressive degree of "catch-up" in global cognitive functioning (Judge, 2003; Rutter et al., 2001), in a majority of children. For instance, in the Rutter et al. (2001) European and Romanian Adoptees (ERA) study sample, only 14 percent of Romanian adoptees continued to evidence global cognitive impairment at assessment several years after adoption. Subsequent studies of the ERA sample have indicated a substantial degree of continuity, though, through at least early adolescence, in terms of global cognitive outcomes (Beckett et al., 2006). Our work as well reveals significant effects of early deprivation on neurocognitive outcomes that persist over time (Behen et al., 2008).

On a much larger sample than that presented in Behen et al. (2008), we revisited the effect of early deprivation on global and specific cognitive outcomes. Table 12.2 presents the neurocognitive characteristics for the full sample. As can be seen, mean full-scale IQ (FSIQ) or global IQ for the full sample (FSIQ = 93) was measured in the average range approximately one-half of a standard deviation (SD) below the normative mean (see Figure 12.1). With regard to the incidence of global cognitive *impairment,* 8 percent (*n* = 13) of the sample had measured FSIQ in the impaired range (FSIQ < 70). Twenty-two percent of the sample (*n* = 35) had FSIQ < 78 (more than 1.5 SDs below the mean), and one-third of the sample (33 percent, *n* = 51) of the sample had measured FSIQ < 85 (1 SD below the mean).

These results suggest that, as a group, children with histories of early deprivation show reduced global intellect compared to their nonadopted typically developing peers. Further, the data are generally consistent with those from samples presented in other studies of internationally adopted children (Nelson et al., 2007; Beckett et al., 2006; Ames, 1997). Beckett et al. (2006) investigated global cognitive outcomes in a random sample of children adopted from Romanian orphanages followed as part of the ERA study and reported that the global cognitive scores for the age six to twenty-four months and more than twenty-four months adoption groups were measured in the borderline to low average ranges on assessments at age six and eleven years. Global cognition in the Ames (1997) report on 157 children adopted after eight months (mean duration = seventeen months) was

TABLE 12.2. Neurocognitive Characteristics for the Full Group (*N* = 156)

Domain	Mean	Standard Deviation
Full-scale IQ	93.15	19.35
Verbal Comprehension Index	95.79	17.76
Perceptual Organizational Index	95.65	18.89
Freedom from Distractibility Index	88.88	18.03
Processing Speed Index	97.86	20.08
Verbal Memory Index	87.39	18.51
Visual Memory Index	91.43	16.47
Reading	96.65	18.11
Spelling	95.64	16.84
Mathematics	92.38	20.12
Expressive Language Processing	99.76	19.49
Receptive Language Processing	88.58	23.64
Sustained Attention	81.68*	35.40
Behavioral Control	75.83*	41.64
Manual Dexterity—dominant hand	89.40	25.61
Manual Dexterity—nondominant hand	85.21	27.59

*Significant relative weaknesses (relative to FSIQ).

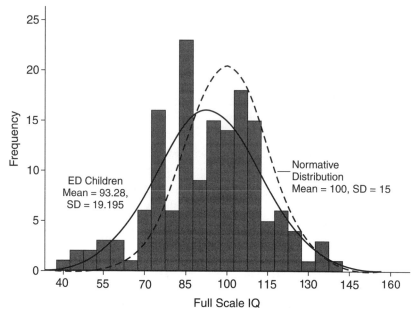

FIGURE 12.1. Distributions of global IQ in a full sample of children with histories of early deprivation (solid line) and normative distribution (dashed line). As can be seen, the distribution of scores for the children with histories of early deprivation is shifted to the left of the normative group.

measured at 90. Global cognition in the present sample was measured in the average range (FSIQ=93). Additionally, the incidence of global cognitive impairment (FSIQ<70) in Rutter, Kreppner, and O'Connor's (2001) large number, randomly selected sample using a cutoff of two standard deviations below the mean was 14 percent, compared to 8 percent in our sample. These studies provide strong empirical support for the notion that early deprivation is associated with reduced global cognitive functioning and increased incidence of impaired global cognition.

Also, our data have suggested that even where global intellect is measured well within normal limits, relative weaknesses are evident in specific neurocognitive areas, including sustained attention, impulse control, manual dexterity, and language processing (Behen et al., 2008). To date, there has been much less work addressing the effects of early deprivation on specific neurocognitive functions (i.e., receptive language, sustained attention, motor dexterity), particularly in children who are measured to be within normal limits on global cognitive measures. Therefore, we were interested in examining the incidence of *specific* neurocognitive impairment in a group of children who experienced early deprivation but who were globally intellectually intact (FSIQ ≥ 85) either by virtue of recovery/catch-up or resilience of basic intellectual functioning.

Specific Neurocognitive Impairment

Although the full sample was measured in the average range (standard score between 90 and 110) on most domains assessed, relative weaknesses (borderline range scores, i.e., standard score of 70–79) were found on measures of sustained attention and impulsivity/behavioral control (see Table 12.2). Additionally, for the globally intact group (FSIQ ≥ 85), most domains were measured in the average range with exceptions found for relatively weaker sustained attention and impulsivity, both measured in the low average range (standard score between 80 and 89). In fact, an inattentive-overactive phenotype has been evident in the literature on outcomes in samples with such histories. Rutter et al. (2010) have referred to an inattentive-overactive phenotype as a "deprivation-specific pattern" that is frequently identified in orphanage-reared children. Indeed, increased incidence of problems in executive behavior (e.g., inattentive/overactive behavioral difficulties) and language in children with histories of early deprivation have also been reported by others (Stevens et al., 2008; Croft et al., 2007). Additionally, there have been several recent studies showing specific deficits on laboratory measures of executive functions in children with histories of early deprivation (Loman et al., 2013 Bos et al., 2009). Thus, there is some evidence for specific neurocognitive impairment in children with histories of early deprivation. We were interested in determining the incidence of specific neurocognitive deficit, particularly in children who have been measured well within normal limits on measures of global cognition.

In order to assess the incidence of specific neurocognitive impairment in our sample, we derived summary scores for the following neurocognitive domains: receptive and expressive language processing, verbal and visual memory, sustained attention, impulsivity, and manual dexterity (for the dominant and nondominant hands). We then examined each individual's neurocognitive profile for areas of absolute impairment, defined as a domain standard score 2 or more SD below the mean of the normative sample (Standard score, SS ≤ 70). Incidence of impairment across these domains was calculated for both the full sample and the globally intact sample. We also assessed internalizing and externalizing behavior difficulties and autism-spectrum symptoms via caregiver report with the Behavioral Assessment System for Children, Second Edition (Reynolds, 2004) and Social Communication Questionnaire (Rutter et al., 2003), respectively.

For the full sample of 156 children assessed in the study, as noted above, 8 percent had impaired global intellect (FSIQ<70). Thirty-seven percent of the sample had no area of impairment. Nearly 40 percent of the sample evidenced impairment in executive function (either sustained attention, behavioral control, or both), approximately 24 percent impairment in either receptive or expressive language processing (or both), 24 percent impairment in manual dexterity, and 23 percent memory impairment.

For the 104 children measured to be globally intact (FSIQ≥85), 54 percent evidenced no area of absolute impairment, while 46 percent of the sample showed at least one area with absolute impairment. Of the globally intact children with area(s) of absolute impairment, 29 percent had impairment in one domain; 17 percent had impairment in two or more domains. The domains most commonly affected in this sample were executive functions (sustained attention, impulsivity) (30 percent), language (12 percent), fine motor dexterity (12 percent), and verbal memory (9 percent).

Behavioral Problems

In addition to neurocognitive impairment, a substantial proportion of children with exposure to early deprivation also evidence problems within the behavioral domain. Early studies by Tizard and Hodges (1978; Hodges & Tizard, 1989) revealed anomalous or absent attachment and elevated rates of behavioral problems in children with histories of institution rearing, particularly in late-adopted children, but also revealed that many children (again especially those adopted earlier) appear to be rather problem free. More recent studies of children with histories of severe and early deprivation have generally replicated these studies, with many reporting increased incidence of insecure and/or anomalous (i.e., absent or disorganized attachment, indiscriminate friendliness) attachment, again particularly in late-adopted children (Zeanah et al., 2005; O'Connor et al., 2003; Chisolm, 1998), as well as increased rates of behavioral problems (Wiik et al., 2011; Sonuga-Barke et al., 2010; Gunnar & van Dulmen, 2007; Maclean, 2003; Rutter et al., 2001) and/or psychiatric diagnoses (Nelson, Fox, & Zeanah, 2013). With regard to the incidence of insecure or anomalous attachment, in the Chisolm (1998) study, 37 percent of children who experienced institution rearing for more than eight months demonstrated secure attachments. In the O'Connor et al. (2003) study, slightly more than 30 percent of late-adopted (six to twenty-four months) were measured to have secure attachments. In Zeanah et al. (2005), less than 20 percent of institution-reared children had a secure classification; almost

13 percent of children in this group were "unclassifiable." Importantly, a subsequent study by Zeanah and colleagues (Smyke et al., 2010) revealed rather striking improvement (in terms of attachment security) following placement in foster care, especially for children placed prior to twenty-four months of age.

With regard to specific quality of behavioral problems, a large number of studies have revealed increased incidence of internalizing (i.e., anxiety, depressed mood) and externalizing (i.e., overactivity, conduct problems, aggressive behavior) behavioral problems or psychiatric conditions in children with histories of early deprivation (Nelson, Fox, & Zeanah, 2013; McGoron et al., 2012; Wiik et al., 2011; Merz & McCall, 2010; Sonuga-Barke et al., 2010; Gunnar & van Dulmen, 2007; Maclean, 2003; Rutter et al., 2001). In the Nelson et al. (2013) study, by five years of age, approximately 62 percent of the children were measured to have a psychiatric diagnosis; most prevalent were anxiety disorders (44 percent) and attention-deficit hyperactivity disorder (ADHD) (23 percent). In Gunnar and van Dulmen (2007), 49 percent of children with histories of institution rearing evidenced as least one area (subscale) of borderline or clinical elevation; 11 percent had five or more of the clinical scales measured in the clinical range. Thirty-three percent of children with histories of institution rearing were reported to have elevated externalizing problems and 18 percent elevated internalizing problems. The domains most commonly affected in this group of children were attention problems (42 percent), thought problems (33 percent), and social problems (33 percent).

Of note is that there is substantial evidence that institution rearing per se is associated with a more specific (rather than pervasive) set of behavioral problems involving problems with attention and social problems (Wiik et al., 2011; Merz & McCall, 2010; Gunnar & van Dulmen, 2007; Juffer & van Ijzendoorn, 2005; Rutter et al., 2001; Tizard & Hodges 1978—see also Stevens et al., 2008). For instance, Gunnar & van Dulmen (2007) reported that while age at adoption was associated with increased incidence of and more pervasive behavioral difficulties for both institution-reared and comparison children, the groups differed (institution reared > comparison) only on measures of attention, thought problems, and social problems (see also Wiik et al., 2011), which may suggest a specific pattern of behavioral difficulty associated with early institutional rearing. Additional evidence for specific behavioral patterns associated with early institutional rearing is found in the work of Rutter et al. (2010), who in their work with the ERA sample have identified four behaviorally defined phenotypes or "deprivation-specific patterns" (DSPs) that are commonly found in institution-reared children, with durations of institutionalization that extend beyond their first six months and are very rare in comparison children. These DSPs include quasi-autism, cognitive impairment, disinhibited attachment, and an inattentive/overactive phenotype. Subsequent studies with this sample have revealed an increased incidence of behavioral problems (at ages eleven and fifteen years), including emotional and conduct problems, but importantly, these behavioral problems only occurred in the presence of a DSP (Sonuga-Barke et al., 2010).

In our study, 46 percent of the sample was reported to have a secure attachment. With regard to the incidence of behavioral problems, 26 percent of the full sample evidenced externalizing and 15 percent internalizing problems rated in the clinical range ($\geq$85th percentile) by their caregiver(s). Those behavioral domains most frequently measured at clinical levels included hyperactivity (29 percent), attention problems (26 percent), and atypicality (21 percent). As noted above, 8 percent evidenced global cognitive impairment, and 12 percent exceeded the cutoff on a caregiver reported measure assessing the presence of an autism-spectrum condition. Combined with the above work on specific neurocognitive impairments, which suggest a very increased incidence of impairment in executive functions (i.e., sustained attention, behavioral control), and along with findings of others (i.e., Gunnar & van Dulmen et al., 2007), these data suggest that rather specific domains are affected by early and severe social deprivation, mostly involving attention, social difficulties, and atypical behavior.

In sum, despite substantial catch-up in global cognitive functioning in children exposed to early severe deprivation and impressive resilience in terms of behavioral functioning in many children, even among those who are measured to be globally intact, a substantial proportion appear to experience enduring effects in specific domains of neurocognitive and behavioral functioning. Our studies, consistent with numerous others, have showed reduced mean global IQ and increased incidence of global cognitive impairment in children with histories of orphanage rearing, as well as increased incidence of specific neurocognitive impairment, especially involving executive functions, but also, to a much lesser degree, including language, motor, and memory. Behaviorally, children with histories of early deprivation evidence increased incidence of insecure and anomalous attachment, as well as increased incidence of behavioral problems and psychiatric conditions, especially involving attention problems, and social difficulties. Important to note is that both functional and structural brain imaging studies (see below) have indicated that early deprivation is associated with alteration/abnormality in specific brain regions and/or pathways as well. The neurocognitive and behavioral problems most frequently affected are those thought to be subserved by these regions/pathways.

Functional Imaging

FDG-PET

In order to examine whether brain dysfunction might underlie the persistent neurocognitive and behavioral deficits reported above, we applied functional neuroimaging with FDG-PET in a group of children ($N = 10$; mean age 8.8 years) adopted from Romanian orphanages. All children had been raised from birth in Romanian orphanages and had spent an average of thirty-eight months in the institution prior to being adopted into families within the United States. The average duration of time spent in their adoptive homes was 67.2 months (Chugani et al., 2001).

In this study, we were interested in evaluating whether there were any focal abnormalities of brain glucose metabolism in order to assess brain regions putatively involved in the persistent areas of impairment, identified above, associated with early and global deprivation.

We used a rigorous analytic approach that involved both the objective and automated determination of focal differences (using Statistical Parametric Mapping, SPM96; Friston et al., 1995),[1] followed by a subjective confirmation using manual definition (i.e., drawing) of brain regions of interest (ROIs) that had been identified as abnormal with the objective automated method (Chugani et al., 2001). Further, we compared the group of children with histories of early deprivation with two control groups: (1) normal adults and (2) the normal hemisphere of children with new-onset focal epilepsy who were typically developing according to neurocognitive testing and psychiatric assessment.[2]

The main results of the study were that early global deprivation was associated with dysfunction in a number of brain regions, including the orbital frontal cortex, prefrontal infralimbic cortex, lateral temporal cortex, medial temporal structures, and brainstem (Plate 6). The findings suggested that the neurocognitive and behavioral problems commonly identified in children with histories of early deprivation may be associated with abnormal functioning of cortical and subcortical brain regions. We further hypothesized that chronic stress endured in the orphanages during infancy and early childhood in these children resulted in altered development of these limbic structures and that altered functional connections in these circuits may represent the mechanism underlying persistent behavioral disturbances in these orphans.

EEG/ERP STUDIES

Several recent studies by the Bucharest Early Intervention Project (BEIP) group have also demonstrated functional abnormality in children with histories of deprivation compared to children raised in foster care, again implicating abnormalities in frontal and temporal brain regions consistent with both our FDG-PET study and the cognitive patterns of deficit widely reported in samples of children with histories of early deprivation. Using EEG, Marshall and Fox (2004) demonstrated decreased high-frequency power at frontal and temporal lobe sites, as well as increased low-frequency power in posterior sites in children living in institutions versus non-institution-raised children. A later study showed that age at placement into foster care from an institution predicted EEG coherence (alpha power and short distance coherence) (Marshall et al., 2008). Additional studies by this group examined ERPs in response to facial recognition (Parker & Nelson, 2005a) and affect discrimination (Parker & Nelson, 2005b) tasks; these studies revealed atypical ERP patterns in children with histories of institutionalization compared to controls. Such findings, the authors suggest, are consistent with a "general cortical hypoactivation" associated with early institutional rearing.

Children with histories of institutionalization have also been found to be less likely to correctly identify emotional facial expressions (Fries & Pollak, 2004) and have also shown hypoactivation to faces (Moulson et al., 2009). Moreover, Parker and Nelson (2005b) found that ever-institutionalized children (age thirty months) demonstrated greater amplitudes to fearful faces while never-institutionalized children exhibited larger amplitudes in response to sad faces. However, event-related potentials did not differ across groups in their sample when participants were administered the task at follow-up (forty-two and fifty months).

Overall, the EEG and facial recognition data provide additional support for frontal and temporal cortical abnormality, brain regions thought to be most affected in children with histories of early deprivation. Elevations in theta relative power and decrements in alpha relative power have also been shown to mediate the relationship between early deprivation and inattentive-overactive (I/O) symptoms (McLaughlin et al., 2010). The authors hypothesize that abnormal EEG in children with histories of institutionalization may be due to decreases in white matter during a possible sensitive period of development (Sheridan et al., 2010); decreased white matter volumes have been demonstrated by other laboratories (Hanson et al., 2013; Rutter, 1998; see below).

fMRI

Regions identified as functionally abnormal on FDG-PET included inferior frontal and lateral temporal cortical brain regions. Given that these regions are known to be involved in language functions, and further, given that language delays (Scott et al., 2011; Windsor et al., 2007) and impairment

(Croft et al., 2007) are commonly reported to occur in children with histories of early deprivation, we were interested in assessing whether children with histories of early deprivation evidenced atypical activations during the performance of language tasks and, in particular, whether children with such histories *and* language difficulties evidenced atypical patterns of language activations. Therefore, we used fMRI to examine activation patterns during language tasks in children who were raised with histories of early deprivation. Specifically, we compared children with histories of early deprivation and language impairment with children with similar histories but no language difficulties and also to a normal control group on functional activations during expressive and receptive language tasks.

The sample included thirty-eight children with histories of early deprivation. The mean age of this overall group at the time of testing was ten years. The average length of stay in the orphanage was twenty-three months; average length of time in the adoptive home was ninety-six months. Fourteen of the children had been adopted from Southeast Asia (China, Vietnam), eleven from Eastern Europe (Romania, Poland, Ukraine), and thirteen from Northern Asia (Russia).

Eighteen of the thirty-eight children with histories of early deprivation were measured to have language impairment (Helder et al., 2013). This group of children with language impairment did not significantly differ from children with similar histories but no language impairment or the group of typically developing, nonadopted children on age at testing, time in adoptive home, gender, handedness, maternal education, body mass index, head circumference, or full-scale IQ.

In order to assess expressive language, participants were asked to covertly generate words that fit into categories (animals, first names, foods, clothing, jobs/occupations). Thus, there were five word generation trials, each separated by periods of rest. For receptive language, participants listened to five simple stories; again, stories were interspersed with periods of rest. Contrasting the signal (blood flow) during performance of the language tasks with the signal during periods of rest yields the areas in the brain that are active during performance of the task. The above tasks have been used extensively in both adults and children and have been shown to activate classical language areas consistently (Hertz-Pannier et al., 1997).

For receptive language activations, between-group comparisons revealed that the children with histories of early deprivation and language impairment had more extra-perisylvian cortical activations than either controls or the early deprivation group with no language difficulties, suggesting increased involvement of nonclassical language regions during this task.

Additionally, the children with histories of early deprivation and normal language evidenced increased activity in classical language (i.e., left superior temporal lobe) regions than both the nonadopted typically developing controls and the early deprivation children with language impairments. Similarly, for the expressive language task, the children with histories of early deprivation and language impairment showed more diffuse activation patterns than either the early deprivation group with no language difficulties and/or the normal controls. The typically developing, nonadopted children also showed increased left inferior frontal activations compared to the early deprivation group with language impairment.

Overall, these fMRI results reliably distinguished among groups; children with histories of early deprivation and language impairment showed atypical patterns of language activations compared to healthy nonadopted children, including a more diffuse pattern of activation on both receptive and expressive tasks, as well as reduced activation in classical language areas during performance of these tasks. These results support abnormal functioning of some of the cortical areas previously shown to be abnormal with FDG-PET. The findings also suggest a neural correlate to the neurocognitive findings, which show an increased incidence of language delay and impairment in children with histories of early deprivation.

Structural Brain Imaging Correlates

MRI Volumetric Studies

Despite a number of studies indicating functional neurological abnormality in children with histories of early deprivation, there have been relatively fewer studies of brain anatomy, perhaps due to the lack of suitable noninvasive methodologies for such investigation. Those that have been done suggest that early deprivation is not only associated with functional brain abnormalities but may also involve structural changes. A study on a subsample of the ERA children showed increased amygdala volumes in children with histories of early deprivation (Mehta et al., 2009). A subsequent study on a larger sample of children with such histories similarly found increased amygdala volumes in a sample of children having spent more than fifteen months in institutional care versus children spending less than fifteen months in orphanages and nondeprived controls (Tottenham et al., 2010). Duration of time in the institution was linearly related to amygdala volumes as well, with later adoption associated with increased volumes. More recently, a study on a subsample of the children in the Bucharest Early

Intervention Project revealed reduced cortical thickness across prefrontal, parietal, and temporal cortices. Specifically, thickness in the lateral orbito-frontal cortex, insula, inferior parietal cortex, precuneus, superior temporal cortex, and lingual gyrus was found to mediate the relationship between institutionalization and inattention and impulsivity (McLaughlin et al., 2014).

Overall, these studies of neural structure have supported that those brain regions identified as functionally abnormal are structurally abnormal as well. A small number of studies have also found reduced whole-brain gray and white matter volumes (Hanson et al., 2013; Mehta et al., 2009).

MRI/Diffusion Tensor Imaging

DTI 1: FIBER TRACTOGRAPHY

While both functional and structural MRI studies have revealed abnormalities in cortical brain regions hypothesized to be involved in neurocognitive (i.e., language) and social and emotional (i.e., amygdala) functions, evaluation of pathways that interconnect these brain regions would further elucidate the mechanisms by which early deprivation might influence the function and structure of such regions. The advent of diffusion tensor imaging (DTI) allows a sensitive and noninvasive measure of diffusion characteristics of cerebral white matter, which reflects the microstructural integrity of white matter. The strength of DTI and, in particular, fiber tractography, which is a technique used to visually represent and quantify diffusion properties of specific white matter tracts, is the ability to differentiate white matter pathways from each other noninvasively and pinpoint abnormalities that are associated with specific fiber tracts. Initially, we used DTI and fiber tractography to investigate whether or not the white matter pathways that link the regions shown to be abnormal on functional and structural imaging studies above were characterized by aberrant connectivity.

In our initial study, we examined several limbic white matter pathways in a small sample of children with histories of early deprivation compared to nondeprived, nonadopted typically developing controls (Eluvathingal et al., 2006). Results revealed reduced integrity of the uncinate fasciculus, a limbic pathway known to be involved in social and emotional functions, but no between-group differences on other limbic pathways. This finding was intriguing, given previous work showing abnormal frontal and medial temporal abnormality; however, we could not be certain whether negative results on other limbic pathways might not be due to the very small sample size ($N = 7$) employed in the study. Thus, in a subsequent study, we utilized a much larger sample (thirty-six children with histories of early deprivation; sixteen nonadopted, nondeprived controls), and in addition, given the incidence of language impairment in children with histories of early deprivation, we also examined the integrity of the arcuate fasciculus, a pathway known to be involved in language functions, as well as several limbic tracts, and the corticospinal tract, a tract important for motor functions (Kumar et al., 2013).

This sample of children had resided in the institution for an average of twenty-six months prior to being adopted into the United States and had been residing in their adoptive homes for an average of ninety-four months. The sample included children from Russia, China, Vietnam, Romania, Ukraine, Poland, Armenia, and Slovakia. Neurocognitively, this group of children was functioning well within the average range in most domains assessed, with relative (to FSIQ) weaknesses in behavioral control, sustained attention, and verbal memory.

Results of this study showed significant differences in the microstructural architecture of several white matter pathways in children with histories of early deprivation. For instance, fractional anisotropy (FA) and mean diffusivity (MD), indices of the integrity of white matter tracts, for several limbic and paralimbic white matter pathways differed for children with histories of early deprivation compared to control children (see Plate 7). Specifically, MD was increased in the arcuate fasciculus in children with histories of early deprivation compared to controls, and MD increased, and FA reduced, in the uncinate fasciculus and several other limbic pathways (i.e., cingulum, fornix). These results suggest some structural alterations of these tracts in children with histories of early deprivation. Additionally, the findings were associated with both duration of time in the orphanage (increased time in the orphanage was associated with reduced integrity of white matter) and duration of time in the adoptive home (as time in the adoptive home increased, integrity of white matter increased) (see Figure 12.2). Finally, correlations between these metrics and neurocognitive and behavioral functions revealed that integrity of white matter for the arcuate fasciculus was positively associated with language functions, and integrity of the uncinate fasciculus and cingulum was inversely correlated with behavioral functioning.

These findings provide neural bases for the neurocognitive and behavioral difficulties so commonly observed in children with such histories. Also, the findings did not appear to affect tracts globally, as there were no between-group differences on microstructural integrity for the corticospinal tract. We hypothesized that such findings might be due to either (or both) the lack of experience-expectant stimuli during critical or sensitive periods of development and/or the deleterious effects of unmitigated stress during

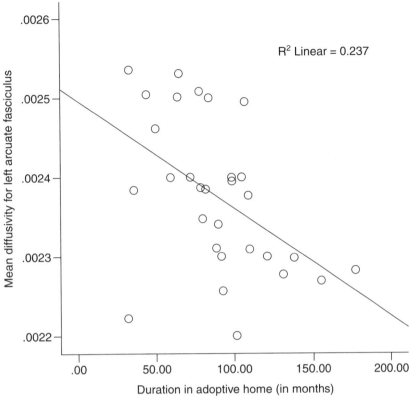

FIGURE 12.2. Scatterplot showing relationship between duration in the adoptive home and mean diffusivity for the left arcuate fasciculus. As can be seen, as duration of time in the adoptive home increases, mean diffusivity is reduced.

early development (see below). The notion that lack of exposure to certain stimuli during brain development can result in a loss of microstructural integrity of selective white matter pathways as measured by DTI is not novel. For example, inadequate exposure to experience-expectant visual stimuli has been shown to reduce FA in the optic radiation in humans suffering from early blindness (Shu et al., 2009; Shimony et al., 2006). In particular, the finding in the arcuate fasciculus of increased diffusivity, in the absence of reduced FA (directionality), may be most consistent with the notion that the lack of experience-expectant stimulation results in a lack of or abnormal pruning (Behen et al., 2009).

DTI 2: TRACT-BASED SPATIAL STATISTICS

Given that fiber tractography involves a priori determination of fiber tracts, the approach left unaddressed the question of whether or not there were white matter differences elsewhere in the brain, for instance, in white matter tracts that we had not chosen to evaluate. To further evaluate this possibility, we used tract-based spatial statistics (TBSS), a technique that offers an automated, objective, and unbiased method for evaluating the integrity of white matter in the *whole* brain (Smith et al., 2006). A number of published studies in recent years have used TBSS to evaluate white matter integrity in a wide variety of neurological and psychiatric conditions such as Alzheimer disease, multiple sclerosis, substance abuse, bipolar disorder, and parental verbal abuse (Choi et al., 2009; Roosendaal et al., 2009; Stricker et al., 2009; Versace et al., 2008).

In this study, we compared seventeen right-handed children with a mean age of ten years who were raised from birth in Eastern European or Central Asian/Russian orphanages with fifteen right-handed typically developing nonadopted children (mean age = eleven years) on white matter integrity. This group of children had spent an average of thirty-two months in the orphanage and an average of ninety-two months in their adoptive homes at the time of the study (Govindan et al., 2010).

Results of the study revealed multiple regions of reduced integrity (decreased FA) in white matter tracts of the children with histories of early deprivation compared to healthy nonadopted children. These regions involved the bilateral uncinate fasciculus with extensive involvement of the right uncinate fasciculus, including the white matter region adjacent to the right amygdala, and regions involving the bilateral superior longitudinal fasciculus, a white matter tract that contains the arcuate fasciculus. Additionally, we found that the *magnitude* of white matter disorganization in these regions was significantly negatively correlated with duration of stay in the orphanage, as well as other neuropsychological outcomes (i.e., hyperactivity, attention problems) previously reported to be commonly present in children with such histories (Stevens et al., 2008).

These findings are consistent with and extend the observations from previous studies, using volumetric MRI (Tottenham et al., 2010), FDG-PET (Chugani et al., 2001), ERPs (Marshall & Fox, 2004; Marshall et al., 2008), and magnetic resonance (MR)–DTI tractography (Kumar et al., 2013). Of note is that the similar findings with divergent methodologies (i.e., FDG-PET, DTI fiber tractography, and DTI with an automated nonbiased method such as TBSS) increase the confidence of findings.

DTI 3: PROBABILISTIC DTI

Finally, given the elevated incidence of the inattentive-overactive phenotype in children with histories of early deprivation (Stevens et al., 2008; Behen et al., 2008), we used MR-DTI to evaluate the potential neural correlates of this phenotype. While it is assumed that such findings are reflective of abnormal neurologic development resulting from early deprivation, the neural substrate(s) or brain regions most affected are poorly understood. In particular, there have been no studies that have evaluated potential neural correlates of the inattentive-overactive phenotype in children with histories of early deprivation.

Research on idiopathic or developmental ADHD has strongly implicated frontostriatal brain regions and/or circuitry as involved in the disorder. Volumetric MRI studies have shown abnormal caudate and prefrontal gray matter volumes (Shaw et al. 2007; Giedd et al., 2001). Studies using DTI have identified reduced white matter integrity (decreased fractional anisotropy) in frontostriatal circuitry in children with ADHD (Pavuluri et al., 2009). Therefore, evaluation of this neural substrate in children with the I/O phenotype was of interest.

The objective of this study was to apply probabilistic fiber tracking to frontostriatal pathways and determine whether the connectivity pattern differed between children with histories of early deprivation and nonadopted, typically developing controls. Probabilistic tractography is a technique that allows for a quantification of the magnitude of structural connectivity of white matter projections between a manually defined seed region (i.e., the caudate nucleus) and a target region(s) (i.e., the frontal lobe). We also were interested in evaluating whether the I/O behavioral characteristics were associated with patterns of frontostriatal connectivity.

We compared the pattern of frontostriatal connectivity in fifteen children raised from birth in Eastern Europe, Northern Asia, or South Asia with twelve nonadopted, typically developing control children. The average duration of orphanage stay was thirty-five months, and average time in the adoptive home was eighty-nine months (Behen et al., 2009).

Specifically, we evaluated the probability of connection or the connectivity strength between the caudate nucleus (seed region) and several targets, including the whole cortex, the dorsolateral prefrontal cortex, and the frontal pole, for both hemispheres. The connectivity strength between the caudate and these cortical targets was compared between groups (Behen et al., 2009). Results indicated aberrant connectivity in frontostriatal projections in children with histories of early deprivation. Specifically, the early deprivation group had significantly increased probability of connection for striatal projections terminating in the cortex, however, with a concomitant reduced probability of connection to the frontal pole in the right hemisphere (see Plate 8). Further, increased frontostriatal connectivity was associated with increased externalizing behavioral problems. These findings suggest a plausible neural substrate for symptoms associated with the

inattentive-overactive behavioral phenotype often described in children
with histories of early deprivation (Stevens et al., 2008).

Stevens et al. (2008) presented functional support for similarities between
the idiopathic ADHD phenotype and expression of inattentive-overactive
in children who had experienced early deprivation. Given the findings from
imaging studies of neural correlates of idiopathic ADHD, which have demonstrated abnormalities in the frontostriatal circuit (Shaw et al., 2007;
Giedd et al., 2001), findings from the present study provide some structural
support for similarities between the inattentive-overactive phenotype and
idiopathic ADHD. Shaw and colleagues (2007) speculated that the delayed
pattern of heteromodal cortical maturation identified in idiopathic ADHD
might reflect a lack of normal pruning. The findings of excessive frontostriatal connectivity in the present study may also be consistent with an
abnormal pruning process, perhaps associated with lack of experience-
expectant stimulation (e.g., language stimulation, caregiver regulation of
emotional states) during orphanage rearing (see also Hanson et al., 2013).
Chatterjee et al. (2007) showed elevations in the number of neurons and
supporting astroglial cells and reduced indices of functionality in cortical
regions in rat pups subjected to maternal deprivation. Reduced functionality
was associated with reduced neuronal pruning and apoptosis (Chatterjee
et al., 2007).

Taken together, results of the MR-DTI studies have demonstrated abnormalities in pattern of connectivity of frontostriatal connections and abnormalities in the integrity of neural pathways that putatively support language
and behavioral functions. Importantly, the structural findings presented here
(and elsewhere) are relatively specific to a few brain regions and connections between these regions: neural circuits that are associated with language functions and emotional/behavioral processing/regulation, including
inattentive/overactive behavior—those functions most frequently reported
to be disturbed in children with histories of early deprivation.

Predictors of Functional and Structural Outcomes

Predictors of Neurocognitive Outcomes

Length of institutionalization has been established as a robust predictor
of functional outcomes (Rutter et al., 1998; Nelson et al., 2007). Our work
as well has supported duration of time in the institution as a robust predictor of cognitive outcomes (Behen et al., 2008). In order to further evaluate which factors were associated with outcome in the present sample, we

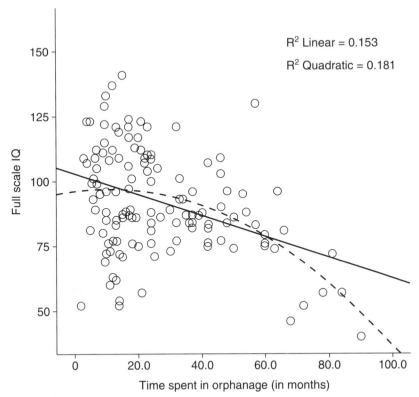

FIGURE 12.3. Scatterplot showing the correlation between duration of time in the orphanage and global (full-scale IQ [FSIQ]) intellectual functioning for the full sample of children with histories of deprivation. As can be seen, global IQ decreases inversely with time in the orphanage. Additionally, the nonlinear (inverted U) relationship is also significant, which suggests that beyond three years or so, FSIQ decreases rather dramatically.

examined correlations between demographic (age, gender, handedness, number of years of adoptive mother and father education, medication use) and orphanage-specific variables (body mass index, duration of time in the orphanage, and adoptive home, region of adoption) with global cognitive outcome (FSIQ) in the full sample of children studied to date. Only duration of time in the orphanage ($r = -0.37$, $p < .001$, see Figure 12.3) and region of adoption ($p < .001$) were significantly related to FSIQ. Specifically, longer duration of time in the orphanage and being from an orphanage in Eastern Europe were associated with lower full-scale IQs. It is noteworthy that region of adoption was perfectly confounded with duration of time in the institution, with children from Eastern European orphanages having longer durations than children from other regions.

The same correlations were also run within the globally intact (FSIQ > 84) group. Again, only duration in the orphanage ($p = .041$) and region of adoption ($p = .012$) were associated with FSIQ.

Prediction of Specific Neurocognitive Impairment

In order to evaluate whether any of the above variables were predictive of the incidence of *specific* impairment and/or number of impairments, the sample was divided into the following groups: no impairment ($n = 56$), specific impairment in one domain ($n = 30$), impairments in multiple domains ($n = 18$), and globally impaired (FSIQ < 85; $n = 51$). These groups were compared on the above demographic and orphanage-specific variables. In order to control for multiple comparisons, Bonferroni correction for multiple comparisons was applied. Since there were ten total comparisons, the adjusted alpha level for between-group analyses was $p = .005$.

Again, the only significant findings were for duration of stay in the orphanage ($p < .001$) and region of adoption ($p = .001$). Post hoc tests revealed that the no-impairment and single-impairment groups spent less time in the orphanage than did the globally impaired group. For region of adoption, children from South/East Asia were less likely to be measured in the impaired range than either the Eastern Europe or Northern Asia groups ($p = .018$).

In order to evaluate potential sensitive periods, we examined incidence of impairment at varying periods of duration; duration of time in the orphanage was categorized as follows: six months or less, seven to twenty months, twenty-one to thirty-six months, and more than 36 months. In the full sample, the likelihood of impairment generally increased as duration of stay in the orphanage increased. Specifically, if orphanage exposure was less than or equal to six months, approximately 30 percent of children evidenced at least one area of impairment (it is important to note that there were few children, $n = 10$, in the present sample in this cell). After six months and up to three years in the orphanage, the likelihood of impairment increased to nearly 60 percent. Beyond three years, the incidence of impairment in at least one domain was greater than 80 percent. The difference across groups was statistically significant ($p = .001$). Removing the globally impaired children and examining the data shows similar relationships across these categories; at orphanage stays up to six months, there was less than a 20 percent chance of at least one area of impairment; for stays of seven to thirty-six months, slightly over 40 percent had evidence at least one area of impairment; and finally, beyond thirty-six months, more than 60 percent

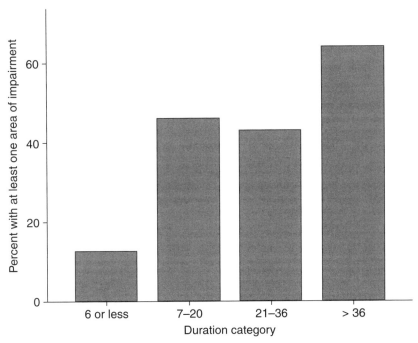

FIGURE 12.4. Bar graph depicting the percentage of the globally intact sample with at least one area of impairment. As can be seen, the incidence nearly doubles from six months or less to the seven- to thirty-six-month category, and then increases to greater than 60 percent incidence beyond thirty-six months.

of children had at least one area of impairment (see Figure 12.4). The association between incidence of impairment and category of duration of stay was also tested without the globally impaired children; the group difference was significant ($p = .034$).

A dose-response effect, which involves increased incidence of impairment as duration of time in the orphanage increases, has been reported by others (Nelson et al., 2007; O'Connor et al., 2000). O'Connor and Rutter (2000) found a linear relationship between duration of orphanage experience and global cognitive functioning in children adopted from zero to forty-two months from Romanian orphanages. However, more recently, Beckett et al. (2006) reported that although greater than six months' duration of orphanage experience was associated with poorer outcome, when the lowest functioning (bottom 15 percent) children were removed from analyses, the linear effect for cognitive functioning in children with durations between six and forty-two months (O'Connor & Rutter, 2000) was no longer present. Croft et al. (2007) reported a similar absence of a dose-response relationship for language functioning in the same sample. These authors report that being in an orphanage for six months represents the limit of safe exposure, after which impairment is significantly more likely, but additional orphanage experience does not appear to further increase the likelihood of impairment (Becket et al., 2006; Croft et al., 2007). Alternatively, studies from the BEIP group have supported a potential threshold for age at adoption of twenty to twenty-four months; children removed from institutional care to foster care prior to twenty-four months had significantly higher global IQ than children placed later (Nelson et al., 2013).

Our data demonstrate that exposures shorter than six months are associated with a low likelihood of any impairment but suggest that risk nearly doubles beyond six months of exposure. This nonlinear association reflects a six-month threshold, which is generally consistent with work from the ERA group. However, our data also suggest a second threshold, with exposures greater than thirty-six months representing a highly increased likelihood of at least one area of neurocognitive impairment.

Overall, results from our own and others' work have supported duration of time in the institution as a robust moderator of cognitive outcomes. The exact nature of the relationship between duration and outcome and/ or whether there is any threshold (and the exact timing of a threshold) is less clear. The differences in absolute threshold between these groups are likely attributable to differences in the sensitivity of measurement (i.e., global vs. specific) and/or to differences in sample characteristics. Given these differences, cross-validation of the findings presented here for specific impairment would be essential before any firm conclusions can be drawn regarding safe exposure or sensitive periods.

With regard to behavioral problems, the association between age of adoption and outcomes is less clear. Findings from the ERA group have suggested that children removed from adverse conditions prior to age six months do not differ from nondeprived children. Other studies have suggested eighteen-month (Mertz & McCall, 2010) to twenty-four-month (Gunnar & van Dulmen, 2007) cutoffs for behavioral problems; still others have found more linear, dose-response, associations with outcome (Wiik et al., 2011), and others fail to find associations between duration of neglect and behavioral outcomes. In our own sample, duration of institutionalization/age at adoption is positively associated with attention problems; there was no significant relationship to any other domain. Of note, however, was that duration of institutionalization was strongly correlated with global intellect, which is in turn highly correlated with behavioral outcome, suggesting an indirect influence on behavioral functioning. Nelson et al. (2013) have noted, in their work on the BEIP sample, that "a sensitive period for mental health was not detected." Importantly, though, their work has shown strong associations between age at adoption and attachment, with children removed from adverse conditions prior to twenty-four months having a greater likelihood of secure attachment (Nelson et al., 2013), which should theoretically offer protection from poor behavioral outcomes. Other variables that have shown associations with behavioral problems in the present sample include country of adoption (children from Eastern Europe and Russia evidencing increased behavioral problems compared to children adopted from South/Eastern Asia, even after controlling for duration of institutionalization), duration of time in the adoptive home (positive correlation between time in the adoptive home and internalizing behavioral problems and withdrawn behavior), and global intellect (negatively correlated with both internalizing and externalizing behavioral problems). Similar findings have been reported elsewhere (Gunnar & van Dulmen, 2007).

With regard to functional brain imaging outcomes, studies from the BEIP group have indicated that age at adoption from the institution was associated with neural function as assessed by EEG (above). EEG patterns were somewhat normalized in children who were placed into foster care intervention at younger ages compared to children who remained in institutions (Marshall et al., 2008). In our own studies (FDG-PET, language fMRI activations), functional imaging correlates were not associated with time in the orphanage. However, the small sample size in both of these studies precludes any meaningful conclusions in these studies.

Predictors of Structural Brain Imaging Findings

As with functional outcomes, duration of time in the institution has consistently (and nearly exclusively) been related to structural brain imaging outcomes. Tottenham et al. (2010) found that time in the institution was positively associated with amygdala volumes and, further, that children adopted before fifteen months had normalized amygdala volumes. In our own work, only duration of exposure (and duration of time in the adoptive home; see below) was associated with outcomes. Longer times in the orphanage were associated with arcuate and uncinate fasciculi integrity, as assessed by MR-DTI (Govindan et al., 2010; Kumar et al., 2013). Importantly, these data too may hint at a threshold of approximately three years, beyond which white matter anatomy is likely to be affected. Further research on this possibility with larger sample sizes is warranted and ongoing in our laboratory.

Interestingly, we also found that length of time in the adoptive home was associated with microstructural integrity of several pathways (Kumar et al., 2013). These findings are not unexpected given research that has demonstrated the often direct impact of the environment on microstructural integrity (e.g., Bengtsson et al., 2005). Further, we know children improve over time in the adoptive home in terms of development (Judge, 2003) and cognition (Rutter, 1998) and that early intervention (i.e., placement into foster care) is associated with increased cognitive functioning (Fox et al., 2011). Animal research has documented resolution of neural abnormalities secondary to early maternal separation or deprivation following exposure to high-level maternal stimulation (i.e., "stroking"; Chatterjee et al., 2007). Importantly, though, previous studies have not supported strong links between time in the adoptive home and functional outcomes but rather have documented the presence of persistent neurocognitive and behavioral impairments in a proportion of children (Rutter et al., 2007; Behen et al., 2008; Croft et al., 2007). Of note, however, is the work of the BEIP group, which showed positive effects of placement in foster care versus children who remained in institutions (Nelson et al., 2007; see also Fox et al., 2011), especially for children placed prior to twenty-four months, and which has had significant effects for global cognition, attachment, internalizing behavioral problems, and EEG power and ERPs as well. Of note is that despite significant and meaningful improvement, it is not clear that children improve to normal levels in the above domains (Nelson et al., 2013). Theoretically, it is possible that for children adopted after a sensitive period, improvements in neural structural organization (or reorganization) are less likely to occur or less complete, leading to persistent impairments (or reduced levels of functioning, even if not to the impaired level), despite normalization of the caregiving environment. At this time, it is unknown whether the microstructural integrity of white matter pathways will undergo further organization if a child is exposed to enriched stimulation after a period of deprivation or if there is a point at which prolonged deprivation results in permanently reduced integrity. Bates has discussed potential limitations in plasticity in children with brain injury, suggesting plasticity is not without cost, and "some price must be paid for wholesale reorganization of the brain to compensate for early injuries" (Bates, 1999, p. 214).

Mechanisms for Altered Function and Structure following Early Deprivation

Potential mechanisms for the observed functional and structural deficits include the absence of experience-expectant stimulation associated with the deprivation experience, chronic stress associated with inadequate caregiving, and exposure to poor pre-, peri-, and postnatal factors that are known to affect development (e.g., malnutrition, illness, toxic substances, e.g., lead).

Early Experience and Brain Development

The human nervous system undergoes substantial development postnatally, and there is growing evidence that sufficient external experience is necessary for the human brain to develop properly. Human infants are born with an overabundance of neurons. This overabundance of neurons in the infant's brain allows adaptation of the brain in response to environmental demands (Nelson, 2002). Those synapses that are activated through frequent use are reinforced and strengthened; those that are not used and/or activated are "pruned." Thus, one's early experiences determine those neural pathways that become permanent and those that will be eliminated. However, for this process to result in normal brain development, the infant "must interact with a living and responsive environment" (Balbernie, 2001, p. 253).

Prolonged exposure to environments that failed to provide adequate experience-expectant stimulation during specific sensitive periods of development is thought to result in abnormal neurodevelopment (Greenough, Black, & Wallace, 1987). Thus, lack of exposure to adequate domain-specific and experience-expectant stimuli during sensitive period(s) of development is expected to be related to abnormal structural development (Nelson, 2002). For instance, presumed reduced language stimulation in the orphanage, particularly during the months and years during which language stimulation is expected to occur, is hypothesized to alter the neural pathways/structures that subserve language functions and presumably underlie impaired language function. Domain-specific stimulation/experience guides selective pruning, which underlies the normal organization of neural substrates that subserve any particular function, serving to increase efficiency of processing (Nelson, 2002). In the absence of sufficient stimulation (which guides pruning or organization of the central nervous system [CNS]), abnormal structural and/or functional organization of such substrates occurs, which may underlie such specific functional impairments as those found in children who have experienced early deprivation.

Deprivation of sensory, motor, and social stimulation has profound effects on both function and structure of the developing nervous system and in domain-specific systems. Hofer (see Hofer, 1994) has experimentally demonstrated that absence of discrete aspects of the mother (i.e., touch) has specific effects on nervous system physiology (see also Hofer, 1996), and there is now substantial support in the animal literature for the notion that early postnatal neglect and deprivation may be associated with both short-term and long-term changes in brain function (reviewed in Suomi, 1997; Hofer, 1996; Kaufman et al., 2000) and structure (Chatterjee et al., 2007). For instance, visual deprivation, especially over a sensitive period, has been shown to result in an altered visual cortex (Nakadate, 2001). At sufficiently prolonged durations in animals, such deprivation leads to irreversible neural alteration (Nakadate, 2001). Such experience-expectant effects have been shown as well for auditory, language, and motor cortex (Lee et al., 2005; Sharma et al., 2005; Vandermeeren et al., 2003). Therefore, it is suspected that a major source of the functional and structural brain imaging findings is the lack of experience-expectant care associated with the absence of a consistent caregiver during early development.

Alternatively, the findings could be secondary to adverse and chronic experience of stress. Dysregulation of stress response as a result of social deprivation has been demonstrated in post-institutionalized children (Carlson & Earls, 1997; Gunnar et al., 2001). Further, prolonged stress is known to have adverse (typically focal) consequences for the developing central nervous system (Bremner & Vermetten, 2001). Importantly, the brain areas and pathways identified in the above studies as functionally and/or structurally abnormal are those known to be damaged as a result of prolonged stress. Infralimbic and orbital cortices are reciprocally connected with the amygdala and hippocampus (Barbas & Pandya, 1989; Barbas & De Olmos, 1990; Morecraft et al., 1992; Barbas, 1993) and are also known to project to subcortical autonomic centers (Neafsy, 1990; Hurley et al., 1991). The infralimbic cortex has been called the autonomic motor cortex (Hurley et al., 1991) and plays a role in regulating visceral responses to emotional stimuli (Freedman et al., 2000); dysfunction of this circuit has been implicated in impaired autonomic response to emotionally significant stimuli (Chu et al., 1997). Rinaman et al. (2000) demonstrated significant postnatal maturation of limbic forebrain projections to central autonomic neurons in rats and hypothesized a critical period during which experience might affect synapse formation of limbic-autonomic circuits.

The interconnected brain regions shown to be functionally and structurally abnormal also are integrally involved in the brain response to stress (reviewed by Lopez et al., 1999). The presence of stress activates a series of pathways involving the brain and the endocrine system. Within the brain, a group of regions, including the neocortex, allocortex, hippocampus, nucleus accumbens, lateral septum, hypothalamus, amygdala, dorsal raphe, locus coeruleus, and brainstem nuclei, are activated in response to different types of stressors (Campeau & Watson, 1997; Cullinan et al., 1995, 1996).

The integration of the brain and endocrine stress response is mediated via the limbic-hypothalamic-pituitary-adrenal axis (Selye, 1936; McEwen et al., 1974), the activation of which results in a series of events leading to glucocorticoid release. There is evidence that chronic elevations of glucocorticoids may cause damage to limbic brain regions (Kaufman et al., 2000; McEwen, 2000; Sapolsky, 2000). Further, stress and glucocorticoids have been implicated in dendritic remodeling (McEwen & Sapolsky, 1995) and inhibition of neurogenesis in the hippocampus (Gould et al., 2000). Stress and adrenal steroids cause reversible impairments in episodic and spatial memory in animals and humans (de Quervain et al., 2000; Lupien & McEwen, 1997), and repeated stress can result in cognitive dysfunction (McEwen & Sapolsky, 1995).

There is also considerable evidence from animal studies that stressors applied early in development can affect behavior in adulthood (for review, see Lopez et al., 1999; Card et al., 2005). Similarly, early adverse experiences in humans are associated with elevated rates of major depression and other psychiatric disorders in adulthood (for review, see Kaufman et al., 2000). Maternal separation is a potent stressor, as evidenced by behavior (Harlow et al., 1969; Harlow, 1969; Suomi, 1997; Newman & Bachevalier, 1997) and neuroendocrine response (Kuhn et al., 1990; Higley et al., 1992; Pihoker et al., 1993), and has been linked to structural abnormalities in animals, including reduction in Purkinje cell size (Floeter & Greenough, 1979), decreases in cortical dendritic branching (Struble & Riesen, 1978), alterations in neurofilament protein immunoreactivity in the dentate gyrus granule cell layer of the hippocampus (Siegel et al., 1993), and reduced number of preautonomic limbic forebrain neurons (Card et al., 2005). Prolonged maternal separation of rat pups resulted in increased limbic-hypothalamic-pituitary-adrenal axis activity (Kuhn et al., 1990; Pihoker et al., 1993) and increased reactivity to stressors during adulthood (Plotsky & Meaney, 1993). Of note is that different strains of rats show different sensitivity to early stress, suggesting that long-term effects of stress are mediated by both exposure and genetic variables (reviewed by Anisman et al., 1998).

In summary, we hypothesize two co-occurring factors that combine to place socially deprived children at risk for cognitive and socioemotional deficits that are mediated by structural and functional brain abnormalities. On one hand, children exposed to early social deprivation may lack sufficient quality or quantity of environmental stimulation associated with the absence of a consistent caregiver hypothesized to be critical to normal postnatal neurodevelopmental events (i.e., pruning). Additionally, these children may also endure negative experience (i.e., chronic unmitigated stress), without the buffering benefit of attachment to a consistent caregiver. These factors, as we have seen, are associated with dysfunction and abnormal structure in a group of limbic and brain regions and pathways that connect them, which are also known to be activated by stress and damaged by prolonged stress. We suggest that lack of expected stimulation and chronic unmodulated stress endured in orphanage-reared children resulted in altered development of these limbic and paralimbic structures and that altered functional and structural connections in these circuits may represent a potential mechanism underlying some of the persistent cognitive and behavioral disturbances in children with histories of early deprivation.

In addition to a lack of experience-expectant stimulation and chronic unmitigated stress, it is important to point out that it was not possible to definitively rule out the presence of pre- and perinatal factors as contributors to functional and/or structural outcomes, despite efforts made to exclude children based on these factors (e.g., low birth weight, knowledge of prematurity, and/or identified suspicion of alcohol exposure prenatally). As with most studies of institutionally adopted children, historical records were poor, and it is likely that we had not completely excluded these confounds from the sample.

Poor prenatal nutrition has been linked to poor myelination and neurotransmission (Lozoff, 2007). Additionally, substantial and impressive data have supported links between maternal stress during pregnancy and altered stress responsivity and limbic structural abnormality (Van den Bergh et al., 2005). Exposure to alcohol has also been shown to be associated with reductions in gray and white matter, including the frontal and temporal lobe (see Spadoni et al., 2007). In addition to pre- and perinatal factors, some degree of malnutrition is known to have occurred in a majority (if not all) of the participants, as is evidenced by small physical stature and head circumference. Postnatal malnutrition has been shown to be associated with structural brain changes, including frontal and temporal cortices (Cordero et al., 1993; Granados-Rojas et al., 2004; Kirksey et al., 1990). Although the findings of the above studies were not associated with head circumference, in at least one of the above studies (DTI, TBSS), findings were associated with body mass index, suggesting that malnutrition may have contributed to the observed structural findings. However, statistical control for body mass index did not substantially alter the findings. Given the research that has shown effects of malnutrition on the developing nervous system (Guerrini et al., 2007), further research is warranted to further evaluate potential associations between malnutrition and neural abnormalities in limbic and paralimbic structures/tracts in children with histories of early deprivation. It is likely that the neural abnormalities reported in the present study are due, at least in part, to a mixture of the above mentioned pre- and postnatal factors. The greater degree of abnormality in participants with longer duration of exposure would be due to a greater "dose" of these multiple factors.

Conclusion

In conclusion, studies in our own and others' laboratories investigating the effects of early and severe social deprivation reveal an increased incidence of neurocognitive and behavioral deficits. Our work has indicated both reduced global cognition for the sample of children raised from birth in international orphanages and increased incidence of specific neurocognitive impairments (i.e., language impairment, inattention/overactive difficulties) and behavioral difficulties, even in children with intact global cognition. Behavioral problems appear to involve specific domains as well, particularly including problems with attachment, attention, social functioning, and atypicality, supporting the notion of deprivation-specific psychological patterns previously proposed by Rutter and Sonuga-Barke (2010). Importantly, research is emerging that such deficits are associated with altered neural structure and function, including prefrontal and medial temporal regional abnormalities, and the pathways (i.e., arcuate, uncinate fasciculi) that reciprocally project to them. These regions/pathways identified to date, both in our and others' laboratories, primarily involve those that are thought to be involved in executive, socioemotional, and language functions.

The age at which the child emerges from the institution (in our sample, since all the children entered institutional care at birth, this equates to the duration of time spent in the institution) is a rather robust indicator of the likelihood of both functional and structural outcomes. Children with exposures (who leave the orphanage) at less than six months of age have a low likelihood of any impairment, but risk increases (nearly doubles) beyond six months for the neurocognitive domain. This nonlinear association appears to reflect a six-month sensitive period for safe exposure. There is also evidence for a twenty-four-month threshold (BEIP group) for improvement in attachment and global cognition, although it is not clear that improvement to this age is to normal levels. Our data may suggest an additional threshold; exposures greater than thirty-six months appear to represent a highly increased likelihood of at least one area of impairment in neurocognitive functions. Additionally, recent work has also indicated that time in the adoptive home or exposure to an enriched environment is also associated with neurologic (e.g., white matter integrity) outcomes as well, although it is not yet clear whether there is a point at which prolonged deprivation (i.e., beyond a sensitive period) results in permanently reduced structural integrity. Further research on timing variables and their associations with functional and structural neural outcomes is warranted and ongoing in our laboratory.

We suggest that such functional deficits and the associated alterations in neural structure and function are due to multiple factors, including (1) insufficient experience-expectant stimulation (i.e., touch, language) associated with the lack consistent care and that alters normal neurodevelopment; (2) exposure to chronic and unmitigated stress associated with a lack of consistent caregiving, which alters normal development and/or results in abnormal neural structure and/or function; and (3) exposure to teratogens (e.g., poor prenatal nutrition, alcohol) early (i.e., prenatally) in life, many of which are also known to have insidious effects on neurodevelopment.

Overall, the findings from our own and others' work provide strong support for the idea that orphanage rearing, as well as the associated absence of consistent caregiving, has deleterious effects on neurocognitive and socioemotional functioning and on functional and structural neurological development. While we and others have presented evidence that, for many individuals with such histories (particularly if extended), such negative outcomes may be persistent, some individuals emerge from such histories with unimpaired functioning; timing of exposure to the deprived environment is the most robust predictor of outcome. However, additional work is necessary to determine if there exists, and/or to more completely outline parameters for, safe exposure to institutional rearing. We have also presented some data that may indicate that at least some of the effects (i.e., microstructural integrity of white matter, intellect) may improve or normalize as time in the adoptive home increases or in response to early intervention (i.e., placement into foster care). However, to what extent, and to what degree, the effects can be reversed is not yet clear. Future work should attempt to determine if subsequent exposure to enriched environments can reverse (in part or in whole) the effects of inadequate early care and, if so, what the timing (or treatment) parameters that permit, allow, or incite such improvement might be.

Notes

1. The application of statistical parametric mapping (SPM) in children older than six years has been validated in our previous study using the same adult control group (Muzik et al., 2000).

2. We had shown previously (Muzik et al., 2000) that the pattern of glucose metabolism in the hemisphere contralateral to the epileptic focus in this control group did not differ from the pattern in the adult control group.

References

Ames, E. W. (1997). *The development of Romanian orphanage children adopted into Canada.* Final Report to Human Resources Development, Canada. Burnaby, Canada: Simon Fraser University.

Anisman, H., Zaharia, M. D., Meaney, M. J., & Merali, Z. (1998). Do early-life events permanently alter behavioral and hormonal responses to stressors? *International Journal of Developmental Neuroscience, 16,* 149–164.

Balbernie, R. (2001). Circuits and circumstances: The neurobiological consequences of early relationship experiences and how they shape later behaviour. *Journal of Child Psychotherapy, 27,* 237–255.

Barbas, H. (1993). Organization of cortical afferent input to orbitofrontal areas in the rhesus monkey. *Neuroscience, 56,* 841–864.

Barbas, H., & Pandya, D. N. (1989). Architecture and intrinsic connection of the prefrontal cortex in the rhesus monkey (*Macaca mulatta*). *Journal of Comparative Neurology, 286,* 353–375.

Barbas, H., & De Olmos, J. (1990). Projections from the amygdala to basoventral and mediodorsal prefrontal regions in the rhesus monkey. *Journal of Comparative Neurology, 301,* 1–23.

Bates, E. (1999). Plasticity, localization and language development. In S. H. Broman & J. M. Fletcher (Eds.), *The changing nervous system: Neurobehavioral consequences of early brain disorders* (pp. 214–253). New York: Oxford University Press.

Beckett, C., Maughan, B., Rutter, M., Castle, J., Colvert, E., Groothues, C., Kreppner, J., Stevens, S., O'Connor, T. G., & Sonuga-Barke, E. J. (2006). Do the effects of early severe deprivation on cognition persist into early adolescence? Findings from the English and Romanian adoptees study. *Child Development, 77,* 696–711.

Behen, M. E., Helder, E., Rothermel, R., Solomon, K., Chugani, H. T. (2008). Incidence of specific absolute neurocognitive impairment in globally intact children with histories of early severe deprivation. *Child Neuropsychology, 14,* 453–469.

Behen, M. E., Muzik, O., Saporta, A. S., et al. (2009). Abnormal frontostriatal connectivity in children with histories of early deprivation: A diffusion tensor imaging study. *Brain Imaging and Behavior, 3,* 292–297.

Bengtsson, S. L., Nagy, Z., Skare, S., Forsman, L., Forssberg, H., & Ullen, F. (2005). Extensive piano practicing has regionally specific effects on white matter development. *Nature Neuroscience, 8,* 1148–1150.

Bos, K. J., Fox, N., Zeanah, C. H., & Nelson, C. A., III. (2009). Effects of early psychosocial deprivation on the development of memory and executive function. *Frontiers in Behavioral Neuroscience, 3,* 1–17.

Bremner, J. D., & Vermetten, E. (2001). Stress and development: Behavioral and biological consequences. *Developmental Psychopathology, 13*, 473–490.

Campeau, S., & Watson, S. J. (1997). Neuroendocrine and behavioral responses and brain pattern of c-fos induction associated with audiogenic stress. *Journal of Neuroendocrinology, 9*, 577–588.

Card, J. P., Levitt, P., Gluhovsky, M., & Rinaman, L. (2005). Early experience modifies the postnatal assembly of autonomic emotional motor circuits in rats. *Journal of Neuroscience, 25*, 9102–9111.

Carlson, M., & Earls, F. (1997). Psychological and neuroendocrinological sequelae of early social deprivation in institutionalized children in Romania. *Annals of the New York Academy of Sciences, 807*, 419–428.

Chatterjee, D., Chatterjee-Chakraborty, M., Rees, S., Cauchi, J., de Medeiros, C. B., & Fleming, A. S. (2007). Maternal isolation alters the expression of neural proteins during development: 'Stroking' stimulation reverses these effects. *Brain Research, 1158*, 11–27.

Chisholm, K. (1998). A three year follow-up of attachment and indiscriminate friendliness in children adopted from Romanian orphanages. *Child Development, 69*, 1092–1106.

Choi, J., Jeong, B., Rohan, M. L., Polcari, A. M., & Teicher, M. H. (2009). Preliminary evidence for white matter tract abnormalities in young adults exposed to parental verbal abuse. *Biological Psychiatry, 65*, 227–234.

Chu, C. C., Tranel, D., Damasio, A. R., & Van Hoesen, G. W. (1997). The autonomic-related cortex: Pathology in Alzheimer's disease. *Cerebral Cortex, 7*, 86–95.

Chugani, H. T., Behen, M. E., Muzik, O., Juhasz, C., Nagy, F., & Chugani, D. C. (2001). Local brain functional activity following early deprivation: A study of postinstitutionalized Romanian orphans. *NeuroImage, 14*, 1290–1301.

Cordero, M. E., D'Acuna, E., Benveniste, S., Prado, R., Nunez, J. A., & Colombo, M. (1993). Dendritic development in neocortex of infants with early postnatal life undernutrition. *Pediatric Neurology, 9*, 457–464.

Croft, C., Beckett, C., Rutter, M., et al. (2007). Early adolescent outcomes of institutionally-deprived and non-deprived adoptees: II. Language as a protective factor and a vulnerable outcome. *Journal of Child Psychology and Psychiatry, 48*, 31–34.

Cullinan, W. E., Herman, J. P., Battaglia, D. F., Akil, H., & Watson, S. J. (1995). Pattern and time course of immediate early gene expression in rat brain following acute stress. *Neuroscience, 64*, 477–505.

Cullinan, W. E., Helmreich, D. L., & Watson, S. J. (1996). Fos expression in forebrain afferents to the hypothalamic paraventricular nucleus follow swim stress. *Journal of Comparative Neurology, 368*, 88–99.

de Quervain, D. J., Roozendaal, B., Nitsch, R. M., McGaugh, J. L., & Hock, C. (2000). Acute cortisone administration impairs retrieval of long-term declarative memory in humans. *Nature Neuroscience, 3*, 313–314.

Eluvathingal, T. J., Chugani, H. T., Behen, M. E., et al. (2006). Abnormal brain connectivity in children after early severe socioemotional deprivation: A diffusion tensor imaging study. *Pediatrics, 117*, 2093–2100.

Floeter, M. K., & Greenough, W. T. (1979). Cerebellar plasticity: Modification of Purkinje cell structure by differential rearing in monkeys. *Science, 206,* 227–229.

Fox, N. A., Almas, A. N., Degnan, K. A., Nelson, C. A., & Zeanah, C. H. (2011). The effects of severe psychosocial deprivation and foster care intervention on cognitive development at 8 years of age: Findings from the Bucharest Early Intervention Project. *Journal of Child Psychology and Psychiatry, 52,* 919–928.

Freedman, L. J., Insel, T. R., & Smith, Y. (2000). Subcortical projections of area 25 (subgenual cortex) of the macaque monkey. *Journal of Comparative Neurology, 421,* 172–188.

Fries, A. B. W., & Pollak, S. D. (2004). Emotion understanding in postinstitutionalized Eastern European children. *Development and Psychopathology, 16,* 355–370.

Friston, K. J., Holmes, A. P., Worsley, K. J., et al. (1995). Statistical parametric maps in functional imaging: A general approach. *Human Brain Mapping, 2,* 189–210.

Giedd, J. N., Blumenthal, J., Molloy, E., & Castellanos, F. X. (2001). Brain imaging of attention deficit/hyperactivity disorder. *Annals of the New York Academy of Sciences, 931,* 33–49.

Gould, E., Tanapat, P., Rydel, T., & Hastings, N. (2000). Regulation of hippocampal neurogenesis in adulthood. *Biological Psychiatry, 48,* 715–720.

Govindan, R. M., Behen, M. E., Helder, E., Makki, M., & Chugani, H. T. (2010). Altered water diffusivity in cortical association tracts in children with early deprivation identified with Tract-based Spatial Statistics (TBSS). *Cerebral Cortex, 20,* 561–569.

Granados-Rojas, L., Aguilar, A., & Diaz-Cintra, S. (2004). The mossy fiber system of the hippocampal formation is decreased by chronic and postnatal but not by prenatal protein malnutrition in rats. *Nature Neuroscience, 7,* 301–308.

Greenough, W. T., Black, J. E., & Wallace, C. S. (1987). Experience and brain development. *Child Development, 58,* 539–559.

Guerrini, I., Thomson, A. D., & Gurling, H. D. (2007). The importance of alcohol misuse, malnutrition and genetic susceptibility on brain growth and plasticity. *Neuroscience and Biobehavioral Reviews, 31,* 212–220.

Gunnar, M. R., Morison, S. J., Chisholm, K., & Schuder, M. (2001). Salivary cortisol levels in children adopted from Romanian orphanages. *Developmental Psychopathology, 13,* 611–628.

Gunnar, M. R., & van Dulmen, M. (2007). Behavior problems in post-institutionalized internationally-adopted children. *Development & Psychopathology, 19,* 129–148.

Hanson, J. L., Adluru, N., Chung, M. K., Alexander, A. L., Davidson, R. J., & Pollak, S. D. (2013). Early neglect is associated with alterations in white matter integrity and cognitive functioning. *Child Development, 84*(5), 1566–1578.

Harlow, H. F. (1969). Age-mate or peer affectional system. In D. S. Lehrman, R. A. Hinde, & E. Shaw (Eds.), *Advances in the study of behavior* (Vol. 2, pp. 333–383). New York: Academic Press.

Harlow, H. F., Dodswort, R. O., & Harlow, M. K. (1969). Total social isolation in monkeys. *Proceedings of the National Academy of Sciences USA,* 54, 90–96.

Helder, E., Behen, M. E., Wilson, B., Muzik, O., & Chugani, H. T. (2013). Language difficulties in children adopted internationally: Neuropsychological and functional neural correlates. *Child Neuropsychology.* 20(4), 470–492.

Hertz-Pannier, L., Gaillard, W., & Mott, S., et al. (1997). Non invasive assessment of language dominance in children and adolescents with functional MRI: A preliminary study. *Neurology,* 48, 1003–1012.

Higley, J. D., Suomi, S. J., & Linnoila, M. (1992). A longitudinal study of CSF monoamine metabolite and plasma cortisol concentrations in young rhesus monkeys. *Biological Psychiatry,* 32, 127–145.

Hodges, J., & Tizard, B. (1989). Social and family relationships of ex-institutionalized adolescents. *Journal of Child Psychology and Psychiatry,* 30, 77–97.

Hofer, M. A. (1994). Early relationships as regulators of infant physiology and behavior. *Acta Paediatric Supplement,* 397, 9–18.

———. (1996). On the nature and consequences of early loss. *Psychosomatic Medicine,* 58, 570–581.

Hurley, K. M., Herbert, H., Moga, M. M., & Saper, C. B. (1991). Effect projections of the infralimbic cortex of the rat. *Journal of Comparative Neurology,* 308, 249–276.

Judge, S. (2003). Developmental recovery and deficit in children adopted from Eastern European orphanages. *Child Psychiatry and Human Development,* 34, 49–62.

Juffer, F., & van Ijzendoorn, M. H. (2005). Behavior problems and mental health referrals of international adoptees: A meta-analysis. *JAMA,* 293, 2501–2515.

Kaufman, J., Plotsky, P. M., Nemeroff, C. B., & Charney, D. S. (2000). Effects of early adverse experiences on brain structure and function: Clinical implications. *Biological Psychiatry,* 48, 778–790.

Kirksey, A., Morre, D. M., & Wasynczuk, A. Z. (1990). Neuronal development in vitamin B6 deficiency. *Annals of the New York Academy of Sciences,* 585, 202–218.

Kuhn, C., Paul, J., & Schanberg, S. (1990). Endocrine responses to mother–infant separation in developing rats. *Developmental Psychobiology,* 23, 395–410.

Kumar, A., Behen, M. E., Singsoonsud, P., Veenstra, A. L., Wolfe-Christensen, C., Helder, E., & Chugani, H. T. (March 2013). Microstructural abnormalities in language and limbic pathways in orphanage-reared children: A diffusion tensor imaging study. *Journal of Child Neurology,* 29(3), 318–325.

Lee, H. J., Kang, E., Oh, S. H., et al. (2005). Preoperative differences of cerebral metabolism relate to the outcome of cochlear implants in congenitally deaf children. *Hearing Research,* 203, 2–9.

Loman, M. M., Johnson, A. E., Westerlund, A., Pollak, S. D., Nelson, C. A., & Gunnar, M. R. (2013). The effect of early deprivation on executive attention in middle childhood. *Journal of Child Psychology and Psychiatry.* 54, 37–45.

Lopez, J. F., Akil, H., & Watson, S. J. (1999). Role of biological and psychological factors in early development and their impact on adult life. *Biological Psychiatry, 46*, 1461–1471.

Lozoff, B. (2007). Iron deficiency and child development. *Food and Nutrition Bulletin, 28*, S560–S571.

Lupien, S. J., & McEwen, B. S. (1997). The acute effects of corticosteroids on cognition: Integration of animal and human model studies. *Brain Research Reviews, 24*, 1–27.

Maclean, K. (2003). The impact of institutionalization on child developmental. *Developmental Psychopathology, 15*, 853–884.

Marshall, P. J., & Fox, N. A. (2004). A comparison of the electroencephalogram between institutionalized and community children in Romania. *Journal of Cognitive Neuroscience, 16*, 1327–1338.

Marshall, P. J., Reeb, B. C., Fox, N. A., et al. (2008). Effects of early intervention on EEG power and coherence in previously institutionalized children in Romania. *Developmental Psychopathology, 20*, 861–880.

McEwen, B. S. (2000). Effects of adverse experiences for brain structure and function. *Biological Psychiatry, 48*, 721–731.

McEwen, B. S., Wallach, G., & Magnus, C. (1974). Corticosterone binding to hippocampus: Immediate and delayed influences of the absence of adrenal secretion. *Brain Research, 70*, 321–334.

McEwen, B. S., & Sapolsky, R. M. (1995). Stress and cognitive function. *Current Opinion in Neurobiology, 5*, 205–216.

McGoron, L., Gleason, M. M., Smyke, A. T., Drury, S. S., Nelson, C. A., Gregas, M. C., Fox, N. A., & Zeanah, C. H. (2012). Recovering from early deprivation: Attachment mediates effects of caregiving on psychopathology. *Journal of the American Academy of Child Psychiatry, 51*, 683–693.

McLaughlin, K. A., Fox, N. A., Zeanah, C. H., et al. (2010). Delayed maturation in brain electrical activity partially explains the association between early environmental deprivation and symptoms of attention-deficit/hyperactivity disorder. *Biological Psychiatry, 68*, 329–336.

McLaughlin, K. A., Sheridan, M. A., Winter, W., Fox, N. A., Zeanah, C. H., & Nelson, C. A. (2014). Widespread reductions in cortical thickness following severe early-life deprivation: A neurodevelopmental pathway to attention-deficit/hyperactivity disorder. *Biological Psychiatry, 76*(8), 629–638.

Mehta, M. A., Golembo, N. I., Nosarti, C., et al. (2009). Amygdala, hippocampal and corpus callosum size following severe early institutional deprivation: The English and Romanian Adoptees study pilot. *Journal of Child Psychology and Psychiatry, 50*, 943–951.

Merz E. C., & McCall R. B.(2010). Behavior problems in children adopted from psychosocially depriving institutions. *Journal of Abnormal Child Psychology. 38*, 459–470.

Miller, L. C., Chan, W., Litvinova, A., et al. (2006). Fetal alcohol spectrum disorders in children residing in Russian orphanages: A phenotypic study. *Alcoholism: Clinical and Experimental Research, 30*, 531–538.

Morecraft, T. J., Geula, C., & Mesulam, M. M. (1992). Cytoarchitecture and neural afferents of orbitofrontal cortex in the brain of the monkey. *Journal of Comparative Neurology, 323*, 341–358.

Moulson, M. C., Fox, N. A., Zeanah, C. H., & Nelson, C. A. (2009). Early adverse experiences and the neurobiology of facial emotion processing. *Developmental Psychology, 45*, 17–30.

Muzik, O., Chugani, D. C., Juhász, C., Shen, C., & Chugani, H. T. (2000). Statistical parametric mapping: Assessment of application in children. *NeuroImage, 12*, 538–549.

Nakadate, K., Imamura, K., & Watanabe, Y. (2001). Effects of monocular deprivation on the expression pattern of alpha-1 and beta-1 adrenergic receptors in the kitten visual cortex. *Neuroscience Research, 40*, 155–162.

Neafsey, E. J. (1990). Prefrontal cortical control of the autonomic nervous system: Anatomical and physiological observations. *Progress in Brain Research, 85*, 147–165.

Nelson, C. A. (2002). Neural development and life-long plasticity. In R. M. Lerner, F. Jacobs, & D. Wetlieb (Eds.), *Promoting positive child, adolescent, and family development: Handbook of program and policy interventions.* Thousand Oaks, CA: Sage.

Nelson, C. A., Zenah, C. H., Fox, N. A., et al. (2007). Cognitive recovery in socially deprived young children: The Bucharest Early Intervention Project. *Science, 318*, 1937–1940.

Nelson, C. A., Fox, N. A., & Zeanah, C. H. (2013). Growing up in institutions: How deprivation impacts brain and behavioral development. *Scientific American, 308*, 62–67.

Newman, J. D., & Bachevalier, J. (1997). Neonatal ablations of the amygdala and inferior temporal cortex alter the vocal response top social separation in rhesus macaques. *Brain Research, 758*, 180–186.

O'Connor, T. G., & Rutter, M. (2000). Attachment disorder behavior following early severe deprivation: Extension and longitudinal follow-up. *Journal of the American Academy of Child and Adolescent Psychiatry, 39*, 703–712.

O'Connor, T. G., Marvin, R. S., Rutter, M., Olrick, J. T., & Britner, P. A. (2003). English and Romanian Adoptees Study Team: Child-parent attachment following early institutional deprivation. *Developmental Psychopathology, 15*, 19–38.

Parker, S. W., & Nelson, C. A. (2005a). An event-related potential study of the impact of institutional rearing on face recognition. *Developmental Psychopathology, 17*, 621–639.

———. (2005b). Bucharest Early Intervention Project Core Group. The impact of early institutional rearing on the ability to discriminate facial expressions of emotion: an event-related potential study. *Child Development, 76*, 54–72.

Pavuluri, M. N., Yang, S., Kamineni, K., et al. (2009). Diffusion tensor imaging study of white matter fiber tracts in pediatric bipolar disorder and attention-deficit/hyperactivity disorder. *Biological Psychiatry, 65*, 586–593.

Pihoker, C., Owens, M. J., Kuhn, C. M., Schanberg, S. M., & Nemeroff, C. B. (1993). Maternal separation in neonatal rats elicits activation of the hypothalamic-pituitary-adrenal axis: A putative role for corticotropin-releasing factor. *Psychoneuroendocrinology, 18*, 485–493.

Plotsky, P. M., & Meaney, M. J. (1993). Early postnatal experience alters hypothalamic corticotropin-releasing factor (CRF) mRNA, median eminence CRF content and stress-induced release in rats. *Molecular Brain Research, 18*, 195–200.

Reynolds, C. R., & Kamphaus, R. W. (2004). *BASC-2: Behavior assessment system for children, second edition manual.* Circle Pines, MN: American Guidance Service.

Rinaman, L., Levitt, P., & Card, J. P. (2000). Progressive postnatal assembly of limbic-autonomic circuits revealed by central transneuronal transport of pseudorabies virus. *Journal of Neuroscience, 20*, 2731–2741.

Roosendaal, S. D., Geurts, J. J., Vrenken, H., Hulst, H. E., Cover, K. S., Castelijns, J. A., Pouwels, P. J., & Barkhof, F. (2009). Regional DTI differences in multiple sclerosis patients. *NeuroImage, 44*, 1397–1403.

Rutter, M. (1998). Developmental catch-up, and deficit, following adoption after severe global early privation. English and Romanian Adoptees (ERA) Study Team. *Journal of Child Psychology and Psychiatry, 39*, 465–476.

Rutter, M., Bailey, A., & Lord, C. (2003). Social Communication Questionnaire. Los Angeles, CA: Western Psychological Services.

Rutter, M., Beckett, C., & Castle, J. (2007). Effects of profound early institutional deprivation: An overview of findings from a UK longitudinal study of Romanian adoptees. *European Journal of Developmental Psychology, 4*, 332–350.

Rutter, M., & Sonuga-Barke, E. J. (Eds.). (2010). Deprivation-specific psychological patterns: Effects of institutional deprivation. *Monographs of the Society for Research in Child Development, 75*, 1–252.

Rutter, M. L., Krepner, J. M., O'Connor, T. J., & the English and Romanian Adoptees (ERA) Study Team. (2001). Specificity and heterogeneity in children's responses to profound institutional privation. *British Journal of Psychiatry, 179*, 97–103.

Sapolsky, R. M. (2000). Glucocorticoids and hippocampal atrophy in neuropsychiatric disorders. *Archives of General Psychiatry, 57*, 925–935.

Schore, A. N. (1994). *Affect regulation and the origin of the self: The neurobiology of emotional development.* Mahwah, NJ: Erlbaum.

Scott, K., Roberts, J., & Glennen, S. (2011). How well do children who are internationally adopted acquire language? A meta-analysis. *Journal of Speech, Language, and Hearing Research, 54*, 1153–1169.

Selye, H. (1936). A syndrome produced by diverse nocuous agents. *Nature, 138*, 32.

Sharma, A., Dorman, M. F., & Kral, A. (2005). The influence of a sensitive period on central auditory development in children with unilateral and bilateral cochlear implants. *Hearing Research, 203*, 134–143.

Shaw, P., Eckstrand, K., & Sharp, W. (2007). Attention-deficit/hyperactivity disorder is characterized by a delay in cortical maturation. *Proceedings of the National Academy of Sciences USA, 104*, 19649–19654.

Sheridan, M., Drury, S., McLaughlin, K., & Almas, A. (2010). Early institutionalization: neurobiological consequences and genetic modifiers. *Neuropsychology Review, 20,* 414–429.

Shimony, J. S., Burton, H., Epstein, A. A., McLaren, D. G., Sun, S. W., & Snyder, A. Z. (2006). Diffusion tensor imaging reveals white matter reorganization in early blind humans. *Cerebral Cortex, 16,* 1653–1661.

Shu, N., Liu, Y., Li, J., Li, Y., Yu, C., & Jiang, T. (2009). Altered anatomical network in early blindness revealed by diffusion tensor tractrography. *PLoS ONE, 4,* e7228.

Siegel, S. J., Ginsberg, S. D., Hof, P. R., et al. (1993). Effects of social deprivation in prepubescent rhesus monkeys: Immunohistochemical analysis of the neurofilament protein triplet in the hippocampal formation. *Brain Research, 619,* 299–305.

Smith, S. M., Jenkinson, M., & Johansen-Berg, H. (2006). Tract-based spatial statistics: Voxelwise analysis of multi-subject diffusion data. *NeuroImage, 31,* 1487–1505.

Smyke, A. T., Zeanah, C. H., Fox, N. A., Nelson, C. A., & Guthrie, D. (2010). Placement in foster care enhances quality of attachment among young institutionalized children. *Child Development, 81,* 212–223.

Sonuga-Barke, E. J., Schlotz, W., & Kreppner, J. V. (2010). Differentiating developmental trajectories for conduct, emotion, and peer problems following early deprivation. *Monographs of the Society for Research in Child Development, 75,* 102–124.

Spadoni, A. D., McGee, C. L., Fryer, S. L., & Riley, E. P. (2007). Neuroimaging and fetal alcohol spectrum disorders. *Neuroscience and Biobehavior Review, 31,* 239–245.

Spitz, R. A. (1945). Hospitalism—an inquiry into the genesis of psychiatric conditions in early childhood. *Psychoanalytic Study of the Child, 1,* 53–74.

Stevens, S. E., Sonuga-Barke, E. J., & Kreppner, J. M. (2008). Inattention/overactivity following early severe institutional deprivation: presentation and associations in early adolescence. *Journal of Abnormal Child Psychology, 36,* 385–398.

Stricker, N. H., Schweinsburg, B. C., & Delano-Wood, L. (2009). Decreased white matter integrity in late-myelinating fiber pathways in Alzheimer's disease supports retrogenesis. *NeuroImage, 45,* 10–16.

Struble, R. G., & Riesen, A. H. (1978). Changes in cortical dendritic branching subsequent to partial social isolation in stumptailed monkeys. *Developmental Psychobiology, 11,* 479–486.

Suomi, S. J. (1997). Early determinants of behavior: Evidence from primate studies. *British Medical Bulletin, 53,* 170–184.

Tizard, B., & Hodges, J. (1978). The effect of early institutional rearing on the development of eight year old children. *Journal of Child Psychology and Psychiatry, 19,* 99–118.

Tottenham, N. H. T., Quinn, B. T., McCarry, T. W., et al. (2010). Prolonged institutional rearing is associated with atypically larger amygdala volume and difficulties in emotion regulation. *Developmental Science, 13,* 46–61.

Van den Bergh, B. R., Mulder, E. J., Mennes, M., & Glover, V. (2005). Antenatal maternal anxiety and stress and the neurobehavioural development of the fetus and child: Links and possible mechanisms. A review. *Neuroscience and Biobehavioral Review, 29,* 237–258.

Vandermeeren, Y., Bastings, E., Good, D., Rouiller, E., & Olivier, E. (2003). Plasticity of motor maps in primates: Recent advances and therapeutical perspectives. *Review of Neurology (Paris), 159,* 259–275.

Versace, A., Almeida, J. R., & Hassel, S. (2008). Elevated left and reduced right orbitomedial prefrontal fractional anisotropy in adults with bipolar disorder revealed by tract-based spatial statistics. *Archives of General Psychiatry, 65,* 1041–1052.

Wiik, K. L., Loman, M. M., Van Ryzin, M. J., Armstrong, J. M., Essex, M. J., Pollak, S. D., & Gunnar, M. R. (2011). Behavioral and emotional symptoms of post-institutionalized children in middle childhood. *Journal of Child Psychology and Psychiatry, 52,* 56–63.

Windsor, J., Glaze, L. E., & Koga, S. F. (2007). Language acquisition with limited input: Romanian institution and foster care. *Journal of Speech, Language, and Hearing Research, 50,* 1365–1381.

Zeanah, C. H., Smyke, A. T., Koga, S. F., & Carlson, E. (2005). Attachment in institutionalized and community children in Romania. Bucharest Early Intervention Project Core Group. *Child Development, 76,* 1015–1028.

13.

Violence, Cognition, and Neighborhood Inequality in America

Patrick Sharkey and Robert J. Sampson

INTERPERSONAL VIOLENCE IS one of the most pressing, and most unique, American public health problems. While petty crimes occur around the world, when it comes to lethal violence, the United States far outpaces other Western nations, with homicide rates many times greater (Zimring & Hawkins, 1999). Moreover, unlike most of the nation's leading causes of mortality, violence disproportionately targets young people. Homicide is the second leading cause of death among all fifteen- to twenty-four-year olds, for example, and it is the leading cause of death among African American young people (Heron, 2012).

But figures on lives lost do not reveal the deeply contextualized nature of violence as a social phenomenon. Violence is divided by place, with sharply uneven distributions across the nation's neighborhoods, towns, and cities (Sampson, 2012). There are some communities where incidents of extreme violence are extremely rare, where serious fights rarely break out in public spaces, the sound of gunshots is unfamiliar, and the sight of a gunshot victim is unknown. In other communities, the potential for violence is a regular part of daily life. In these communities, the threat of violence structures interactions in public spaces such as parks, streets, and schools (Anderson, 2000). The sound of gunshots is familiar to children, and the chaotic aftermath of extreme violence is a common scene. The spatial concentration of violence maps onto the concentration of a range of social phenomena, from poverty to racial segregation to birth weight (Sampson, 2003).

The spatial organization of violence focuses our attention on the way that incidents of interpersonal violence reverberate around communities, a feature that makes violence different from most other public health problems. Although interpersonal violence involves a physical act inflicted by an individual upon another individual, the effects of that act extend well beyond the victim and perpetrator. Individuals who witness extreme acts of violence directly are more likely to experience symptoms of posttraumatic stress disorder and to behave violently themselves (Bingenheimer et al., 2005; Pynoos et al., 1987). In the aftermath of an incident of violence, children in the surrounding residential setting exhibit impaired cognitive functioning and self-regulatory behavior (Sharkey, 2010; Sharkey et al., 2012). Exposure to community violence over an extended period of time has effects that are similar to other traumatic events or stressors in children's lives, with consequences that extend across a range of social-emotional, behavioral, and cognitive domains (Osofsky, 1999; Margolin & Gordis, 2004).

The impact of violence is not limited to the communities where it is concentrated. Violence exacerbates urban inequality by altering social life in the most disadvantaged communities, creating an added layer of risk that amplifies the effects of economic and racial segregation. Avoiding violence and associated problems like gangs and drugs is the most common reason why families living in high-poverty public housing projects sign up for mobility programs that give them the chance to move elsewhere (Kling, Liebman, & Katz, 2007). Rising levels of violent crime are linked with neighborhood and city depopulation, suggesting that violence plays a role in generating neighborhood inequality through processes of sorting and residential mobility (Morenoff & Sampson, 1997). The same processes of sorting serve to concentrate economic and social disadvantage, providing the context for diminished community capacity to contain violent crime (Sampson, Raudenbush, & Earls, 1997).

Violence is thus interwoven with urban inequality and constitutes a central force behind the great urban divide in American cities: violence *generates* urban inequality and is *generated by* urban inequality. It is a phenomenon that is fundamentally corporal and fundamentally social. An incident of violence is a physical act creating bodily harm or death. But the act of violence is only possible when a motivated offender and a vulnerable victim converge in time and in a space that lacks a capable guardian (Cohen & Felson, 1979). The sequence of violence may involve bloodshed and death but occurs within networks of individuals linked to groups that are concentrated in space (Block & Block, 1995; Papachristos, 2011).

The case of violence reveals in a very unique and powerful manner the way that social and biological processes are interwoven together. Violence reveals the limitations of approaches to health and inequality that focus attention on the individual body, without placing the individual in a larger context. At the same time, violence reveals the limitations of sociological efforts to understand social inequality while ignoring the body, the brain, and the biological processes that help to illuminate how social processes work.

In this chapter, we trace the connections between the social and biological dimensions of violence, and we situate the study of violence within the context of individuals, networks, neighborhoods, and cities. We describe the most convincing evidence on the full toll of violence, as well as the physiological and social mechanisms by which its consequences emerge. We proceed by documenting the ways that interpersonal violence is generated by and generates urban inequality. We conclude on a more hopeful note by focusing on one of the most dramatic changes in the nation's public health, and the nation's urban communities, over the past several decades: the decline in violent crime. After describing the scale of the crime decline, we present a series of questions about what the decline in violence might mean for urban inequality in America.

The Full Toll of Violence

What happens when a child is faced with the threat of violence? To move toward an answer requires a more general description of the set of behavioral and physiological responses to any source of environmental stress (McEwen, 1998). Information about external stressors is transmitted to the amygdala, the area of the brain associated with emotional processing, which activates the stress response system. Activation of the sympathetic nervous system leads to a set of physiological changes arising in response to a surge of adrenaline, including elevated heart rate and blood pressure. Activation of the HPA axis, which is composed of the hypothalamus, the pituitary gland, and the adrenal glands, leads to the release of the hormone cortisol, which maintains vigilance in the face of a continuing stressor in the environment. As the threat passes, the parasympathetic nervous system acts to return the body to its normal state.

Although adaptive in the face of an immediate threat, this complex response to stress has costs. Persistent activation of the stress response system leads to long-term changes in the way that the brain and body process information from the external environment and increased "wear and tear" on the body, as represented with the concept of "allostatic load" (Lupien et al., 2009; McEwen and Wingfield, 2003; McEwen 2004). Exposure to chronic environmental stress leads to elevated risk of mental health problems such as anxiety and depression as well as physical health problems such as hypertension, obesity, and compromised immune function (McEwen, 2003; Rodrigues et al., 2009; Sapolsky et al., 2000).

A Biosocial Model of Urban Stratification

What does this mean for children living in violent environments? Extending the literature from developmental psychology and neuroscience on stress response, Massey (2004) proposes a "biosocial" model of social stratification that makes the link between the spatial concentration of violence and the reproduction of racial inequality. There are three elements of Massey's conceptual model.

In the first part of the model, the combination of social inequality and racial and economic segregation allows for the emergence of areas of concentrated disadvantage and violence (Sampson & Wilson, 1995). The works of urban historians and sociologists have documented the ways in which political, social, and economic forces converge to maintain the stratification of urban neighborhoods by race/ethnicity and economic status (Dreier et al., 2001; Massey & Denton, 1993; Sharkey, 2013). Examples reflect explicit attempts to create physical separation between white and nonwhite communities, such as the policy of urban renewal and public housing development that served to concentrate expanding black populations within rigidly constrained sections of cities (Massey & Denton, 1993). Other examples reflect passive policies that have allowed discrimination by race/ethnicity and income to continue in the private housing and lending markets (Goering, 2007; Turner & Ross, 2005).

Although the level of racial segregation in America's urban areas has declined since the 1970s, black Americans remain isolated in communities that feature concentrated poverty and elevated rates of crime and violence. The racial stratification of America's urban neighborhoods is not explained by group differences in income or wealth. For instance, Sharkey (2014) finds that the average level of disadvantage in the neighborhoods of black Americans earning at least $100,000 or more annual income is greater than the level of disadvantage in the neighborhoods of white Americans making $30,000 or less in annual income (see also Logan, 2011). This is possible because of three types of segregation: segregation of all neighborhoods by economic status, segregation of black Americans from other racial and ethnic groups with higher average income, and acute segregation of high-income black Americans from high-income members of other racial and ethnic groups (Quillian, 2012).

Whereas the segregation of black Americans has declined slightly over the past few decades, segregation by income has risen steadily over time (Reardon & Bischoff, 2011). At the bottom of the distribution, this trend has resulted in a new form of concentrated poverty that is most prevalent in central cities but has spread to suburbs as well (Kneebone & Berube, 2008, 2013; Wilson, 1987). As described in more detail in the following section, areas where poverty is concentrated provide a spatial niche where community organization, institutional strength, and the connections between community residents and key institutions like the police begin to break down. In the absence of informal social controls and functioning institutions, spatially concentrated violent crime is likely to emerge.

In the second component of Massey's conceptual model, the spatial concentration of violence creates an environment in which the threat of victimization is constant, creating the conditions for chronic stress among residents within the area. In his ethnographic work in Boston, David Harding (2010) describes how the threat of victimization leads young people to form networks that are designed to provide protection in public space by spanning across age groups. These cross-age networks serve to expose young boys to the risky activities and behaviors more typical among older adolescents and teens. Elijah Anderson (2000) documents the daily challenges faced by youth living in areas of intensely violent sections of Philadelphia during the mid-1990s. In the neighborhoods studied by Anderson, the potential for violence structures routine interactions and forces children to develop adaptive patterns of behavior that provide protection and limit the likelihood of victimization. Where the threat of violent confrontation is always present, a new status system emerges along with a code of behavior that is required in order to navigate urban streets while mitigating the potential for danger.

The role of violence as a source of environmental stress leads us to the third component of Massey's biosocial model. Massey argues that allostatic load associated with life within the chaotic and violent American ghetto translates into elevated rates of physical and mental health problems, deficits in cognitive skill development, and disrupted capacity for learning. A recent strand of research provides evidence in support of this idea by focusing on the way that specific incidents of extreme violence get into the minds of children to affect cognitive functioning and behavior in the school setting, with consequences for short-term academic performance and long-term developmental trajectories.

Evidence on Effects of Exposure to Violence

Identifying the effects of violence is challenging, because violence is not randomly dispersed across urban neighborhoods and cannot be reproduced in a laboratory setting. For this reason, analyses that compare the outcomes of children who live in more or less violent settings are susceptible to the problem of selection bias. Differences in outcomes related to cognitive skills or academic outcomes among children living in neighborhoods with varying levels of violence could be driven by exposure to violence or by unobserved characteristics of families that lead them into certain neighborhoods and that also may affect the outcomes of children.

To confront this problem, a set of recent studies analyzed variation in the timing of exposure to incidents of violence among children living within the same communities. As an example, Sharkey (2010) analyzed African American children's performance on two assessments of verbal and language skills from the Project on Human Development in Chicago Neighborhoods. The study exploits the fact that the sample of children was clustered in a select set of neighborhoods within Chicago and was interviewed over a period of several months, beginning in 1994. Data on local violence, measured with police reports on the timing and location of homicides, were merged together with the survey data based on the location of homicides and the location of children's residential addresses. Using neighborhood fixed effects analysis to make comparisons among children living within the same areas, the study finds that children who were assessed within a week of a homicide that occurred close to the home performed substantially worse on the assessments of cognitive skills. The scores of children exposed to a recent homicide in their census block group were roughly one-half standard deviation lower than those of other children, living in the same block group, who were assessed at a time when no local violence had taken place in the period prior to the interview. This finding was replicated in a second, independent data set conducted over the same timeframe in Chicago but using different assessments of cognitive skills.

Subsequent research using the same approach provides additional evidence indicating that the burden of local violence is brought into the classroom to affect children's behavior and performance in school. In a second study also conducted with a sample of children in Chicago, Sharkey et al. (2012) found that children exposed to a homicide in close proximity to their home exhibited lower levels of attention and impulse control within the classroom setting. A third study conducted with the population of public school students in New York City showed that African American children exposed to a violent crime on their own blockface in the week before city-wide standardized exams were 3 percentage points less likely to pass the English/language arts exam compared with African American students exposed to a violent crime on their blockface that occurred in the week after the exam (Sharkey et al., 2013).

This research provides more concrete evidence demonstrating that specific incidents of violent crime alter children's capacity to regulate their behavior, to maintain attention, and to succeed on high-stakes assessments of academic achievement. The research does not reveal the specific mechanisms leading to compromised functioning within the school setting. The literature on stress response described previously suggests that exposure to acute violence affects performance in the school setting through several possible mechanisms arising from physiological, social, and emotional responses to acute environmental stress (McEwen & Sapolsky, 1995; LeDoux, 2000). These responses to acute environmental stress may be linked with outcomes related to cognitive functioning and academic functioning through their impact on symptoms of acute stress disorder (e.g., inability to concentrate, difficulty sleeping), psychosocial effects (e.g., internalizing or externalizing behaviors, aggression), or other coping mechanisms (e.g., substance abuse or dissociation) (Buka et al,. 2001; Martinez & Richters, 1993; Pynoos et al., 1987).

The result is students who are unable to regulate their behavior and perform at a high level when they enter the classroom. The consequences are not limited to the days or weeks after an incident of violence occurs but accumulate to alter children's academic trajectories. Extended exposure to community violence is associated with deficits in the development of cognitive skills and reading achievement (Delaney-Black et al., 2002), along with lower grades, elevated levels of nonattendance (Hurt et al., 2001; Bowen & Bowen, 1999), and lower rates of high school graduation and college attendance (Grogger, 1997).

The effects of violence are not limited to academic or cognitive outcomes of children. But the evidence generated on these outcomes provides a concrete example of how violence in the community makes its way into the school setting, altering children's capacity to learn and impeding the development of cognitive skills that are essential for a successful transition into early adulthood. As a result of this process, the disadvantaged position of children raised in areas of concentrated violence is reproduced.

Violence and Neighborhood Inequality

A cornerstone of our argument is that violence generates urban inequality and is generated by urban inequality. These twin forces reinforce the spatial segmentation of American cities and, in turn, cognitive inequalities. The evidence on the clustering of violence and indicators of urban disadvantage is vast and has been reviewed at length elsewhere. The following facts will suffice for present purposes: first, there is considerable social inequality between neighborhoods, especially in terms of socioeconomic position and racial/ethnic segregation. Second, these factors are connected in that concentrated disadvantage often coincides with the geographic isolation of racial minority and immigrant groups. Third, violence and a number of health-related problems tend to come bundled together at the neighborhood level and are predicted by neighborhood characteristics such as the concentration of poverty, racial isolation, single-parent families, and, to a lesser extent, rates of residential and housing instability. Fourth, a number of social indicators at the upper end of what many would consider progress, such as affluence, computer literacy, and elite occupational attainment, are also clustered geographically (Sampson, 2012; Sampson, Morenoff, & Gannon-Rowley, 2002).

Concentrated inequality undermines neighborhood social organization, especially the collective efficacy of residents. Sampson et al. (1997) define collective efficacy as the combination of shared expectations for informal social control and social cohesion. While concentrated poverty is directly related to lower collective efficacy, in communities that are otherwise similar in demographic and economic composition, those with higher levels of collective efficacy exhibit lower rates of violence (Sampson et al., 2002; Sampson, 2012). There is also evidence that collective efficacy predicts future variations in violence, adjusting for the aggregated characteristics of individuals and traditional forms of neighbor networks. Although more infrequently studied, highly efficacious communities seem to do better along a number of other dimensions besides crime, such as birth weight, teen pregnancy, asthma, and mortality, suggesting a link to the general concept of population well-being. In brief, the evidence suggests that indicators of neighborhood social organization, such as collective efficacy, partially mediate the effects of urban inequality on rates of violence and general well-being. But as we now examine, there is evidence of a kind of "reverse" effect of violence on inequality and neighborhood social organization.

The Role of Crime and Violence in Generating Urban Inequality

Beginning about 1965, which Robert Putnam argues is the point of decline of American civic life (Putnam, 2000), crime rates began a rapid ascent in American cities. Violence in particular rose to unprecedented heights and fluctuated at high levels in the 1970s and 1980s and again in the early 1990s, a period that saw considerable increases in the concentration of poverty. Yet violence and disorder, unmentioned as major suspects by Putnam, have been overlooked in the feedback processes that helped to perpetuate poverty traps, especially in precipitating selective outmigration from central cities burdened with high rates of victimization. In particular, violence has been argued to trigger the withdrawal of businesses and middle-class families from inner-city areas, which may have fueled more violence and a deepening of poverty and neighborhood inequality. As Sampson (2012, p. 143) argues, neighborhoods with highly visible signs of physical disorder are especially prone to developing reputations as places to be avoided. The consequences of such stigmatization combine with the historical legacy in U.S. cities, where racial segregation and poverty are bound up with patterns of disinvestment. A form of self-fulfilling prophecy takes place: residents acting on their perceptions of crime and disorder undertake actions that have the effect of increasing that disorder and crime.

The result is a reinforcing cycle of urban inequality, violence, and disorder. Studying Chicago neighborhoods, Bursik (1986, p. 73) found that "although changes in racial composition cause increases in the delinquency rate, this effect is not nearly as great as the effect that increases in the delinquency rate have in minority groups being stranded in the community." In a study of forty neighborhoods in eight cities, Skogan (1990) found that high rates of crime and disorder were associated with higher rates of fear, neighborhood dissatisfaction, and intentions to move out. Morenoff and Sampson (1997) showed that increases in violent crime and proximity to violence contributed to population loss and decline of neighborhoods in Chicago. The effect of crime on population loss is also observed at the city level. In a study conducted over twenty years ago, Sampson (1986) showed that increases in homicide were strongly associated with population decline and increases in the poverty of the black population in major U.S. cities. A later study found that robbery rates played a significant role in white flight from central cities, in turn increasing racially segregated poverty (Liska & Bellair, 1995). These results are independent of the usual demographic predictors of urban change. More recent evidence shows that collective perceptions of disorder are related to increases in later poverty, independent of rates of observed disorder and even prior rates of poverty itself (Sampson, 2012, p. 145).

Collective efficacy also appears to be bound up with cycles of urban change. For example, Sampson (2012, pp. 176–177) found that collective efficacy was significantly lower in neighborhoods characterized by concentrated disadvantage and high crime rates (controlling for numerous other neighborhood characteristics). Controlling for prior collective efficacy, prior crime continued to be important, suggesting that *changes* in collective efficacy over time are in part a response to prior experiences with crime and exposure to violence.

We have described community violence, collective efficacy, disorder, concentrated poverty, and racial segregation as reciprocally related in a kind of feedback loop. In the following section, we turn to a converging strand of research that provides further insight on the mechanisms by which the cycle of violence and social disadvantage represents a consistent source of toxic stress that impairs children's functioning and behavior and alters everyday activities and interpersonal interactions in public streets, parks, and schools.

Violence as a Mechanism for Neighborhood Effects

Ronald Wilson and Brent Mast (2014) recently reviewed evidence on the most common reasons for neighborhood dissatisfaction among low-income families. In virtually every study they reviewed, Wilson and Mast found that concerns about crime and violence were the primary reasons why families wanted to leave their communities.

The sentiments of families are consistent with the empirical literature on why growing up in a highly disadvantaged environment affects the behaviors, networks, and developmental outcomes of youth. To supplement ethnographic data collected in Boston, Harding (2009) drew on data from the National Longitudinal Study of Adolescent Health (Add Health) to assess the degree to which neighborhood violence mediates the relationship between structural disadvantage and key developmental outcomes like high school graduation or teenage pregnancy. Neighborhood violence was found to be a strong predictor of each outcome for girls and for boys, after adjusting for an array of individual- and family-level controls. Violence in the neighborhood also was found to mediate the effects of neighborhood disadvantage, particularly in models of high school graduation. For boys, about half of the conditional association between neighborhood disadvantage and high school graduation was explained by neighborhood violence.

For girls, the relationship between disadvantage and graduation was almost entirely explained by neighborhood violence.

One of the important insights arising from Harding's analysis is that the impact of violence is not limited to the groups most directly linked with violent activity and victimization. Despite the fact that boys are much more likely to be involved with violent activity and victimized, Harding found that community violence may be even more salient for girls than for boys. This result is consistent with findings from the Moving to Opportunity (MTO) program, a social experiment that randomly offered vouchers to public housing residents in five cities that allowed them to move to low-poverty neighborhoods. Across numerous domains of child development, the experiment produced the largest changes in the lives of girls, not boys. In particular, girls in families that moved to low-poverty neighborhoods reported feeling safer in their new communities, and ethnographic research suggested that "freedom from fear" was the most important change experienced by girls (Clampet-Lundquist et al., 2011; Popkin et al., 2008).

The conclusion from Harding's analysis is that "violence is a critical social characteristic of disadvantaged neighborhoods, explaining a sizable portion of the effects of such neighborhoods" (Harding, 2009, p. 11). This conclusion is reinforced by evidence from a very different analysis that exploits a set of observational and experimental studies to understand why neighborhood disadvantage has been found to be harmful for youths' developmental trajectories in some studies but not others.

The analysis was the result of a collaborative effort designed to review evidence from several mobility experiments and one major observational study, all focusing on the effects of exposure to neighborhoods with concentrated disadvantage or poverty on children's cognitive skills (Burdick-Will et al., 2011). A summary of the core findings of the study is shown in Figure 13.1. The figure displays results from five roughly comparable estimates of the effect of moving out of a highly disadvantaged or poor neighborhood on children's verbal, reading, or language skills, all of which are displayed on a common metric.

The estimate on the far left of the figure is based on data on African American youth from the Project on Human Development in Chicago Neighborhoods (PHDCN), an observational study of child development within neighborhoods of Chicago (Sampson, Sharkey, & Raudenbush, 2008). In this study, moving out of highly disadvantaged neighborhoods within Chicago was found to improve black children's verbal ability by roughly .25 standard deviations, a positive and substantively large effect. The second estimate, labeled "CHAC Public Housing," is based on data from a natural experiment arising when the firm administering Chicago's

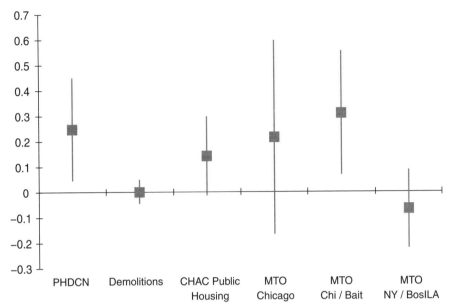

FIGURE 13.1. Summary of effects of different studies on children's verbal test scores. Source: Burdick-Will et al. (2011, p. 61).

housing voucher program opened their wait list for housing and randomized applicants for housing vouchers to positions on the wait list (Ludwig et al., 2010). Families receiving vouchers made moves that led to declines in neighborhood poverty very similar to those made through the MTO program. The estimated effect on language/reading scores (the y-axis reflects the effect size in terms of standard deviations of the test score distribution) of moving to lower-poverty neighborhoods in this experiment was just under .2 standard deviations.

The third estimate is based on data from the Chicago sample of MTO. Previously published research from MTO that pooled data from all five sites (Baltimore, Boston, Chicago, Los Angeles, and New York) found no statistically significant impacts on reading or math test scores measured four to seven years after the program was implemented (Sanbonmatsu et al., 2006). One possible reason why MTO might have produced discrepant results compared to other studies is that MTO was conducted in five very different cities. The third estimate in Figure 13.1 shows that when the sample is limited to MTO families in Chicago, the estimated effects are very similar to the estimates from the two other studies. The small sample from Chicago leads to a less precise estimate, but the magnitude of the effect size is very close to the effect sizes in the other two studies. Subsequent analysis has showed that the estimated effects of moving out of high-poverty neighborhoods were similarly large in the Chicago and Baltimore sites, but there were no effects for families in the Boston, Los Angeles, or New York sites (Burdick-Will et al., 2011).

To assess *why* moving out of high-poverty neighborhoods seemed to improve children's cognitive skills development in some cities and not others, an additional set of exploratory analyses was conducted using variation in program effects across the five sites of MTO (Burdick-Will et al., 2011). Two findings emerged from this analysis. First, children who showed the largest improvements in cognitive skills were those who moved out of the most severely disadvantaged environments. Out of the five cities in which Moving to Opportunity was conducted, Baltimore and Chicago featured neighborhoods that had a level of concentrated poverty and racial segregation on a different scale than in Boston, New York, and Los Angeles, the other MTO sites.

Second, and more relevant for the purposes of this chapter, children's test scores improved most when their mobility led to major changes in their exposure to local violent crime, as measured by police beats or districts. Baltimore and Chicago, the two MTO cities that produced the largest effects on cognitive test scores, have much higher levels of violent crime than the other three MTO cities: 1998 homicide rates per 100,000 equaled 47.1 in Baltimore and 25.6 in Chicago, compared with 6.1 in Boston, 11.8 in Los Angeles, and 8.6 in New York City. Figure 13.2 shows the average effect size generated by the experiment on tests of reading skills for fifteen different groups—three groups within each of the five cities of MTO. These effect sizes are plotted against the average change in community violent crime generated by the experiment, which is displayed on the x-axis. The shape of these data points shows very clearly that the groups of youth who experienced the largest declines in exposure to local violent crime were the groups that experienced the largest improvements in cognitive skills. In this sense, the finding that families in the Baltimore and Chicago sites experienced the largest changes in community levels of violent crime may be crucial to understanding why the children in these families experienced such improvements in their performance on tests of cognitive skills.

Evidence from MTO is based on fifteen data points representing the different configurations of two treatment groups and one control group from five cities across the country and should be seen as suggestive, not definitive. Still, the argument for violence as a primary mechanism linking neighborhood disadvantage with children's developmental trajectories is supported not only with data from MTO but also with Harding's (2009) analysis of a nationally representative data set and with several rich ethnographic studies of everyday life in the most disadvantaged urban neighborhoods.

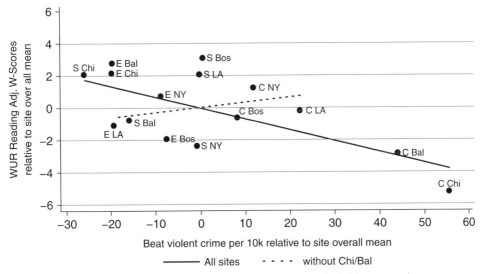

FIGURE 13.2. Relationship between violent crime and children's reading test scores across MTO demonstration cities and randomized mobility groups. Source: Burdick-Will et al. (2011, p. 271).

The conclusion from this research is that one primary way that neighborhood disadvantage becomes salient in the lives of youth is by exposing them to high levels of community violence.

Neighborhood Effects in a Less Violent Nation

In this chapter, we have argued that community violence is a primary reason why growing up in in a neighborhood characterized by poverty, segregation, low collective efficacy, and physically disorder is linked with negative developmental outcomes. Exposure to incidents of extreme violence impairs self-regulatory behavior, cognitive functioning, and academic performance. Over an extended period, living within an intensely violent neighborhood affects child health, brain development, cognitive skills development, and academic performance. Further, we have pointed to evidence suggesting that moving out of violent environments has substantial developmental consequences for young people. When children in the Moving to Opportunity experiment exited extremely violent neighborhoods, their scores on tests of cognitive skills improved substantially.

If our argument is valid, then one would think that dramatic changes in the level of violent crime within a community, a state, or the nation as a whole should have important implications for child development and for childhood inequality in America. Over the past twenty years, the United States has experienced exactly this type of change in the level of violence. According to data from the Federal Bureau of Investigation's (FBI's) Uniform Crime Reports, there were about 25,000 homicides in the United States in 1991. In 2010, there were about 15,000 homicides across the entire nation. Over the same timeframe, the population in the United States increased, meaning the rate of homicides per 10,000 people declined by more than half, dropping from 9.8 in 1991 to 4.8 in 2010 (FBI, 2013). Similar declines have occurred for every type of violent crime, from robbery to rape. Although there have been other large drops in crime that have taken place over the past forty years or so in the United States, what distinguishes the most recent crime drop is its duration (Zimring, 2007). Crime began dropping in the early 1990s and has continued to decline, at a steady pace, through the end of the 2000s.

Data on reported crime from the FBI are reinforced by national surveys of victimization. In 1993, 80 out of every 1,000 Americans were the victims of violent crimes, according to the National Crime Victimization Survey. By 2011, the rate of violent victimization had dropped to about 23 out of every 1,000 Americans. Violent victimization has dropped for every racial and ethnic group at all levels of income. Among individuals in households making less than $7,500 per year, the rate of violent victimization has dropped from 123 victims per 1,000 individuals in 1993 to 53 victims per 1,000 individuals in 2011 (Bureau of Justice Statistics, 2013).

The crime decline has occurred across most of the country, but not in a uniform fashion. Ingrid Gould Ellen and Katherine O'Regan (2009) show that the largest drops in crime occurred in large cities with relatively high levels of poverty and high concentrations of racial and ethnic minorities, as well as in places where crime was highest in the early 1990s. The implication is that the impact of the crime decline has been most pronounced in places where the problem of violent crime was most severe in the 1990s. At the start of the 1990s, the average African American and Hispanic city-dweller lived in a city with a substantially higher rate of crime than the average white city-dweller. By 2000, the average Hispanic city-dweller lived in a city with a slightly *lower* crime rate than the average white city-dweller, and the city crime rate for the average African American was only slightly higher (Ellen & O'Regan, 2009).

All of the data on crime and victimization indicate that American children are now growing up in a nation that is much less violent than it was two decades ago. This development should have major implications for child development, academic achievement, neighborhood effects, and childhood inequality. Yet virtually all of the research on America's crime decline has focused on the magnitude and the causes of the national drop in crime and not on its consequences. In addition, although violence has declined, it remains sharply divided in its spatial distribution. Relative variations in the experience of traumatic violent events may also still be consequential, especially for children. Imagine, for example, how the worldviews of children and adolescents living in a distressed Chicago neighborhood may have changed after thirteen people were gunned down playing in a public park, including a three-year-old shot in the face by a gunman wielding an assault rifle (Davey & Williams, 2013). Violence in Chicago may be down in the aggregate, but events like this, which are out of sight and out of mind for most communities, cannot be ignored.

We therefore argue that a new research agenda is necessary to understand the implications of the crime decline for inequality in America. This agenda begins with empirical questions at multiple levels of analysis, including the following: How is cross-national variation in crime trends linked with cross-national changes in academic achievement? Are the states that experienced the largest declines in crime the states that experienced the greatest gains in academic achievement and the largest declines in achievement gaps? Looking at communities within cities, have children in the neighborhoods where crime has declined the most achieved the largest improvements in cognitive skills and academic achievement? In cities experiencing the largest declines in crime, have the negative effects of growing up in the most disadvantaged neighborhoods become weaker over the past two decades? Or are relative variations what count, such that the magnitude of decline is less important than continuing spatial inequality in violence and fear?

The logic of our argument also stresses the importance of examining how policy interventions, especially place-based initiatives (e.g., the Harlem Children's Zone or the Obama administration's "Promise Zones") and voucher-based interventions (e.g., MTO), interact with the crime decline. For example, do children whose families move to areas declining in crime do better than children who move to otherwise similar areas where violence remains entrenched? What role does exposure to violence play in our understanding of the effects of the Harlem Children's Zone on learning outcomes? Attention to these questions will go a long way toward addressing and potentially ameliorating the cognitive inequalities that have for too long characterized the urban landscape in American cities.

References

Anderson, E. (2000). *Code of the street: Decency, violence, and the moral life of the inner city.* New York: W. W. Norton.

Bingenheimer, J. B., Brennan, R. T., & Earls, F. J. (2005). Firearm violence exposure and serious violent behavior. *Science, 308*(5726), 1323–1326.

Block, R., & Block, C. R. (1995). Space, place and crime: Hot spot areas and hot places of liquor-related crime. In J. E. Eck & D. Weisburd (Eds.), *Crime and place* (Crime Prevention Studies, Vol. 4, pp. 145–183). Washington, DC: Criminal Justice Press.

Bowen, N. K., & Bowen, G. L. (1999). Effects of crime and violence in neighborhoods and schools on the school behavior and performance of adolescents. *Journal of Adolescent Research, 14*, 319–342.

Buka, S. L., Stichick, T. L., Birdthistle, I., & Earls, F. J. (2001). Youth exposure to violence: Prevalence, risks and consequences. *American Journal of Orthopsychiatry, 71*, 298–310.

Burdick-Will, J., Ludwig, J., Raudenbush, S., Sampson, R., Sanbonmatsu, L., & Sharkey, P. (2011). Converging evidence for neighborhood effects on children's test scores: An experimental, quasi-experimental, and observational comparison. In G. Duncan & R. Murnane (Eds.), *Whither opportunity? Rising inequality, schools, and children's life chances* (pp. 255–276). New York: Russell Sage.

Bureau of Justice Statistics. (2013). Rates of violent victimizations, 1993–2011. http://www.bjs.gov/index.cfm?ty=nvat.

Bursik, R. J. (1986). Delinquency rates as sources of ecological change. In J. M. Byrne & R. J. Sampson (Eds.), *The social ecology of crime* (pp. 63–76). New York: Springer-Verlag.

Cohen, L. E., & Felson, M. (1979). Social change and crime rate trends: A routine activity approach. *American Sociological Review, 44*, 588–608.

Clampet-Lundquist, S., Edin, K., Kling, J. R., & Duncan, G. J. (2011). Moving teenagers out of high-risk neighborhoods: How girls fare better than boys. *American Journal of Sociology, 116*, 1154–1189.

Davey, M., & Williams, T. (2013, September 21). Violence flares anew on Chicago's South Side. *New York Times*, p. A13.

Delaney-Black, V., Covington, C., Ondersma, S. J., Nordstrom-Klee, B., Templin, T., Ager, J., Janisse, J., & Sokol, R. J. (2002). Violence exposure, trauma, and IQ and/or reading deficits among urban children. *Archives of Pediatrics & Adolescent Medicine, 156*(3), 280–285.

Dreier, P., Mollenkopf, J. H., & Swanstrom, T. (2001). *Place matters: Metropolitics for the twenty-first century*. Lawrence: University of Kansas Press.

Ellen, I. G., & O'Regan, K. (2009). Crime and U.S. cities: Recent patterns and implications. *Annals of the American Academy of Social and Political Science: The Shape of the New American City, 626*, 22–38.

Federal Bureau of Investigation. (2013). Crime in the United States. http://www.fbi.gov/about-us/cjis/ucr/crime-in-the-u.s/2011/crime-in-the-u.s.-2011/tables/table-1.

Goering, J. (2007). The effectiveness of Fair Housing programs and policy options. In J. Goering (Ed.), *Fragile rights within cities: Government, housing, and fairness* (pp. 253–286). Lanham, MD: Rowman & Littlefield.

Grogger, J. (1997). Local violence and educational attainment. *Journal of Human Resources, 32*, 659–682.

Harding, D. J. (2009). Collateral consequences of violence in disadvantaged neighborhoods. *Social Forces, 88,* 757–782.

———. (2010). *Living the drama: Community, conflict, and culture among inner-city boys.* Chicago: University of Chicago Press.

Heron, M. (2012). Deaths: Leading causes for 2009. CDC National Vital Statistics Reports. http://www.cdc.gov/nchs/data/nvsr/nvsr61/nvsr61_07.pdf.

Hurt, H., Malmud, E., Brodsky, N. L., & Giannetta, J. (2001). Exposure to violence: Psychological and academic correlates in child witnesses. *Archives of Pediatrics & Adolescent Medicine, 155,* 1351–1356.

Kling, J. R., Liebman, J. B., & Katz, L. F. (2007). Experimental analysis of neighborhood effects. *Econometrica, 75,* 83–119.

Kneebone, E., & Berube, A. (2008). *Reversal of fortune: A new look at concentrated poverty in the 2000s.* Washington, DC: Brookings Institution Metropolitan Policy Program.

———. (2013). *Confronting suburban poverty in America.* Washington, DC: Brookings Institution Press.

LeDoux, J. E. (2000). Emotion circuits in the brain. *Annual Review of Neuroscience, 23,* 155–184.

Liska, A. E., & Bellair, P. E. (1995). Violent-crime rates and racial composition: Convergence over time. *American Journal of Sociology, 101,* 578–610.

Logan, J. (2011). *Separate and unequal: The neighborhood gap for blacks, Hispanics and Asians in metropolitan America.* US2010 Project, Brown University American Communities Project and The Russell Sage Foundation, Providence and New York.

Ludwig J., Jacob, B., Duncan, G., Rosenbaum, J., & Johnson, M. (2010). *Neighborhood effects on low-income families: Evidence from a housing-voucher lottery in Chicago.* Working paper, University of Chicago.

Lupien, S. J., McEwen, B. S., Gunnar, M. R., & Heim, C. (2009). Effects of stress throughout the lifespan on the brain, behaviour and cognition. *Nature Reviews Neuroscience, 10,* 434–445.

Margolin, G., & Gordis, E. B. (2004). Children's exposure to violence in the family and community. *Current Directions in Psychological Science, 13,* 152–155.

Martinez, P., & Richters, J. E. (1993). The NIMH community violence project: II. Children's distress symptoms associated with violence exposure. *Psychiatry, 56,* 22–35.

Massey, D. S. (2004). Segregation and stratification. *DuBois Review, 1,* 7–25.

Massey, D. S., & Denton, N. (1993). *American apartheid: Segregation and the making of the underclass.* Cambridge, MA: Harvard University Press.

McEwen, B. S. (1998). Stress, adaptation, and disease: Allostasis and allostatic load. *Annals of the New York Academy of Sciences, 840,* 33–44.

———. (2004). Protection and damage from acute and chronic stress: Allostasis and allostatic overload and relevance to the pathophysiology of psychiatric disorders. *Annals of the New York Academy of Sciences, 1032,* 1–7.

McEwen, B. S., & Sapolsky, R. M. (1995). Stress and cognitive function. *Current Opinion in Neurobiology, 5,* 205–216.

McEwen, B. S., & Wingfield, J. C. (2003). The concept of allostasis in biology and biomedicine. *Hormones and Behavior, 43,* 2–15.

Morenoff, J. D., & Sampson, R. J. (1997). Violent crime and the spatial dynamics of neighborhood transition: Chicago, 1970–1990. *Social Forces, 76,* 31–64.

Osofsky, J. D. (1999). The impact of violence on children. *The Future of Children, 9,* 33–49.

Papachristos, A. V. (2011). The coming of a networked criminology? *Advances in Criminological Theory, 17,* 101–140.

Popkin, S., Theodos, B., Roman, C., & Guernsey, E. (2008). *The Chicago Family Case Management Demonstration: Developing a new model for serving 'Hard to House' public housing families.* Washington, DC: The Urban Institute.

Putnam, R. (2000). *Bowling alone: The collapse and renewal of American community.* New York: Simon & Schuster.

Pynoos, R. S., Frederick, C., Nader, K., Arroyo, W., Steinberg, A., Eth, S., Nunez, F., & Fairbanks, L. (1987). Life threat and posttraumatic stress in school-age children. *Archives of General Psychiatry, 44,* 1057.

Quillian, L. (2012). Segregation and poverty concentration the role of three segregations. *American Sociological Review, 77,* 354–379.

Reardon, S., & Bischoff, K. (2011). Income inequality and income segregation. *American Journal of Sociology, 116,* 1092–1153.

Rodrigues, S. M., LeDoux, J. E., & Sapolsky, R. M. (2009). The influence of stress hormones on fear circuitry. *Annual Review of Neuroscience, 32,* 289–313.

Sampson, R. J. (1986). The contribution of homicide to the decline of American cities. *Bulletin of the New York Academy of Medicine, 62,* 562–569.

———. (2003). The neighborhood context of well-being. *Perspectives in Biology and Medicine, 46,* S53–S64.

———. (2012). *Great American city: Chicago and the enduring neighborhood effect.* Chicago: University of Chicago Press.

Sampson, R. J., & Wilson, W. J. (1995). Toward a theory of race, crime, and urban inequality. In J. Hagan & R. D. Peterson (Eds.), *Crime and Inequality* (pp. 37–56). Stanford, CA: Stanford University Press.

Sampson, R. J., Raudenbush, S. W., & Earls, F. (1997). Neighborhoods and violent crime: A multilevel study of collective efficacy. *Science, 277*(5328), 918–924.

Sampson, R. J., Morenoff, J. D., & Gannon-Rowley, T. (2002). Assessing 'Neighborhood Effects': Social processes and new directions in research. *Annual Review of Sociology, 28,* 443–478.

Sampson, R. J., Sharkey, P., & Raudenbush, S. (2008). Durable effects of concentrated disadvantage on verbal ability among African-American children. *Proceedings of the National Academy of Sciences, 105,* 845–852.

Sanbonmatsu, L., Kling, J., Duncan, G., & Brooks-Gunn, J. (2006). Neighborhoods and academic achievement: Results from the Moving to Opportunity experiment. *Journal of Human Resources, 41,* 649–691.

Sapolsky, R. M., Romero, L. M., & Munck, A. U. (2000). How do glucocorticoids influence stress responses? Integrating permissive, suppressive, stimulatory, and preparative actions. *Endocrine Reviews, 21,* 55–89.

Sharkey, P. (2010). The acute effect of local homicides on children's cognitive performance. *Proceedings of the National Academy of Sciences, 107,* 11733–11738.

——. (2013). *Stuck in place: Urban neighborhoods and the end of progress toward racial equality.* Chicago: University of Chicago Press.

——. (2014). Spatial segmentation and the black middle class. *American Journal of Sociology,* 119, 903–954.

Sharkey, P., Strayer, N., Papachristos, A., & Raver, C. (2012). The effect of local violence on children's attention and impulse control. *American Journal of Public Health,* 102, 2287–2293.

Sharkey, P., Schwartz, A. E., Ellen, I. G., & Lacoe, J. (2013). *High stakes in the classroom, high stakes on the street: The effects of community violence on students' standardized test performance.* Working Paper 03-13, New York University Institute for Education and Social Policy.

Skogan, W. (1990). *Disorder and decline: Crime and the spiral of decay in American cities.* Berkeley: University of California Press.

Turner, M. A., & Ross, S. L. (2005). How racial discrimination affects the search for housing. In X. d. S. Briggs (Ed.), *The geography of opportunity: Race and housing choice in metropolitan America* (pp. 81–100). Washington, DC: Brookings.

Wilson, R. E., & Mast, B. D. (2014). Housing choice vouchers and escaping neighborhood crime. In G. Bruinsma & D. Weisburd (Eds.), *Encyclopedia of Criminology and Criminal Justice* (pp. 2363–2371). New York: Springer.

Wilson, W. J. (1987). *The truly disadvantaged: The inner city, the underclass, and public policy.* Chicago: University of Chicago Press.

Zimring, F. E. (2007). *The great American crime decline.* New York: Oxford University Press.

Zimring, F. E., & Hawkins, G. (1999). *Crime is not the problem: Lethal violence in America.* New York: Oxford University Press.

14.

The Normal Pain of the Social Brain

Confusing Depressive Disorder with Normal Sadness

Allan V. Horwitz

THE BRAIN is an intensely social organ that is biologically designed to respond to its environment. Brain-based mental structures are inherently sensitive to social contexts so they cannot be understood through reducing them to organic substrates. "Our inner faculties," psychologist William James (1900) famously observed, "are adapted in advance to the features of the world in which we dwell" (p. 4). Many of these features involve suffering from diseases that ravage our bodies, natural disasters, or the pain of losing valued human relationships. Normal brains respond to such adverse circumstances with negative feelings, including sadness, fear, and anger. Intensely distressing emotions that respond to losses, threats, and other stressors are natural reactions to the taxing circumstances in which they emerge.

This chapter uses two extended examples to illustrate the importance of social context in determining whether emotions are normal or pathological. The first is grief and the controversy over when this emotion should be considered a disorder. Grief is perhaps the paradigmatic case of an intensely painful emotion that nevertheless is often an appropriate response to a genuine loss. Indeed, the general definition of mental disorder in the *DSM-5* uses "the death of a loved one" to illustrate the difference between a painful but normal emotion and a mental disorder:

> A mental disorder is a syndrome characterized by clinically significant disturbance in an individual's cognition, emotion regulation, or behavior that re-

flects a dysfunction in the psychological, biological, or developmental processes underlying mental functioning. Mental disorders are usually associated with significant distress or disability in social, occupational, or other important activities. An expectable or culturally approved response to a common stressor or loss, such as the death of a loved one, is not a mental disorder. (American Psychiatric Association [APA], 2013, p. 20)

Yet, grieving processes can also go wrong and indicate the presence of a mental disorder when they involve especially severe or long-lasting symptoms. Examining when grief is normal and when it becomes pathological can illuminate some fundamental issues regarding not just distinctions between normality and abnormality but also the relationship between the brain and the social environment. Grief is not a unique stressor but is comparable to other stressors such as the loss of valued relationships, jobs, health, or goals. The *DSM-5* definition implies this when it uses grief as an example, not as an exclusive exemption to diagnosis.

As a second example, I examine one well-known study of depression that illustrates the pitfalls of conflating sadness that stems from external stressors with symptoms of major depression. I conclude that the current bereavement exclusion should be extended to symptoms that arise as a result of environmental stressors and dissipate when these stressors go away. My argument, however, directly contradicts current trends in psychiatry and, in particular, the current changes that psychiatry's diagnostic manual, the *DSM-5,* recently enacted.

A central challenge for the mental health disciplines is to distinguish natural emotional responses to stressful contexts from symptomatically similar conditions that indicate mental disorders. Indeed, the most fundamental distinction in medicine is between the normal and the pathological. Mental disorders are not simply distressing or impairing conditions but indicate that some mental process is not functioning as it is biologically designed to function. To understand when a psychological mechanism is not operating appropriately requires understanding when it is working properly. Psychiatrists and other mental health professionals, however, rarely consider what appropriate psychological functioning involves. "It is indeed astonishing," neurologist Antonio Damasio (1994) exclaims, "to realize that (medical) students learn about psychopathology without ever being taught normal psychology" (p. 255). This means that pathology cannot be equated with the sheer presence of negative emotions, since bad feelings can often exist for good reasons and be normal (Nesse, 1990). Adequate conceptions of normality are foundational for accurate knowledge about what is pathological.

Making an adequate distinction between depressive disorders and normal sadness has become particularly important as knowledge about the human genome grows. Major breakthroughs in genetic research since the 1990s have allowed researchers to associate gene clusters with the presence of symptoms. Yet, despite these advances, current research on the genetics of depression remains handicapped by its failure to distinguish under what circumstances genetic factors lead to natural sadness in response to loss or to depressive disorder. Current *DSM* symptom-based definitions of depression do not adequately distinguish intense normal sadness from disorder, yet much important genetic research relies on population-based samples that are likely to be composed of predominantly normal individuals. Thus, researchers are in jeopardy of mistakenly identifying findings about the roots of normal sadness as discoveries about the causes of depressive disorder.

The mind—and the brain, which is the organ in which most mental processes occur—has many special features, such as learning, cultural shaping, plasticity in taking on new tasks, and interpreting the meanings of contextual events, which makes the health/disorder distinction more complex in psychiatry than in physical medicine. Nevertheless, the ultimate benchmark for health and disorder is the same in psychiatry as it is in physical medicine, namely, whether the individual's mental processes are performing the functions they were biologically designed to perform. Evolution designed the eyes to see, the heart to pump blood, the kidneys to eliminate waste, and the lungs to enable us to breathe. These structures are healthy when they are carrying out their evolutionarily intended functions. Conversely, they are diseased when they are unable to accomplish these purposes. The definition of mental dysfunction is conceptually analogous to the definition of physical dysfunctions: mental disorders exist when a psychological mechanism is unable to perform its evolutionarily designed function.

There are, however, fundamental distinctions between the normal and abnormal functioning of physical and mental processes. First, physical medicine typically possesses biological markers that can indicate the presence of a disease and confirm or refute a diagnosis: cardiologists use positron emission tomography (PET) scans to see if a heart has tissue damage, nephrologists take X-rays to find the presence of a kidney stone, or oncologists employ laboratory tests to detect cancerous cells. Psychiatrists and other mental health professionals rarely have these tools. It is the case that some forms of dementia have characteristic brain lesions, and the dexamethasone suppression test can sometimes detect a particular type of depression known as "melancholia" (Shorter, 2013, p. 84). These tests, however, are exceptions in psychiatry. More commonly, patient self-reports and, sometimes, clinician observation constitute the sole diagnostic resources for mental health professionals. At present, no independent criteria exist that might verify the accuracy of a clinician's assessment of nearly all mental disorders. Therefore, diagnostic criteria, in themselves, are particularly important for the mental health professions because they are typically the only tool available to separate abnormal from normal conditions.

In addition, bodily systems do not turn on and off but must constantly function. A lung that stopped breathing, a heart that stopped pumping blood, or kidneys that cannot discharge waste lead to certain death. In contrast, as philosophers since Aristotle have emphasized, psychological mechanisms are *contextual*. Natural emotions "may be felt both too much and too little, and in both cases not well; but to feel them at the right times, with reference to the right objects, towards the right people, with the right motive, and in the right way is what is both intermediate and best, and this is characteristic of virtue" (Aristotle, 1980, p. 30). They are inherently designed to adjust to context so that definitions of normal and abnormal conditions must take into account situational factors. For example, people naturally become anxious when they confront dangerous situations or sad when they face losses. Conversely, anxiety and sadness are not naturally present in the absence of contexts in which they would be appropriate. Distressing emotions that arise in the kinds of circumstances they were designed to respond to are natural and not disordered.

Despite the necessity to consider context in making judgments about mental disorder, current biological views assume that brain functioning in itself can indicate the presence of a mental disorder. These perspectives assume that examining brain circuitry and identifying biological differences that signify disorder versus normality allows us to distinguish normal from disordered conditions. Notwithstanding the lack of biological markers that can aid in making diagnoses of most mental disorders, psychiatrists often assert that such conditions are brain diseases. "People who suffer from mental illness," according to psychiatrist Nancy Andreasen (1984), "suffer from a *sick or broken brain*, not from weak will, laziness, bad character, or bad upbringing" (p. 8). Reflecting this view, a common approach in psychiatry is to try and pinpoint the genes or other markers that are presumably responsible for various mental disorders. For example, the National Institute of Mental Health has launched an initiative, the Research Domain Criteria Project (RDoC), which strives to classify mental disorders based on their neurobiological correlates (Insel & Cuthbert, 2009). Examining brain functioning, however, is not as straightforward as it seems as a way to answer the conundrum of which mental symptoms are normal and which disordered.

The reason is simple: *normal* painful emotions as well as disordered ones are associated with certain forms of brain activity. Thus, discovering a difference in biological processes between two groups does not in itself tell you whether you have discovered a difference that signifies disorder versus nondisorder as opposed to two normal variations or two disorders. One cannot directly leap from observing that there is a brain process that produces, say, depression or anxiety to a conclusion about what is normal versus disordered. Natural distress is just as likely as mental disorder to be related to neurological underpinnings, so correlations of a group of symptoms with certain brain states do not indicate whether the condition is a normal or a pathological one.

For example, the brain scans of depressed patients strongly resemble the brain scans of actors asked to pretend that they feel intensely sad because they both are generating intense feelings of sadness (Mayberg et al., 1999). Or, imagine looking at brain scans of soldiers going out on patrol in an Afghan neighborhood in which there has been recent violence and in which hypervigilance is essential. These scans might reveal brain activity in anxiety-generating centers at the same or higher levels as among people with anxiety disorders, yet this anxiety would be an entirely normal response to extraordinarily threatening circumstances. The brain scans themselves, however, would not reveal whether the condition is a natural response to an extreme environment or an anxiety disorder. The same configuration of neurochemicals or electrical activity that might be normal in the face of a direct threat might indicate a disorder when no danger exists.

Mental disorders and normal intense distress thus share a major characteristic—intense distress. The brain activity underlying some emotional condition does not in itself indicate a disorder because extremely disturbing emotions that arise because of a severe loss or threat are normal. In such cases, heightened levels of brain activity and perhaps special brain circuitry might come into play as part of a normal, biologically designed response. Therefore, looking at the intensity of activity of any part of the brain is not a way to diagnose disorder. Except in cases of gross trauma to the brain or other rare cases where we already know there is brain pathology, to search for a "broken brain," we have to know how to recognize the kind of brain state correlated with disorder. To do that, we have to go outside of the biological level and consider the circumstances to which the intense distress respond so that we can judge whether the brain-generated emotional state is likely normal or not. At least for the time being, only consideration of the context in which emotions emerge allows one to judge whether it is a normal reaction or a psychiatric disorder.

The Contextual Nature of Normal Sadness

Since the earliest known medical writings, commentators have emphasized the grounding of both normal and pathological emotions in states of the brain. The Hippocratics noted that

> men ought to know that from the brain, and from the brain only, arise our pleasures, joys, laughter, and jests, as well as our sorrows, pains, griefs and tears.... It is the same thing which makes us mad or delirious, inspires us with dread and fear, whether by night or by day, brings sleeplessness, inopportune mistakes, aimless anxieties, absentmindedness, and acts that are contrary to habit. (Porter, 2002, p. 7)

At the same time, Hippocratic writings rejected any sharp dichotomy between internal and environmental forces and considered disease a disruption of a holistic relationship between individuals and their surroundings.

Diagnosticians from the earliest times to the present have also routinely distinguished normal sadness that is a contextually appropriate emotion from depressive mental disorder. In the fifth century B.C., Hippocratic writings defined the symptoms of melancholia in a way that is remarkably similar to current definitions of depression: "aversion to food, despondency, sleeplessness, irritability, restlessness" (Hippocrates, 1923–1931, p. 185). Yet, their definition of melancholia made clear that symptoms alone were not sufficient indicators of a mental disorder: "If fear or sadness last for a long time it is melancholia" (Hippocrates, 1923–1931, p. 263). Natural fear and sadness persist proportionately to their generating context: only symptoms that "last for a long time" indicate disorder.

Several centuries later, the renowned Greek physician Aretaeus of Cappadocia (ca. A.D. 150–200) specified the distinction between normal and disordered conditions: "(Melancholic) patients are ... dejected or unreasonably torpid, without any manifest cause; such is the commencement of melancholy. And they also become peevish, dispirited, sleepless, and start up from a disturbed sleep. Unreasonable fear also seizes them" (Jackson, 1986, p. 39). Aretaeus' definition indicates the importance of social context in definitions of disorder. The criterion of "without any manifest cause" differentiated disorders that are "unreasonable" from normal sadness, indicating how normal conditions could be misdiagnosed as disorders when symptoms alone were taken into account.

Hippocratic-based definitions of depression prevailed for millennia. The most celebrated work on depression, Robert Burton's *Anatomy of Melancholy,* published in 1621, provided a profound distinction between contextually appropriate sadness and depressive disorder. Normal sadness was a ubiquitous aspect of the human condition:

> Melancholy . . . is either in disposition or habit. In disposition, it is that transitory melancholy which goes and comes upon every small occasion of sorrow, need, sickness, trouble, fear, grief, passion, or perturbation of the mind, any manner of care, discontent, or thought, which causeth anguish, dullness, heaviness, and vexation of spirit. . . . And from these melancholy dispositions, no man living is free, no Stoic, none so wise, none so happy, none so patient, so generous, so godly, so divine, that can vindicate himself; so well composed, but more or less, some time or other, he feels the smart of it. Melancholy, in this sense is the character of mortality. (Burton, 1621/2001, pp. 143–144)

In contrast to such natural melancholic feelings that arise after losses, which are the "character of mortality," melancholic disorders arise "without any apparent occasion" (Burton, 1621/2001, p. 331). As well, Burton emphasized how the normal response to deaths of intimates need not be mild but often reached intense extremes: "This is so grievous a torment for the time, that it takes away their appetite, desire of life, extinguisheth all delights, it causeth deep sighs and groans, tears, exclamations . . . howling, roaring, many bitter pangs . . . brave discreet men otherwise oftentimes forget themselves, and weep like children many months together" (Burton, 1621/2001, pp. 358–359).

Writing much later, and from a thoroughly different perspective, Sigmund Freud nevertheless made a comparable distinction between normal grief and melancholic disorder:

> Although grief involves grave departures from the normal attitude to life, it never occurs to us to regard it as a morbid condition and hand the mourner over to medical treatment. We rest assured that after a lapse of time it will be overcome, and we look upon any interference with it as inadvisable or even harmful. (Freud, 1917/1957, p. 165)

While Freud asserted that symptoms associated with mourning are both intense and "grave departures from the normal," he nevertheless insisted that grief is not a "morbid" condition. Indeed, he emphasized that it would "never occur to us" to provide medical treatment to the bereaved. In addition, he stressed that grief is naturally self-healing, so that with time the mourner would return to a normal psychological state. Medical intervention, he suggested, could actually harm the grieving person through interfering with natural healing processes.

Diagnostic criteria in psychiatric manuals up to the present have also separated contextually appropriate grief from depressive disorders. For example, the *DSM-II* (1968) defined depressive neurosis as follows: "This disorder is manifested by an excessive reaction of depression due to an internal conflict or to an identifiable event such as the loss of a love object or cherished possession" (APA, 1968, p. 40). This definition clearly recognizes that psychiatrists should not consider reactions that are proportionate and not "excessive" to their contexts as mental disorders.

The criteria for major depressive disorder (MDD) in the *DSM-IV-TR* (2000), the manual that preceded the current *DSM-5*, also recognized the normality of grief. Both the *DSM-IV* and *DSM-5* diagnoses of MDD require that five symptoms out of the following nine be present during a two-week period (the five must include either depressed mood or diminished interest or pleasure): (1) depressed mood, (2) diminished interest or pleasure in activities, (3) weight gain or loss or change in appetite, (4) insomnia or hypersomnia (excessive sleep), (5) psychomotor agitation or retardation (slowing down), (6) fatigue or loss of energy, (7) feelings of worthlessness or excessive or inappropriate guilt, (8) diminished ability to think or concentrate or indecisiveness, and (9) recurrent thoughts of death or suicidal ideation or suicide attempt (APA, 2000, p. 356; APA, 2013, pp. 160–161).

These symptom criteria form the heart of the definition of MDD, but there was one further important clause in the *DSM-IV* definition: "The symptoms are not better accounted for by Bereavement, i.e., after the loss of a loved one, the symptoms persist for longer than 2 months or are characterized by marked functional impairment, morbid preoccupation with worthlessness, suicidal ideation, psychotic symptoms, or psychomotor retardation" (APA, 2000, p. 356). Patients are exempt from diagnosis if their symptoms are due to what the *DSM* defines as a normal period of bereavement after the death of a loved one, lasting no more than two months and not including especially serious symptoms, such as psychosis or thoughts about suicide. In other words, a patient whose bereavement does not exceed a two-month duration or involve particularly severe features such as suicidal ideation or psychotic symptoms are considered to be undergoing a normal period of grief. This "bereavement exclusion" acknowledged that some instances of normal intense sadness might satisfy the symptomatic criteria but still not be a disorder.

The *DSM-IV* criteria also recognized that bereavement could sometimes "go wrong" and become pathological depression. Such "complicated" disorders involve symptoms such as marked functional impairment, morbid preoccupation with worthlessness, or psychomotor retardation that go beyond normal grief. Complicated grief also extends beyond the two-week period of normal grief and must last for at least two months. The criteria thus recognized that, while most bereaved people do not have mental disorders, in some cases the severity and length of the grieving process can indicate a disorder.

At least for the specific case of grief, an unbroken history of medical thought up to and including the diagnostic manuals before the *DSM-5* recognized that biological and psychological states that might otherwise seem to indicate a mental disorder but that emerge as a response to the context of the death of an intimate are natural, rather than pathological. Indeed, this 2,500-year history seems to be no more than a reflection of common sense. What, then, makes grief reactions an interesting lens into the interaction between biological and social contexts?

Example One: The Equivalence of Bereavement and Other Losses

While medical thought has always recognized that grief after the death of an intimate is a natural phenomenon, it typically viewed grief as just one example of a normal response rather than a distinctive form of loss. As Burton's description emphasized, normal sadness can arise as a reaction to a multitude of "every small occasion of sorrow, need, sickness, trouble, fear, grief, passion, or perturbation of the mind, any manner of care, discontent, or thought, which causeth anguish, dullness, heaviness, and vexation of spirit" (Burton, 1621/2001, p. 143). The *DSM-5* definition of mental disorder, quoted above, also uses bereavement as an example of "an expectable and culturally approved response to a common stressor or loss," not as the sole type of appropriate reaction to a stressor.

Yet, in the *DSM-IV*, bereavement was the *only* stressful context that excludes someone from diagnosis when his or her symptoms would otherwise meet the criteria for major depression. This seemingly contradicts not only millennia of psychiatric thought but also the *DSM*'s own general definition of mental disorder that used grief as just one possible example of a nondisordered state. The logic of the bereavement exclusion seems to indicate that symptoms resulting from and persisting in stressful contexts other than bereavement, such as the loss of a valued job or relationship, the diagnosis of a life-threatening physical illness in oneself or an intimate, or the failure to achieve a long sought-after goal, should similarly be excluded from diagnosis even if they result in a two-week period of symptoms that meet the MDD criteria.

Considerable empirical evidence does indicate that the distress arising from bereavement is not unique but instead is comparable to the pain stemming from other kinds of losses. For example, Wakefield et al. (2007; see also Wakefield & Schmitz, 2012, 2013) used data from the first wave of the National Comorbidity Survey (NCS), a nationally representative community-based epidemiological survey of over 8,000 persons conducted from 1990–1992. First, they divided this sample into two groups: those who met MDD criteria but were excluded from diagnosis because their symptoms emerged just after the death of an intimate and so met the criterion for the bereavement exclusion. They also examined a comparable group who reported that their symptoms arose after some type of loss other than bereavement. They then excluded these two groups from an MDD diagnosis because of an "uncomplicated" loss.

As noted above, the *DSM-IV* also qualified the bereavement exclusion: if post-bereavement symptoms were either especially severe, involving "morbid preoccupation with worthlessness, suicidal ideation, marked functional impairment or psychomotor retardation," or lasted longer than two months, they are considered to indicate "complicated bereavement." Wakefield et al. (2007) then further subdivided the NCS sample into those with complicated bereavement and those who had either a particularly serious or prolonged episode after some loss other than bereavement. They were thus able to compare the four groups of uncomplicated and complicated bereavement-triggered losses and uncomplicated and complicated other-triggered losses.

Their findings indicated almost no differences between the bereaved and other-loss groups. Symptoms from uncomplicated bereavement- and uncomplicated other-triggered losses were comparable on eight of nine indicators of possible disorder, including number of depressive symptoms, melancholic features, suicide attempts, duration of longest episode, seeing a mental health professional for depression, going to a hospital because of depression, taking a medication for depression, and number of depressive episodes. The only significant difference was that respondents with bereavement-triggered episodes were less likely than those with other-triggered episodes to say that their condition created a lot of interference with their lives. Likewise, they found no differences in the bereavement- and other-triggered groups in eight of nine possible symptom groups; the only difference was that the bereaved were more likely to say they had "thought about death" after their loss. Finally, Wakefield et al. (2007) found that uncomplicated bereavement- and other-triggered groups were generally lower on disorder indicators than the two complicated types of cases. In another study using different data, Wakefield and Schmitz (2013) showed not only that uncomplicated forms of bereavement were similar to non-bereavement-related episodes but that all stressor-related conditions were more similar to normal distress than to depressive disorder.

These findings indicate that bereavement is not a unique stressor that differs from other types of losses but instead that depressive symptoms arising after all kinds of losses are comparable. They also show that the criteria for complicated diagnoses are similar for bereavement and other losses. In addition, they demonstrate that the overall prevalence of major depression, as measured by *DSM* criteria, drops by about a quarter when diagnoses after other-triggered losses are excluded from disorder status. Wakefield et al. (2007) conclude that the current bereavement exclusion should be expanded to encompass individuals whose depressive symptoms arise after some loss other than grief. This suggestion corresponds to the long tradition of psychiatric history, which split disorders "with cause" from those "without cause" without singling out bereavement as a special type of loss.

Findings from a number of other studies also indicate the continuity of bereavement and other losses. One important study by Ramin Mojtabai (2011) used prospective data from the National Epidemiologic Survey on Alcohol and Related Conditions (NESARC) to test the validity of the bereavement exclusion. It could thus compare the prognoses of bereaved and non-bereaved people who have had depressive episodes. If the bereavement exclusion is valid, then bereavement-related symptoms should resolve over time and not have the chronic and recurring course that typifies depressive disorders.

Mojtabai's (2011) findings show that three years after an initial episode, bereaved people were no more likely than people who were not depressed at the first period of measurement to have subsequent depressive episodes. The rate of depression among the bereaved group (8.2 percent) was comparable to those who were not initially depressed (7.5 percent) but significantly lower than the depressed group that was not bereaved (14.7 percent). As Freud predicted, the prognosis of bereavement is benign compared to other depressed persons; grieving people are likely to self-heal without treatment. Providing further evidence for the wisdom of the bereavement exclusion, Mojtabai also found that compared to those with other depressive episodes, respondents with bereavement-related episodes were less likely to have impaired role functioning, psychiatric treatment, or comorbid disorders. These findings are likely to understate the differences between the bereaved and others who met MDD criteria because the latter group includes people who met these criteria because of other types of losses. Were this group excluded from the MDD group, the differences between the bereaved and non-bereaved group likely would have been even larger.

Another study that confirms the absence of differences between bereavement and other-loss related depressive episodes stems from the research of Kendler and colleagues, which uses data from the Virginia Twin Study to compare bereavement-related depression to depression related to other stressful life events. Comparable to the Wakefield et al. (2007) findings,

Kendler et al. found that the two groups were not distinctive in most of the duration, severity, and impairment criteria they used to test for differences. They summarize: "The similarities of bereavement-related depression and depression related to other stressful life events far outweigh their differences." (Kendler, Myers, & Zisook, 2008, p. 1454).

Yet, Kendler and colleagues reach a starkly different conclusion than the Wakefield group and Mojtabai. Instead of suggesting that the bereavement exclusion should be maintained or expanded, they state that the exclusion should be eliminated because of the lack of evidence that bereavement is a unique stressor. There is, therefore, no justification for singling bereavement out for exclusion from diagnosis of major depression. Because Kendler was a prominent member of the *DSM-5* working committee, his work was highly consequential for the bereavement exclusion.

The *DSM-5* and the Death of the Bereavement Exclusion

A new edition of the *DSM*, the *DSM-5*, was published in May 2013. While it kept intact the symptom criteria for MDD from the previous *DSM-IV*, it removed the bereavement exclusion from the previous criteria. Instead, it added a note that states,

> Responses to a significant loss (e.g. bereavement, financial ruin, losses from a natural disaster, a serious medical illness or disability) may include the feelings of intense sadness, rumination about the loss, insomnia, poor appetite, and weight loss noted in [the symptom criteria], which may resemble a depressive episode. Although such symptoms may be understandable or considered appropriate to the loss, the presence of a major depressive episode in addition to the normal response to a significant loss should also be carefully considered. (APA, 2013, pp. 125–126)

While the note's language is confusing, in fact, the revised criteria mean that bereaved people who meet the standard MDD criteria noted above are liable to a diagnosis. Someone who has suffered the loss of an intimate would be diagnosed with depression if his or her symptoms, whether severe or not, did not dissipate after a *two-week* period following the death. In light of millennia of psychiatric thought that has distinguished contextually appropriate symptoms from those that are not contextually appropriate as well as empirical findings that show no significant distinctions between bereaved and other-loss groups—not to mention the commonsense notion that it is normal to feel intensely sad for at least two weeks following the death of an intimate—what is the rationale for eliminating the bereavement exclusion?

One reason that the *DSM-5* working group provided for eliminating the bereavement exclusion is the very lack of the difference between bereavement and other losses (Zisook, Shear, & Kendler, 2007). For them, this provides grounds for abolishing, rather than expanding, the exclusion. They state, "The DSM-5 Mood Disorders Work-group has recommended the elimination of the bereavement exclusion criteria from major depressive episodes in light of evidence that 'the similarities between bereavement related depression and depression related to other stressful life events substantially outweigh their differences' (Kendler et al., 2008)" (Coryell, 2012). The president of the American Psychiatric Association, John Oldham, similarly justified the proposal to eliminate the bereavement exclusion as follows:

> (the bereavement exclusion is) very limited; it only applies to a death of a spouse or a loved one. Why is that different from a very strong reaction after you have had your entire home and possessions wiped out by a tsunami, or earthquake, or tornado; or what if you are in financial trouble, or laid off from work out of the blue? In any of these situations, the exclusion doesn't apply. What we know is that any major stress can activate significant depression in people who are at risk for it. It doesn't make sense to differentiate the loss of a loved one as understandable grief from equally severe stress and sadness after other kinds of loss. (www.medscape.com/viewarticle/758788)

Yet, this rationale ignores the *DSM-5*'s own requirement that "an expectable or culturally approved response to a common stressor or loss, such as the death of a loved one, is not a mental disorder" (APA, 2013, p. 20). Kendler also believes that the bereavement exclusion is an anomaly that "was not present in the two major psychiatric diagnostic systems that formed the basis for the DSM-III" (Kendler, 2010, p. 1). Yet, as we have seen, the unbroken record of psychiatric history, including the *DSM-I* and *DSM-II,* would not have viewed "nonexcessive" bereavement as a depressive disorder.

Moreover, advocates of eliminating the bereavement exclusion failed to take into account the findings that the course of the symptoms of the bereaved is more similar to those of nondepressed than of depressed individuals (Mojtabai, 2011; Wakefield & Schmitz, 2013). Most bereaved people who meet MDD criteria after a two-week period no longer meet these criteria after several months, even in the absence of treatment. Finally, it assumes that symptoms in themselves, without regard to the context within which the symptoms develop, indicate the presence of a mental disorder. The conceptual and empirical reasons for extending, or at least maintaining, the exclusion seem to far outweigh those for eliminating it.

The argument for eliminating the bereavement exclusion also does not consider the enormous pathologization that would occur if the criteria for major depression counted all bereaved persons who meet the *two-week* criteria as disordered. Given that about 40 percent of grieving people meet these criteria a month after their loss, it is likely that a majority of the bereaved could be diagnosed with MDD after a two-week period (Clayton, 1982). Because nearly everyone will suffer the loss of an intimate at some point, abandoning the bereavement exclusion could lead most of the population as liable to be diagnosed with a depressive disorder over the course of a lifetime.

Finally, advocates for eliminating the bereavement exclusion urged diagnosis of the bereaved on the grounds that the benefits of treating people who have "suicidal ideation, major role impairment or a substantial clinical worsening" far outweigh the costs of eliminating the exclusion (Kendler, 2010, p. 2). Yet, this argument ignores the fact that the preexisting *DSM-IV* bereavement criteria considered grieving persons with especially severe symptoms or impairment as not meeting the exclusion criteria. All of the indications the working group cite as reasons for abolishing the bereavement exclusion were already grounds for diagnosing MDD among the bereaved. The elimination of the bereavement exclusion in the *DSM-5* has no foundation in good conceptual, empirical, or treatment-related grounds.

Example Two: Confusing Depressive Disorder and Normal Sadness in Community Studies

Studies of the genetics of depression have entered a new era that potentially can help promote understandings of the heritability of this condition. Yet, genetic research is hindered by the failure to indicate when depressive symptoms indicate normal sadness or depressive disorder. To illustrate this problem, I examine the article, "Influence of Life Stress on Depression: Moderation by a Polymorphism in the 5-HTT Gene," by psychologist Avshalom Caspi and colleagues (Caspi et al., 2003). This article's influence on the general scientific community may be greater than that of any genetic study of mental illness that has been conducted to date. *Science* magazine named it, along with two other articles on the genetics of mental illness, as the second most important scientific breakthrough of 2003 (after only an article about newfound insights into the nature of the cosmos). The National Institute of Mental Health's (NIMH) website cited the study as one of the great accomplishments of the agency's focus on the biological basis of mental illness. Thomas Insel, the director of the NIMH, claimed that "what they have done is going to change the paradigm for how we think about genes and psychiatric disorders" (Vedantam, 2003, p. A1). Another

NIMH psychiatrist called the study "the biggest fish yet netted for psychiatry" (Holden, 2003, p. 291). The study's findings were broadly disseminated and featured in both U.S. and worldwide media (Horwitz, 2005).

The research stems from a longitudinal study of a cohort of 847 Caucasians in New Zealand born in the early 1970s and followed from birth into young adulthood. The researchers' central concern was to examine the association between stressful life events, depression, and the 5-HTT gene when cohort members were twenty-six years old. They chose to study the 5-HTT gene because it controls the way that serotonin, itself the focus of much genetic research on depression, passes messages through brain cells. Previous research suggested that the gene is associated with reactions to stressful stimuli in mice, monkeys, and people undergoing brain imaging, although no prior studies had found a direct link between the gene and depression.

The 5-HTT gene has three genotypes: in the New Zealand sample, 17 percent of respondents had two copies of the short allele; 31 percent, two copies of the long allele; and 51 percent, one short and one long allele. The study measured stress through an additive index of fourteen life events, including employment, financial, housing, health, and relationship stressors that participants experienced between ages twenty-one and twenty-six years. It also used the Diagnostic Interview Schedule (DIS), designed to perform *DSM* diagnoses, to determine whether or not participants had experienced an episode of major depression over the preceding year. The researchers' central hypothesis was that people who have one or two of the short versions of the 5-HTT allele might be especially vulnerable to highly stressful environments, whereas those with genes containing the long version might be more resistant to adverse environmental stressors.

The study found that 17 percent of this population sample of twenty-six-year-olds reported episodes of depression severe enough to meet MDD criteria over the preceding year. It showed no association between the 5-HTT gene and those who became depressed. There was, in other words, no direct genetic effect on depression: people with two short alleles, two long alleles, or one of each allele had equivalent chances of becoming depressed. The findings also indicated no relationship between the 5-HTT genotype groups and the number of stressful life events that participants experienced, so the genotype should not account for differential exposure to stressors. That is, it was unlikely that possessing a given genotype would cause the number of stressful life events that respondents reported.

The researchers did find a strong positive relationship between experiencing more stressful life events and developing what they define as "depression." As the number of life stressors increased from zero to four or more, rates of MDD increased from 10 percent to 13, 15, 20, and 33 percent, respectively. Put another way, people who experienced four or more stressful life events were about three and a half times more likely to develop depression than those who experienced no stressful events.

The study's major finding, and the one that generated so much attention, was a significant gene-by-environment interaction. Among the 15 percent of the sample who experienced four or more stressful life events after their twenty-first and before their twenty-sixth birthdays, those with one or two copies of the short allele on the 5-HTT gene were significantly more likely to have MDD, as well as self- and informant-reported depressive symptoms, than those with two copies of the long allele. In the group that faced four or more stressful life events, 43 percent of individuals with two short alleles and 33 percent with one short allele became depressed compared with 17 percent of those with two long alleles who did. Thus, although the study did not find a direct effect of the 5-HTT gene on depression, it did show that the 5-HTT gene interacted with the number of life events to predict depression; at high levels of stressful events, possession of the short gene was associated with more depression.

The authors viewed their finding as confirmation of the "diathesis-stress theory of depression," which predicts that experiences of higher levels of stress will elevate the vulnerability of depression much more among people who are at high genetic risk than among those at low genetic risk (Monroe & Simons, 1991). The short allele on the 5-HTT gene presumably makes people more sensitive to stress, whereas the long allele protects them from the impact of stress. Therefore, the short allele is the stress-sensitive genotype associated with depressive disorder.

But this interpretation of the short allele is open to question. For one thing, this view does not account for the clearest cases of depressive disorder, cases of endogenous depression (depression "without cause") that emerge without any environmental precipitants. The study found that about 10 percent of the 263 people who had experienced no negative life events over the preceding five years developed depression. This 10 percent was the group who most clearly had depressive disorders as opposed to normal intense sadness because their symptoms arose in the absence of any sort of loss, yet there was no impact of the 5-HTT genotype on this group's response to stress. If there is a genetic cause of endogenous depression, it does not seem to show up here, so this particular type of depressive disorder appears unrelated to the 5-HTT gene.

There is a second and more fundamental problem with Caspi et al.'s (2003) interpretation of their findings: it is not clear that the identified gene has much to do with depressive disorder at all. The study used *DSM* criteria for depression, which, aside from the bereavement exclusion, contain no systematic distinction between normal sadness and depressive disorder. The extraordinarily high rate of depression among the young people in this study—17 percent of the entire community sample of twenty-six-year-olds met *DSM* criteria for MDD—itself suggests that many of these cases actually reflected normal intense sadness, not depressive disorder. Nor was there some unusual situation that might explain high rates of disorder: the research took place in a modern and prosperous country during a period of tranquility when there were no wars, major economic downturns, or cultural upheavals, and it excluded the Maori, a deprived ethnic minority that would be expected to have high rates of depression. The fundamental question of whether the measure of disorder was valid and thus whether the observed interaction reflected normal variation or disorder remains unaddressed and unanswerable based on the existing data.

Concluding that the short allele is a genotype for depressive disorders is especially premature because of the particular kinds of stressful life events the Caspi et al. (2003) study measured. Most of the fourteen stressful life events that the study measured were associated with inadequate financial resources, such as problems with debt, not having money for food and household expenses, lacking money for medical expenses, and difficulty paying bills. Consequently, many of these events might be co-occurring results of a single stressor, such as unemployment or long-term poverty. In many cases, reports of four or more stressors would indicate not an additive increase in stressful life events but the experience of a particular kind of financial stressor connected with many of the measures the study uses. The short allele's impact, therefore, might not be associated so much with experiencing *more* stressors as it is with experiencing particular *kinds* of stressors that are linked to financial problems that are especially likely to be related to normal sadness.

Although this study does not report the association of social class with these life events, other studies of similar age groups find strong relationships between low socioeconomic status and the number of major life events that young adults experience (e.g., Turner, 2003). The Caspi et al. (2003) study may actually mainly show how people with limited economic resources are exposed to the kinds of stressors—financial debt, social inequality, and poverty—that might naturally lead people to report symptoms of normal sadness. If correct, this interpretation has important implications for prevention or treatment efforts, because over two-thirds of the population has at least one short allele. The Caspi et al. article focuses on the possibility of medication, noting that "more knowledge about the functional properties of the 5-HTT gene may lead to better pharmacological treatments for those already depressed" (Caspi et al., 2003, p. 389). But if the 5-HTT gene is largely responsible for normal sadness that emerges because of economic problems rather than depressive disorders, effective preventive efforts would address social conditions and not exclusively focus on medicating a presumed internal genetic defect.

In any event, the meaning of the Caspi et al. (2003) findings remains ambiguous. Whether the studied genes interact with certain types of stressors or stressors in general, rather than revealing the genetic underpinnings of depressive disorder, the findings could be equally well interpreted as revealing normal genetic variations in the tendency for people to become sad when they are under intense stress. The study's data are entirely consistent with the possibility that the short and long alleles represent two roughly equal, fitness-enhancing variations on the pattern of sensitivity in normal loss responses. Subsequent attempts to replicate the study's findings display serious discrepancies both among themselves and in relation to the original study, yielding a confusing rather than scientifically congealing picture (e.g., Kendler et al., 2005; Eley et al., 2004; Gillespie et al., 2004; Surtees et al., 2006; Karg et al., 2011, Risch et al., 2009). The resulting ambiguities may stem from the fact that all this research fails to separate natural from dysfunctional conditions and thus likely encompasses some heterogeneous mix of normal and disordered sadness with varying genetic determinants. The use of measures that separate normal sadness from disordered depression could help clarify this problematic situation.

Broadening the Bereavement Exclusion to Encompass More Types of Stressors

A central purpose of psychiatric diagnosis is to distinguish psychological dysfunctions from normal responses to stressful conditions. Bereavement is perhaps the clearest example of a loss where symptoms such as sadness, sleeplessness, restlessness, inability to concentrate, and the like are *natural* rather than disordered. Indeed, the entire history of psychiatric diagnosis until the *DSM-5* recognized that contextually appropriate grief is normal. Calling grief a "depressive disorder," especially when symptoms need only persist for a two-week period, would create a blatantly invalid diagnostic category.

Yet, the logic behind the bereavement exclusion applies not only to grief but to all symptoms that emerge in response to stressors and that naturally dissipate over time or when the stressful conditions disappear. Instead of expanding the bereavement exclusion to cover a broader array of stressors, however, the *DSM-5* moved the exclusion out of the criteria for depression and placed it in a footnote. The virtual abandonment of the bereavement exclusion not only violates the core definition of what a mental disorder is but also pathologizes a natural behavior. Psychiatry loses legitimacy and credibility when it uses such loose and unjustifiable standards for mental disorder.

Substantial evidence indicates that the current criteria for MDD, even with the bereavement exclusion, have major problems of validity (Horwitz & Wakefield, 2007). In particular, the criteria only require that symptoms persist for a mere two-week period, thus risking confounding transitory responses to stressors that dissipate over time or when conditions change with more lasting mental disorders. Indeed, depressive symptoms that arise in many circumstances—the breaking up of a romantic relationship and finding a new attachment, a contingent diagnosis of a possible serious illness that is not confirmed, or a loss of a job with subsequent reemployment—might persist for two weeks but disappear once the situation improves. Only symptoms that become unmoored from their precipitating contexts and persist after the initial circumstances have been resolved are genuine disorders. As the Caspi et al. (2003) study shows, rates of putative depression are extremely high when cases of normal sadness are conflated with depressive disorders.

Abandoning the bereavement exclusion could also have a strong negative impact on research into the causes of depressive disorder. Lumping people who meet MDD criteria because of bereavement or other stressors with those who have genuine depressive disorders creates a heterogeneous group of subjects. All individuals with symptoms that can be diagnosed as MDD might have brain-related conditions, but the symptoms of the bereaved or people reacting to other losses stem from brains that are operating as they are naturally designed to operate. Conflating people with normal symptoms with those whose symptoms stem from a dysfunction can only delay progress in research that strives to find brain-related causes of depression.

In addition, the prognosis—the likely outcome of the future course of symptoms—of people with natural sadness differs from those with depressive disorders. "Diagnosis," according to psychiatrists Robert Woodruff, Donald Goodwin, and Samuel Guze (1974), "is prognosis" (p. ix). Natural responses to disturbing events are far less likely than those that characterize depressive disorders to be prolonged and severe. Symptoms arising from environmental stressors should naturally dissipate over a relatively short period: most grieving people who would otherwise receive an MDD diagnosis are no longer depressed after a period of a few months or so. Likewise, although many residents of Manhattan showed elevated levels of depressive symptoms immediately after the terrorist attacks of 9/11, only a small number remained symptomatic a few months later. The *DSM-IV* bereavement exclusion that diagnosed MDD when symptoms were "complicated" (i.e., severe or prolonged) already took into account the conditions of bereaved people whose conditions were not benign. Similarly, if new criteria broadened the bereavement exclusion to encompass other stressors, a similar "exclusion to the exclusion" would still encompass people who have sufficient severity or duration of symptoms after experiencing severe stressors.

Finally, treatment implications differ for the bereaved and others. Recall Freud's (1917/1957, p. 165) injunction:

> Although grief involves grave departures from the normal attitude to life, it never occurs to us to regard it as a morbid condition and hand the mourner over to medical treatment. We rest assured that after a lapse of time it will be overcome, and we look upon any interference with it as inadvisable or even harmful.

When symptoms of grief or other stress-related depression are especially severe or prolonged, they often require treatment, as the diagnostic criteria recognize. Most people, however, will heal without medical intervention over a period of a few months. Treatment, which typically involves powerful psychoactive medications, is usually unnecessary for normal grief and in some cases can even block natural healing processes (Nesse, 2005).

Conclusion

Aside from unusually severe or persistent conditions, symptoms of most psychiatric disorders in themselves do not necessarily indicate psychological dysfunctions. The brain, as James emphasized, is an intensely social organ that naturally responds to the circumstances in which it operates. Only symptoms that are inappropriate when considered within the social context where they develop and persist are mental disorders. Indeed, the MDD criteria are somewhat unusual among current psychiatric diagnoses for their failure, aside from the bereavement exclusion, to recognize the contextual underpinnings of psychiatric diagnoses. Consider, for example, the *DSM-III-R* criteria for generalized anxiety disorder (GAD) that required

> Unrealistic or excessive anxiety and worry about two or more life circumstances, e.g. worry about possible misfortune to one's child (who is not in

danger) and worry about finances (for no good reason), for a period of six
· months or longer. (APA, 1987 p. 252)

In contrast to the MDD definition, these GAD criteria are thoroughly contextual. They require "unrealistic or excessive" symptoms, implying that
contextually realistic and nonexcessive symptoms are not signs of disorder.
In addition, they provide examples of worries about a child "who is not in
danger" or finances "for no good reason" to clearly separate contextually
appropriate from inappropriate symptoms. Finally, they require that symptoms persist for six months or longer, in contrast to the minimal two-week
required duration of MDD.

Such criteria that place symptoms within their social contexts could be
a model for MDD. The bereavement exclusion could have been extended
to cover other major losses such as valued jobs, relationships, or social
status. The resulting diagnoses would be far more valid and suitable for
psychiatry's mandate to diagnose and treat psychological dysfunctions, not
natural distress that results from the brain's natural reaction to life's mis-
fortunes. Expanding the bereavement exclusion would have recognized that
the brain is an intensely social organ, not a structure that functions in isolation from its environment. The fact that the developers of the *DSM-5* did
not even consider contextualizing and expanding the MDD diagnosis, but
instead abandoned the bereavement exclusion, shows how mainstream psychiatric thought misconstrues how normal brains operate within stressful
social contexts.

The controversy over the bereavement exclusion as well as findings from
community studies of depression indicates the need to merge biological
functioning and social context. When diagnostic criteria only consider
symptoms without regard to context, psychiatric disorder is hopelessly confused with natural functioning. Painful emotions—not only grief and sadness but also fear, jealousy, anger, and so on—are often normal responses
to unpleasant, inequitable, or threatening environments. Calling them
"mental disorders" misunderstands the intrinsic relationship between the
brain and the social context in which it functions.

References

American Psychiatric Association. (1968). *Diagnostic and statistical manual of
    mental disorders* (2nd ed.). Washington, DC: American Psychiatric Association.
    ———. (1987). *Diagnostic and statistical manual of mental disorders* (3rd ed. rev.).
    Washington, DC: American Psychiatric Association.

————. (2000). *Diagnostic and statistical manual of mental disorders* (4th ed. text rev.). Washington, DC: American Psychiatric Association.

————. (2013). *Diagnostic and statistical manual of mental disorders* (5th ed.). Washington, DC: American Psychiatric Association.

Andreasen, N. C. (1984). *The broken brain: The biological revolution in psychiatry.* New York: HarperCollins.

Aristotle. (1980). *The Nicomachean ethics* (Ross, D., Trans.). New York: Oxford World Classics.

Burton, R. (1621 [2001]). *The anatomy of melancholy.* New York: New York Review Books.

Caspi, A., Sugden, K., Moffitt, T. E., Taylor, A., Craig, I. W., Harrington, H., et al. (2003). Influence of life stress on depression: Moderation by a polymorphism in the 5-HTT gene. *Science, 301,* 386–389.

Clayton, P. (1982). Bereavement. In E. S. Paykel (Ed.), *Handbook of affective disorders* (pp. 15–46). London: Churchill Livingstone.

Coryell, W. (2012). Proposal to eliminate the bereavement exclusion criteria from major depressive episode in *DSM-5.* www.dsm5.org/ProposedRevisions/Pages /proposedrevision.aspx?rid=427#.

Damasio, A. (1994). *Descartes' error: Emotion, reason, and the human brain.* New York: HarperCollins.

Eley, T. C., Sugden, K., Corsico, A., Gregory, A. M., Sham, P., McGuffin, P., et al. (2004). Gene-environment interaction analysis of serotonin system markers with adolescent depression. *Molecular Psychiatry, 9,* 908–915.

Freud, S. (1917 [1957]). Mourning and melancholia. In J. Strachey (Ed. & Trans.), *Standard edition of the complete works of Sigmund Freud* (Vol. 14, pp. 237–258). London: Hogarth.

Gillespie, N. A., Whitfield, J. B., Williams, D., Heath, A. C., & Martin, N. G. (2004). The relationship between stress life events, the serotonin transporter (5-HTTLPR) genotype and major depression. *Psychological Medicine, 35,* 101–111.

Hippocrates. (1923–1931). *Works of Hippocrates* (Vols. 1–4, W. H. S. Jones & E. T. Withington, Eds. & Trans.). Cambridge, MA: Harvard University Press.

Holden, C. (2003). Getting the short end of the allele. *Science, 301,* 291–293.

Horwitz, A. V. (2005). Media portrayals and health inequalities: A case study of characterizations of gene × environment interactions. *Journal of Gerontology, 60B,* 48–52.

Horwitz, A. V., & Wakefield, J. C. (2007). *The loss of sadness: How psychiatry transformed normal sorrow into depressive disorder.* New York: Oxford University Press.

Insel, T. R., & Cuthbert, B. N. (2009). Endophenotypes: Bridging genomic complexity and disorder heterogeneity, *Biological Psychiatry, 66,* 988–989.

Jackson, S. J. (1986). *Melancholia and depression: From Hippocratic times to modern times.* New Haven, CT: Yale University Press.

James, W. (1900). *Psychology* (American Science Series, Briefer Course). New York: Henry Holt.

Karg, K., Burmeister, M., Shedden, K., & Sen, S. (2011). The serotonin transporter promoter variant (5-HTTLPR), stress, and depression meta-analysis revisited. *Archives of General Psychiatry, 68,* 444–454.

Kendler, K. S. (2010). Member, DSM-5 Mood Disorder Work Group. *American Psychiatric Association.* http://www.dsm5.org/about/Documents/grief%20exclusion _Kendler.pdf. Accessed 11/26/2014.

Kendler, K. S., Kuhn, J. W., Vittum, J., Presscott, C. A., & Riley, B. (2005). The interaction of stressful life events and a serotonin transporter polymorphism in the prediction of episodes of major depression: A replication. *Archives of General Psychiatry, 62,* 529–535.

Kendler, K. S., Myers, J., & Zisook, S. (2008). Does bereavement-related depression differ from major depression associated with other stressful life events? *American Journal of Psychiatry, 165,* 1449–1455.

Mojtabai, R. (2011). Bereavement-related depressive episodes: Characteristics, 3-year course, and implications for the *DSM-5. Archives of General Psychiatry, 68,* 920–928.

Mayberg, H. S., Liotti, M., Brannan, S. K., McGinnis, S., Mahurin, R. K., Jerabek, P. A., et al. 1999. Reciprocal limbiccortical function and negative mood: Converging PET findings in depression and normal sadness. *American Journal of Psychiatry, 156,* 675–682.

Monroe, S. M., & Simons, A. D. (1991). Diathesis-stress theories in the context of life stress research: Implications for the depressive disorders. *Psychological Bulletin, 110,* 406–425.

Nesse, R. M. (1990). Evolutionary explanations of emotions. *Human Nature, 1,* 261–289.

———. (2005). An evolutionary framework for understanding grief. In D. J. Stein, D. J. Kupfer, & C. B. Wortman (Eds.), *Late life widowhood in the United States* (pp. 195–226). New York: Springer.

Porter, R. (2002). *Madness: A brief history.* New York: Oxford University Press.

Risch, N., Herrell, R., Lehner, T., Liang, K.-Y., Eaves, L., Hoh. J., et al. (2009). Interaction between the serotonin transporter gene (5-HTTLPR), stressful life events, and risk of depression: A meta-analysis. *JAMA, 301,* 2462–2471.

Shorter, E. (2013). *How everyone became depressed: The rise and fall of the nervous breakdown.* New York: Oxford University Press.

Surtees, P. G., Wainwright, N. W., Willis-Owen, S. A., Luben, R., Day, N., & Flint, J. (2006). Social adversity, the serotonin transporter (5-HTTLPR) polymorphism and depressive disorder. *Biological Psychiatry, 59,* 224–229.

Turner, R. J. (2003). The pursuit of socially modifiable contingencies in mental health. *Journal of Health and Social Behavior, 44,* 1–18.

Vedantam, S. (2003, July 18). Variation in one gene linked to depression. *The Washington Post,* p. A1.

Wakefield, J., & Schmitz, M. (2012). Recurrence of depression after bereavement-related depression: Evidence for the validity of *DSM-IV* bereavement exclusion from the epidemiologic catchment area study. *Journal of Nervous and Mental Disorders, 200,* 480–485.

————. (2013). When does depression become a disorder? Using recurrence rates to evaluate the validity of proposed changes in major depression diagnostic thresholds. *World Psychiatry,* 12, 44–52.

Wakefield, J. C., Schmitz, M. F., First, M. B., & Horwitz, A. V. (2007). Extending the bereavement exclusion for major depression to other losses: Evidence from the National Comorbidity Survey. *Archives of General Psychiatry,* 64, 433–440.

Woodruff, R. A., Goodwin, D. W. & Guze, S. B. (1974). *Psychiatric diagnosis.* New York: Oxford University Press.

Zisook, S., Shear, K., & Kendler, K. S. (2007). Validity of the bereavement exclusion criterion for the diagnosis of major depressive episode. *World Psychiatry,* 6, 102–107.

15.

Cognitive Enhancement Therapy for Improving the Social Brain and Cognition in Schizophrenia

Shaun M. Eack and Matcheri S. Keshavan

HUMANS ARE SOCIAL BEINGS who have helped construct a world that is characterized by dynamic and near-continuous social interactions. The success of most individuals hinges upon their ability to engage effectively with others in this social world. There is accumulating evidence that human beings are uniquely equipped with the neurocircuitry needed to meet the high social demands of life (Adolphs, 2003) and that a substantial component of cognitive and neurodevelopment is directed specifically toward the facilitation of our social capabilities (Blakemore & Choudhury, 2006). Despite the biological predisposition that people have for becoming social participants, great heterogeneity exists in trajectories of social development and the ability of individuals to actualize their potential and succeed in the social world. In many cases, psychiatric disorders represent an affliction of social development and participation (American Psychiatric Association, 2000), ranging from the child with autism who is unable to engage in reciprocal play with his peers to the adult with depression who feels a continual sense of self-defeat that biases her social interactions toward negative attributions and interpretations.

For many years, the neurobiological structures involved in social behavior and development were thought to be fixed, and any abnormalities in these fundamental contributors to social functioning could at best be treated palliatively through social inclusion and group reorganization. Recently, however, evidence is emerging of the remarkable plasticity of the human brain (Bruel-Jungerman, Davis, & Laroche, 2007), including the neural circuits supporting social cognition, which directly affect interpersonal functioning. It is possible to remediate congenital impairments in the social brain in childhood or even to jump-start social development well into adulthood after traditional developmental milestones have long since been missed; this possibility is now becoming a clear reality and a target for intervention development. This chapter will provide an introduction to the area of social brain rehabilitation using schizophrenia as an illustrative disorder of social information processing. A brief overview of social cognition and the social brain will be provided (also see chapters in this volume by Nestor, Choate, and Shirai, Chapter 4; Lee, Horan, and Green, Chapter 7; and Hooker, Chapter 5), followed by a presentation of the evidence concerning the presence of developmental social cognitive deficits in adults with schizophrenia that beckon the need for a social and nonsocial cognitive rehabilitation intervention to improve interpersonal functioning. The fundamentals of neuroplasticity and the opportunities they bring for intervention development will then be briefly reviewed (for details, the reader may be referred to the introductory section by Keshavan, Chapter 2, this volume). Finally, an evidence-based cognitive rehabilitation approach, cognitive enhancement therapy (Hogarty & Greenwald, 2006), will be presented to demonstrate the promise of harnessing brain plasticity to improve the social brain and social functioning in individuals with schizophrenia.

Social Cognition

The key cognitive abilities that the brain supports in the processing and interpreting of social information needed to succeed in interpersonal interactions have collectively become known as social cognition. Classically, Thorndike (1920) defined social cognition simply as the ability to "act wisely in human relations." By the mid-1990s, this domain of study had grown considerably and encompassed over 100 different definitions owing to the broad nature of the concept (Wyer & Srull, 1994). A more recent definition of social cognition that is both broad and informative is the ability to process and interpret socioemotional information in oneself and others (Newman, 2001). From this definition, one can see that social cognition includes a number of important components. The first component emphasizes the importance of both social and emotional aspects of experience and social information. The second component recognizes that social cognition includes both the processing and interpretation of information. The processing stream ranges from social cue identification (Corrigan, 1994) and self-referential memory (Mitchell, Banaji, & MacRae, 2005) to social and emotional perception (Allison, Puce, & McCarthy, 2000; Ekman, 1993). Of course, social cognitive abilities include much more than the mere intake and storing of social information; they also include our own interpretation and appraisal of that information. The importance of moving from information gathering to interpretation has been elegantly illustrated by Flavell's (1992) work on perspective taking. The first level of being able to take the perspective of others is a processing level, which includes merely identifying that other perspectives exist that are not one's own. Higher-order perspective taking, however, is far more interpretive and includes the application of social meaning to the perspective of others and the use of this information to guide behavior. A third component involved in social cognition is that of the self. Social cognition is not merely the ability to understand others but also the ability to understand oneself. Sometimes referred to as meta-cognition (Flavell, 1976), the understanding of one's own social strengths and challenges is an important source of information for the selection of social engagements and the identification of opportunities to further develop one's social abilities.

Given the centrality of interpersonal relationships and social situations to everyday life, it is not surprising that disruptions in the social cognitive abilities that allow us to make the most of these encounters result in grave functional consequences. The inability to identify important social cues, to interpret the emotional signals being sent by others, or to manage one's own emotions and sense of self gives rise to many different forms of psychopathology, leading minimally to social awkwardness and at its height to complete social disability. Many psychiatric disorders can be traced to challenges in some form of social cognition. Major depressive disorder, for example, appears to be rooted in an inability regulate negative emotions (Ehring, Tuschen-Caffier, Schnülle, Fischer, & Gross, 2010; also see Hooley, Chapter 9, this volume) and construct appropriate appraisals of the self (Gladstone & Kaslow, 1995). Individuals who experience mania have problems regulating positive emotions (Surguladze et al., 2010). Those with autism have been hypothesized to suffer from mind-blindness (Baron-Cohen, 1990) and often appear unable to understand or account for the perspectives of others. Even individuals who do not fully develop a psychiatric disorder, but experience some impairment in social cognition, also experience substantial challenges. For example, studies of *emotional intelligence* (Salovey & Mayer, 1990) have repeatedly indicated that individuals who are unable to understand, identify, and regulate the emotions of themselves and others are less likely to succeed academically (Brackett & Mayer, 2003) and more likely to encounter challenges in the workplace

(Lopes, Grewal, Kadis, Gall, & Salovey, 2006) and to have an overall poorer quality of life (Lopes, Salovey, & Straus, 2003).

Clearly, social cognition is a central set of abilities needed for succeeding in life, but can its roots be traced to a neurobiologic origin? Given the breadth of the concept of social cognition, many have questioned the possibility of ever locating its biological basis. However, the neural basis of social cognition is becoming increasingly clear with advances in measurement and neuroimaging technologies that allow for innovative methods for probing social and emotional information processing. Broadly, frontotemporal pathways connecting frontal executive circuits to phylogenetically older medial-temporal regions of the brain are now known to support many of the social cognitive abilities that are studied today. The chapters by Nestor, Choate, and Shirai (Chapter 4) and Hooker (Chapter 5) provide an in-depth review of current knowledge regarding the biological basis of social cognition that becomes critical for understanding how social cognitive neural systems have become disrupted in schizophrenia.

Social and Cognitive Challenges in Schizophrenia

Schizophrenia represents a hallmark psychiatric condition for interventions designed to address neurobiologically based impairments in social cognition due to its considerable impact on social disability, the lack of efficacy of current pharmacologic approaches in addressing this disability, marked and pervasive social cognitive impairments, and consistent evidence that these impairments are key rate-limiting factors to functional recovery in the disorder. Schizophrenia is a severe and persistent mental illness that is characterized by hallucinations and delusions that represent the processing of stimuli that is not consistent with reality (American Psychiatric Association, 2000). For example, individuals with paranoid schizophrenia often experience auditory hallucinations (voices) telling them that they are being persecuted by some entity. Such individuals then develop a system of beliefs (delusions) in an attempt to explain their abnormal sensory experiences (e.g., that they have special powers that the government is attempting to suppress). However, beyond hallucinations and delusions, schizophrenia is also characterized by marked social disability. Individuals develop the disorder in late adolescence or early adulthood when critical milestones in social development are being reached, such as beginning to assume adult roles, developing lasting intimate relationships, and learning the rules and norms of the professional workplace. The devastating nature of the condition means that for many individuals, the achievement of these social milestones is never met. Social disability is one of the most marked and persistent problems that individuals with schizophrenia experience and permeates nearly every aspect of their lives. Studies have consistently shown that people with schizophrenia have fragmented and smaller social networks, poorer social skills, and more turbulent social relationships, and they experience high degrees of social withdrawal (Mueser & Tarrier, 1998). Not surprisingly, this social disability has had significant functional consequences for people with this condition, including low levels of employment (Marwaha & Johnson, 2004), high suicide rates (Palmer, Pankratz, & Bostwick, 2005), and poor quality of life (Eack & Newhill, 2007). Sadly, these challenges in social functioning do not appear to remit, even with the stabilization of psychotic symptoms (Robinson, Woerner, Mcmeniman, Mendelowitz, & Bilder, 2004), and once individuals leave the hospital, many find it challenging to reintegrate into the fabric of society.

The causes of social disability in schizophrenia have been an area of intense study for several decades. Although individuals are certainly disabled when they are acutely psychotic and experiencing the height of hallucinatory and delusional symptoms, a puzzling picture has emerged indicating that these "positive" symptoms contribute relatively little to the lasting social disability that people with schizophrenia experience. Key pieces of evidence that have called into question the contribution of the cardinal symptoms of psychosis to social disability in the disorder include stable social deficits after the psychotic phase of the illness (Robinson, Woerner, Mcmeniman, Mendelowitz, & Bilder, 2004), the inability of antipsychotic medications to address impairments in psychosocial functioning (Swartz et al., 2007), and the presence of significant levels of social disability prior to the full onset of psychotic symptoms and the disorder (Eack et al., 2010a; Keshavan, Diwadkar, Montrose, Rajarethinam, & Sweeney, 2005). Such findings have led many investigators to examine other potential contributors to social disability in schizophrenia, and among the many areas that have been studied, impairments in cognition have been shown to be one of the strongest predictors of social and functional disability in the illness. Much like social disability itself, considerable evidence has accumulated that cognitive impairments in schizophrenia are broad (Heinrichs & Zakzanis, 1998; Penn, Corrigan, Bentall, Racenstein, & Newman, 1997), present before the onset of the condition (Eack et al., 2010a; Keshavan et al., 2009), present throughout the course of the illness (Horan et al., 2012; also see Lee, Horan, and Green, Chapter 7, this volume), and are currently unresponsive to antipsychotic medications (Keefe et al., 2007; Sergi et al., 2007).

Cognitive impairments in schizophrenia have been broadly classified into two domains, those concerning neurocognition and those concerning social cognition (Green et al., 2004). Neurocognitive impairments include such domains as speed of processing, attention, working memory, and executive functioning and have shown consistent and large (> 1 standard deviation [SD]) deficits in the disorder (Heinrichs & Zakzanis, 1998). Studies of social cognitive impairment in schizophrenia have primarily focused on deficits in emotional processing (e.g., emotion perception and regulation), social perception (e.g., social cue perception), theory of mind, social understanding (e.g., social knowledge and the development of social schema), and attributional style (Green et al., 2008). Every social cognitive domain studied has at some point demonstrated medium to large levels of impairment across diverse samples of schizophrenia patients, although the greatest evidence has come mostly from studies of emotion perception (Kohler, Walker, Martin, Healey, & Moberg, 2010) and theory of mind (Brune, Abdel-Hamid, Lehmkamper, & Sonntag, 2007), primarily because these have been the two domains that have received the most investigation.

Impairments in social and nonsocial cognition have demonstrated some of the strongest cross-sectional and prospective associations with functional outcome in patients with schizophrenia of any construct under study (Couture, Penn, & Roberts, 2006; Green, Kern, Braff, & Mintz, 2000). It is understandable that the degree of impairment schizophrenia patients experience in cognition would pose significant challenges to their recovery from the disorder. For example, a patient who is unable to focus beyond a short period of time and hold important instructions in working memory is unlikely to be able to maintain employment or remember the ongoing gist of a conversation. The evidence has largely supported these notions, and in a recent meta-analysis (Fett et al., 2011), effect sizes for the association between cognition and functional outcome ranged from small to large and explained nearly a quarter of the variance in patient functioning. Neurocognitive domains particularly associated with functional outcome were verbal learning and memory, which is consistent with an earlier meta-analysis (Green, Kern, Braff, & Mintz, 2000), as well as processing speed and attention. Longitudinal studies have found processing speed and attentional deficits to be robust predictors of such important domains as vocational functioning in multiyear follow-up studies of individuals who developed a first episode of schizophrenia or other psychotic disorder (e.g., Milev, Ho, Arndt, & Andreasen, 2005). Perhaps most important, studies have shown that impairments within these neurocognitive domains are uniquely predictive of patients' functioning, above and beyond psychiatric symptomatology (Milev, Ho, Arndt, & Andreasen, 2005).

Evidence is also accumulating regarding the functional significance of the social cognitive impairments that patients with schizophrenia experience

(Couture, Penn, & Roberts, 2006). In fact, deficits in social cognition might be even more debilitating than those in neurocognitive function, where individuals who are unable to take the perspective of others or pick up on often subtle social cues are likely to find themselves confused by a fast-paced social world, experience repeated difficulties in their interactions, and withdraw from social situations. While studies of social cognition in schizophrenia are relatively newer than those of neurocognitive domains, a growing body of evidence has accumulated within recent years indicating that such deficits are not only present but significant predictors of functional disability in the disorder. Couture and colleagues (2006) found that impairments in social perception were frequently related to difficulties in community functioning and social behavior. Impairments in emotion perception were also consistently associated with difficulties in these functional domains, although to a lesser degree than social perception. Far fewer studies at the time of their review have examined the association between theory of mind and attributional-style deficits with functioning. When comparing the impact of neurocognitive and social cognitive deficits on community functioning in schizophrenia, social cognition has been shown to be a stronger predictor (Fett et al., 2011). Further, findings are increasingly indicating the interconnected nature of neurocognitive and social cognitive impairments, such that neurocognitive deficits may achieve their primary functionally disabling effects through impairing social cognition (Sergi, Rassovsky, Nuechterlein, & Green, 2006). Taken together, these findings support both social and nonsocial cognitive domains as key areas of impairment in schizophrenia and call for the need for comprehensive neuroplasticity-based treatment strategies to address both of these domains to improve functional recovery in the disorder.

Brain Plasticity and the New Window for Intervention

For many years, focal and diffuse brain impairments such as those experienced in patients with schizophrenia were thought to be relatively intractable. Once a biological or physical insult impacted and damaged the brain, restoration was often thought of as a lost cause. With the growth of neuroimaging methods and scientists dedicated to this area, the field has revised its pessimistic view of brain change by increasingly conceptualizing the brain as a highly plastic and malleable organ that can be not only damaged but also shaped in positive directions to improve function, efficiency, and connectivity across a wide range of disorders (Bruel-Jungerman, Davis, & Laroche, 2007). The concept of neuroplasticity is broad and can have several different meanings that bear distinction (see Keshavan, Chapter 2, this volume, for further discussion on this topic). Of course, the notion that the brain is capable of being impaired and physically altered might be considered a classical understanding of neuroplasticity, although such concepts usually fall under the rubric of neurodegeneration, neuronal atrophy, or neurobiologic lesions. Neuroplasticity has most commonly carried a positive connotation that broadly refers to the capacity of the brain to be altered for the development or enhancement of cognitive functions that are supported by specific neural systems. One common meaning of neuroplasticity is that of neurogenesis, or the growing of new brain tissue (Eriksson et al., 1998). During cognitive and neurobiological development, gray matter growth in many areas of the brain is observed, with a systematic pattern of growth occurring across ages of childhood development (Gogtay et al., 2004). In addition, the sprouting of white matter tracts, particularly long-range fiber tracts, also occurs at various milestones of cognitive development, all of which represent some form of neurogenesis. The growing of neurons and neuronal connections, however, is not circumscribed to the early years of life, and several studies have observed neurogenesis in the hippocampus in adults well beyond their primary years of cognitive development (Eriksson et al., 1998; Roy et al., 2000).

The second common meaning of neuroplasticity is that of neuronal reorganization or specialization. While neurogenesis might be thought of as enhancing the brain's capacity for information processing, neuronal reorganization is more akin to the restructuring of brain networks and representations to become more efficient and effective at processing information. For example, as children learn to identify faces from different profiles, the perceptual system becomes increasingly more focused and specialized, such that between the ages of five and eight months, infants begin to activate the fusiform face area when viewing different facial profiles (Nakato et al., 2009). Increasing evidence is indicating that the same type of localization can be identified even for single word processing among healthy adults (Just, Cherkassky, Aryal, & Mitchell, 2010). This concept of neural specialization lays the fundamental theoretical framework for the neurobiologic basis of learning and is one of the earliest forms of neuroplasticity studied. In an experimental animal study, Kleim, Barbay, and Nudo (1998) trained rats in either a skilled (i.e., reaching within a slot to grab a food pellet) or unskilled (i.e., pressing a simple lever to drop a food pellet into the cage) reaching task over the course of ten days and then mapped activity in the motor cortex associated with the coordination of various motor activities. Interestingly, the investigators found significant increases in wrist and digit representations in the motor cortex among the rats who received the skilled reaching training, demonstrating a functional specialization of the motor cortex commensurate with learning to complete a specific task. Such findings have also been demonstrated in humans in such studies as those showing increased digit representations in violinists (Elbert, Pantev, Wienbruch, Rockstroh, & Taub, 1995), increased auditory representations in musicians (Pantev et al., 1998), and functional reorganization of the primary motor cortex during digit sequence training (Karni et al., 1995).

With the increasing and now large evidence base that fundamental areas of the brain involving cognition can both grow and reorganize in response to the demands of learning and cognitive development, many have sought applications of these mechanisms of neuroplasticity in the treatment of various brain disorders. Initial applied intervention work began in the areas of stroke and traumatic brain injury, where studies began to observe that not only could motor function be regained through repetitive practice and strategic motor use but that accompanying these motor improvements were underlying alterations in the motor cortex (Robertson & Murre, 1999). One study by Liepert and colleagues (1998) treated six stroke patients with constraint-induced movement therapy (i.e., constraining the healthy limb and attempting forced movements of the affected limb) and mapped cortical activity on the motor cortex over the course of fourteen days of therapy. Several interesting findings shed light on the possibilities of neuroplasticity as a window of intervention in this study, including evidence that limb movement improved in all patients, that cortical activity was significantly increased after treatment, and that the focus of neural activity moved to locations adjacent to the affected brain areas. Consequently, this study provided important evidence that basic rehabilitation strategies can affect even severely brain-damaged patients, and that in the cases of such damage, functional reorganization appears to occur to compensate for the affected brain region.

Since initial work on traumatic brain injury and stroke, which effectively started cognitive rehabilitation interventions designed to capitalize on brain plasticity, such approaches have been applied to many other cognitive disorders. In particular, cognitive deficits related more to information-processing problems than focal lesions, such as those with dyslexia, began to become important targets for rehabilitation. In the case of dyslexia, investigators found that repeated auditory training improved both language and reading skills in dyslexic individuals (Tallal, Merzenich, Miller, & Jenkins, 1998) and that these improvements reflect an enhancement of phonological brain functions (Temple et al., 2003). Psychiatric disorders have also recently become important targets of cognitive rehabilitation efforts, including mild cognitive impairment (Talassi et al., 2007), Alzheimer disease (Sitzer, Twamley, & Jeste, 2006), attention-deficit hyperactivity disorder (Tamm et al., 2010), and schizophrenia (Hogarty et al., 2004), all of which are presumed to produce underlying changes in the brain, with some emerging evidence of this (e.g., Eack et al., 2010b).

Of course, what about the social brain? As already reviewed, the neural circuitry involved in social cognition is becoming increasingly clear (see Chapters 4 and 5). Should it be expected that such networks are any less plastic than those supporting movement or memory? Emerging evidence is indicating that social cognitive rehabilitation is just as possible as motor and neurocognitive rehabilitation and that here too neuroplasticity appears to play a key role. A holistic analysis of the cognitive rehabilitation literature might suggest that while many diverse intervention approaches have been applied, all represent an attempt to provide an enriched environmental experience to the patient or subject. In the case of stroke rehabilitation, an enriched physical environment is constructed to introduce experiences and exercises that can support the relearning of limb movement. For the treatment of memory loss in aging, targeted memory exercises are provided that help with facial and conceptual recognition and recall. Carrying these principles of providing enriched environmental experiences forward to the social domain suggests that the enhancement of the social environment and/or the introduction of enriched experiences in the social environment could be effective for rehabilitating brain deficits in social cognition.

Similar to work on neurocognitive rehabilitation, efforts to study the neuroplastic mechanisms of social cognitive rehabilitation began in studies of animals. The impact of the environment on social behavior and development had already been established in classic experimental studies (Harlow, 1958). Subsequently, animal studies began to observe the important effects of enriched social environments on the brain and neuroplastic processes. For example, one recent study found that an enriched social environment (i.e., communal nesting) produced not only more prosocial behavior in rats but also increased levels of several neurotrophic factors implicated in brain plasticity (Branchi et al., 2006). Another study by Lu and colleagues (2003) found that rats raised in group-rearing environments both became significantly better learners and demonstrated greater neurogenesis in areas of the hippocampus after learning. Perhaps even more important, the negative effects of isolation rearing on neurogenesis were reversed after introducing a group environment, indicating that environmental enrichment can both enhance neuroplasticity and reverse developmental neuroplastic delays.

Such animal studies have stimulated and supported interventions in humans designed to improve social functioning and the social brain through the enrichment of social environments. One systems-based example of this work has been that of Nelson and colleagues, where institutionalized children in Romania were placed in significantly more enriched social environments (e.g., foster care) with marked improvements in cognition and behavior (Nelson et al., 2007). Not surprisingly, children who remained institutionalized continued to experience cognitive and developmental delays compared to those who were able to be raised in more enriched settings. Further, the earlier individuals were placed in foster care, the greater their level of cognitive improvement. Halperin and colleagues (2013) studied a more individualized intervention designed to provide enriched social and environmental experiences for children with attention-deficit hyperactivity disorder. Their intervention consisted of a unique array of cognitive and physical games conducted in a school setting that were designed to improve behavioral control, planning, attention, and motor skills. While a randomized trial has not yet been completed, early pilot work indicates that that children exposed to the intervention experienced significant reductions in attention problems and impulsivity, as observed by both parents and teachers.

While the studies presented above demonstrate examples of how enriched social environments can have a meaningful impact on the lives of individuals, few investigations have directly examined the impact of such interventions on the social brain. Cognitive enhancement therapy (Hogarty & Greenwald, 2006) is one of the few cognitive rehabilitation approaches whose effects on the social brain have begun to be documented, and this intervention provides a unique illustration of how the development of a targeted treatment designed to provide individuals with enriched environmental and secondary socialization experiences can be used to harness brain plasticity and improve the social brain.

Improving the Social Brain with Cognitive Enhancement Therapy

Overview

Cognitive enhancement therapy (CET; Hogarty & Greenwald, 2006) is a comprehensive developmental approach to the remediation of the social and nonsocial cognitive deficits that limit functional recovery from schizophrenia. The intervention is based on a developmental perspective of schizophrenia that identifies cognitive impairments in the disorder as a neurodevelopmental delay (Hogarty & Flesher, 1999a). A comprehensive review of the cognitive development literature by Hogarty revealed the insight that patients diagnosed with schizophrenia exhibited cognitive profiles similar to typically developing preadolescent children. For example, thinking in schizophrenia is often found to be egocentric, guided by rigid and explicit rules, and context independent. Conversely, hallmark characteristics of adult social cognition, such as an appreciation for the impact of the social context on rules for behavior, the ability to abstract the social "gist" from spontaneous interpersonal interactions to decipher implicit social norms, and the continual assessment of the perspectives of others to negotiate and succeed in social situations, are frequently lacking in schizophrenia. The conceptualization of cognitive impairments in schizophrenia as a developmental delay led to the creation of CET, which is designed to stimulate cognitive development by providing enriched secondary socialization and environmental experiences.

Over the course of eighteen months, CET provides individuals with schizophrenia an enriched environmental experience through two integrated approaches: neurocognitive training and social cognitive group therapy. Neurocognitive training consists of sixty hours of targeted computer-based exercises designed to enhance attention, memory, and problem solving. These fundamental cognitive abilities are critically impaired in schizophrenia and are essential for supporting higher-order social cognition. The social cognitive group therapy component of CET focuses on providing individuals with secondary socialization experiences through a structured forty-five-session social cognitive curriculum containing in vivo cognitive exercises designed to help individuals develop and practice key components of social cognition, such as perspective taking, social context appraisal, reading of nonverbal cues, and emotion regulation. After several initial months of neurocognitive training to help improve attention, the social cognitive groups begin and are subsequently conducted simultaneously with neurocognitive training in an integrated fashion.

Neurocognitive Training

Rationale. The focus of CET is on the enhancement of cognition, particularly social cognition, to facilitate the improvement of meaningful functional outcomes in patients with schizophrenia. Given this focus, one might consider targeting only challenges in social cognition, given their contribution to many different domains of functioning (Fett et al., 2011). However, such an approach would overlook the interrelated nature of neurocognitive and social cognitive deficits in schizophrenia and evidence that enhanced neurocognitive function is likely to be important for facilitating the achievement of higher-order social cognitive abilities in the disorder (Sergi, Rassovsky, Nuechterlein, & Green, 2006). The marked deficits patients with schizophrenia experience in processing speed, attention, memory, and executive function all limit their ability to process, interpret, and act wisely upon social information.

CET not only focuses on but begins with neurocognitive training precisely because of the limitations that impairments in basic components of neurocognition place on the effective use and learning of social cognitive abilities. Of course, the deficits in social cognition that patients with schizophrenia experience are not entirely due to challenges in basic information processing, as has been illustrated by the numerous neurocognitive training programs in schizophrenia that have demonstrated significant benefits on cognition but not social behavior. Many more cognitively capable patients continue to experience significant social deficits, as is often seen in the early course of schizophrenia where neurocognitive impairments are less severe (although certainly not intact) (Braw et al., 2008), but deficits in social cognition continue to be great. The improvement of neurocognitive functions in CET is thus seen as necessary but not sufficient for the improvement of social cognition and functional outcomes. Consequently, CET uniquely integrates an extensive neurocognitive training program with a comprehensive social cognitive group curriculum to arrive at a holistic intervention approach that is greater than the sum of its parts.

Approach. The approach to neurocognitive training in CET is designed to not only facilitate improvements in attention, memory, and problem solving but is also structured to promote social cognition and strategic thinking. Unlike most neurocognitive training programs, which are conducted in isolation and employ a drill-and-practice approach, neurocognitive training in CET is conducted in participant pairs with the aid of a skilled therapist/ coach. The situation of neurocognitive training within the context of two participants who form a computer pair adds to the complexity of the program but also affords the opportunity for socialization experiences that can support social cognition. Participant pairs work together in the neurocognitive training by switching back and forth between completing a cognitive exercise and keeping score for their partner throughout the sixty-minute session. The coach uses this opportunity to begin to teach participants basic social cognitive abilities, such as giving support. Participants are also actively engaged by the coach in helping their partner devise strategies for improving performance on the exercise, thus engaging in strategic thinking regardless of whether they are actively completing the exercise. During the course of the session, several brief breaks are also given to provide some relief from the challenging cognitive exercises and engage in "small talk" among the participants and the coach. Early conversations are almost always directed toward the coach, but gradually the coach encourages participants to spontaneously interact with each other based on what they have learned about shared interests and/or experiences. The fact that most participant pairs will get to know each other well during the several months of computer training prior to starting the social cognitive group also serves to ease participant anxiety about going into a group of strangers, as he or she will already know two people in the group by the time it starts (the computer partner and the coach).

The second key component to the approach toward neurocognitive training taken in CET is that of strategic learning. The field of cognitive rehabilitation has been largely divided into approaches that focus only on repetition to improve cognition (i.e., drill and practice), and those that combine repeated practice with active thinking about strategies that can be used become a more efficient cognitive processor (i.e., strategic learning). CET takes the latter approach of strategic learning through the implementation of a hands-on coach in neurocognitive training. The role of the coach is not to provide solutions for the participants to improve their performance on the cognitive exercises. After all, therapists have been solving problems for their patients for years, and this does little to develop the ability of individuals to think strategically and solve problems for themselves. Rather, the goal of the coach is to stimulate thinking on the part of the participant as to what strategies he or she can use to become better at the exercise. For example, during memory training, participants often become challenged with the amount of information to be stored in memory. The coach will query the participant to ask what strategies he or she might be using to help encode the information. In many cases, participants are relying on rote memory, rather than developing a relational strategy for storing information. The coach then asks the participant what different strategies he or she might use to remember the pictures on the screen. If the participant does not consider a relational approach to encoding, the coach might ask if there is a strategy the participant can use that considers the relationship between the pictures. With coaching, participants often learn that encoding information in a meaningful way that captures the relationship among the items to be remembered is a very helpful device for improving memory performance.

Cognitive Exercises. The core component of neurocognitive training in CET is centered on cognitive exercises designed to improve attention, memory, and problem-solving abilities. In total, there are sixteen cognitive exercises (three attention, seven memory, and six problem solving) employed during the course of CET. The attention exercises were developed by Ben-Yishay (Ben-Yishay, Piasetsky, & Rattok, 1985), and the memory and problem-solving exercises were developed by Bracy (1994), both originally for individuals with traumatic brain injury. Progression through these cognitive exercises proceeds in a hierarchical fashion, beginning with attention training, then moving to memory training, and finally problem-solving training. This structure was developed strategically by Hogarty and colleagues, particularly due to the need for a strong attentional capacity for both memory and problem-solving abilities.

CET begins with two to three months of attention training that occur before the social cognitive groups are formed. The attention exercises are designed to improve speed of processing, lengthen sustained attention, heighten vigilance, and generally increase mental stamina. Plate 9 presents an example attention exercise known as the Attention Reaction Conditioner (ARC). In this exercise, individuals must respond to the center target light when it flashes green by pressing the space bar within a short window of time (e.g., 300 ms). Prior to the target light illuminating, a series of auditory cues (beeps) are given to prepare the participant for the onset of the target light. If the participant responds to the target light within the response window, then all nine of the feedback lights that form a pyramid around the target light will illuminate. If the participant responds slightly outside of the response window, only some of the feedback lights will illuminate, with fewer illuminating the slower the participant is to respond. Initially, participants are given five auditory cues for each second before the target light appears. Gradually, these cues are faded so that individuals have to learn to sustain their attention without external cues, and this becomes a challenging exercise for increasing the speed of processing and sustained attention. After attention training, individuals proceed to memory training, and usually the social cognitive groups will have begun concurrently, although the timeline varies depending on the abilities and needs of the individuals. Memory training focuses on developing a schematization or categorizing capacity, cognitive flexibility, an abstracting attitude, and executive (decision making) functions through the completion of sequential, delayed, spatial, visual, auditory, and verbal memory exercises. Finally, problem-solving training aims to improve analytic logic, effortful executive functions, strategic and foresightful planning, and intuition—abilities that support the gistful, abstract thinking that is fundamental to higher-order social cognition (Hogarty & Greenwald, 2006).

Social Cognitive Training

Rationale. The targeting of social cognition is the cornerstone of CET, and neurocognitive training is utilized as an effective component for supporting higher-order social cognitive abilities. The emphasis on social cognition in CET comes from the foresight of Hogarty and colleagues in predicting that impairments in this domain were driving a substantial component of social functioning deficits in patients with schizophrenia (Hogarty & Flesher, 1999b), a point that was finally confirmed many years later (Fett et al., 2011). Despite adequate antipsychotic treatment, patients with schizophrenia remain markedly socially disabled. Further, interventions focused solely on improving neurocognitive function have had less success at reducing this disability, unless they have been strategically paired with broader psychosocial treatments (McGurk, Twamley, Sitzer, McHugo, & Mueser, 2007). It is now known that patients with schizophrenia experience deficits in social cognition ranging from challenges in taking the perspectives of others to understanding emotional facial expressions to responding to social situations in a context-appropriate manner. All of these challenges have clear logical connections to an inability to function in the adult social world, which have been repeatedly documented (Couture, Penn, & Roberts, 2006). Consequently, CET treats the improvement of social cognition as an important component for functional recovery from schizophrenia, and a large portion of the intervention is dedicated to this effort.

Approach. There are many different approaches one could consider when constructing a social cognitive intervention designed to provide enriched environmental experiences to individuals. Large-scale systems approaches, such as those studied by Nelson and colleagues (2007), can indeed be effective but are less feasible as a targeted cognitive rehabilitation intervention. Computerized approaches are gaining momentum due to their ease of administration but may lack the critical human element that characterizes everyday social interactions. Individual therapy approaches are also potentially attractive, but one-to-one sessions represent a not particularly rich social experience. Hogarty and colleagues decided to develop the social cognitive component of CET using a small group-based curriculum (Hogarty & Greenwald, 2006). Group settings are powerful social environments that can provide a uniquely stimulating experience even beyond the focus of their content. For example, individuals learn from others in the group, practice observing their peers, attempt to give feedback in a tactful manner, and coalesce around the norms of the group.

CET capitalizes on such naturally occurring group experiences to help facilitate the development of social cognition among group members. The ability to abstract the rules and norms of behavior in spontaneous social situations is the cornerstone of secondary socialization (Parsons & Bales, 1956), where individuals begin shifting their learning about the social world from explicit rules (i.e., primary socialization) to an appraisal of the social context, behavior of others, and constituent perspectives in order to identify the implicit norms governing the situation. The CET group embodies this secondary socialization approach both in its content and structure, where individuals are provided with experiential learning opportunities to engage in secondary socialization to facilitate their social and cognitive development. The possibility of providing such a rich socialization experience outside of a group context is difficult to imagine.

Group Content. CET consists of a total of forty-five 1.5-hour group sessions that form its social cognitive curriculum. This curriculum covers a purposively broad array of social cognitive abilities ranging from perspective taking to social context appraisal to emotion perception and management. These social cognitive groups integrate experiential learning opportunities in group exercises designed to facilitate social cognitive development with structured homework assignments, psychoeducation, and coaching. The group curriculum is divided into three modules that begin with "Basic Concepts" to provide foundational psychoeducation on schizophrenia, medication, cognition, and stress/emotion management. Core concepts covered include cognitive flexibility, enhancing motivation, getting the main point or "gist" in communications, learning to recognize early cues of distress, and implementing techniques to manage stress (e.g., diaphragmatic breathing).

The second module, "Social Cognition," covers a focused but comprehensive array of social cognitive abilities that are fundamental to successful interpersonal interactions and encourages their use through homework assignments and in-group cognitive exercises. Perspective taking is the central social cognitive ability around which other aspects of social cognition are taught. For example, when individuals learn about reading nonverbal cues, they learn that eye contact, body language, and facial expressions are all ways to understand what a person is thinking and feeling, that is, a person's perspective. Emotional temperature taking is another social cognitive ability that is covered during the second module of the group, where individuals learn how to pick up on the emotional state of others and use this information to determine how they should interact with that person (e.g., it is probably best not to make requests of a person who has a "hot" emotional temperature). Individuals also learn the importance of providing their own perspective to others when covering such concepts as giving a motivational account and elaborated speech. When learning to give a motivational account, individuals learn to give a realistic account of their behavior and how to ascertain when such an account would be necessary to provide. The critical point is that if an individual misunderstands your intentions, he or she could come to negative conclusions that harms the relationship, and it is important to provide that person with your own perspective and reason for your behavior (e.g., why you were late to work, why you had to turn down a lunch invitation). All too often, patients with schizophrenia will simply use unelaborated speech (e.g., "sorry" when they are late, "I can't" when they cannot accept a lunch invitation) that leaves others wondering about their perspective and often jumping to the conclusion that the individual either does not care or is being rude. Throughout the course of the group, cognitive exercises are conducted to enhance and practice these and other social cognitive abilities, along with psychoeducation on their use and importance.

In the third and final group module, "CET Applications," the emphasis is shifted from learning about and practicing new social cognitive abilities to generalizing and practicing these abilities in everyday life. Generalization to daily life is of course emphasized throughout the program in a variety of ways (e.g., homework, the construction of recovery plans with strategies for solving problems outside of treatment), but in this module, special attention is given to consolidating the knowledge individuals have gained over the previous sessions and developing a plan for using this information in everyday life both during treatment and when treatment ends. Psychoeducation is provided on relevant topics to this area, such as dealing with transitions and addressing common social dilemmas individuals are likely to encounter as they initiate new social and vocational activities, along with exercises that strategically target the transfer and consolidation of learning. For example, one of the first exercises in this module is "Using CET to Help a Friend," where individuals are presented with a scenario of a friend with a common social problem and asked to engage in an interaction with the friend to provide support to him or her and advice using what they have learned in CET that is relevant to the situation. In this manner, the final module of the group ties much of the previous sessions together into applications of CET strategies and social cognitive abilities to promote generalization.

Group Structure. The social cognitive group sessions in CET are small-group sessions consisting of six to eight participants and at least two coaches. The group is highly active and not possible to run effectively with a single coach. The general format of the group sessions is highly structured, with a specific agenda, handouts, and assigned roles (e.g., members who will be participating in this week's exercise, the coach who will be giving the psychoeducation talk). The format lends itself well to the purpose of the group, which is more educational than a traditional psychotherapy group. Many participants consider CET more akin to a class than a group therapy where they discuss their feelings and emotional turmoils. Indeed, an education on social cognition and how to develop its components is precisely what CET aims to provide, and given the comprehensive array of concepts covered, a great deal of structure is needed to accomplish all the tasks that are needed to give individuals the best opportunity to continue their social cognitive development.

Social cognitive group sessions begin with a "Welcome Back" by one of the CET coaches, which reviews the agenda for the day and situates it within the broader context of the curriculum. Subsequently, the coach welcoming the members back asks for one of the participants to volunteer to be the chairperson for the "Homework Presentation." The homework presentation is designed to revisit the previous week's educational topic and participants' application of that topic to their daily life. In addition, the homework presentation aims to provide the opportunity for participants to think more deeply and abstractly about the topic learned and its personal relevance. After a participant presents his or her homework, coaches ask questions to stimulate greater thinking about the concept, facilitate a deeper understanding of the material, and help participants practice "thinking on their feet" in unrehearsed social situations. The homework presentation is chaired not by one of the coaches but by one of the participants. Chairing the homework presentation in itself provides an excellent real-world cognitive exercise, where participants must adhere to the norms of the group, remember the role of the chairperson, keep an online tally of who has presented homework, and act tactfully to respond to common dilemmas (e.g., when multiple people raise their hands to present their homework at the same time). The chairperson is charged not only with calling on his or her fellow group members to present their homework but also on the coaches, who too must raise their hands to be recognized by the chair. This experience then becomes not only a fruitful cognitive exercise that keeps members highly mentally active but also empowers them to take ownership of part of the group and their own recovery process within treatment.

After the homework presentation concludes, selected group members participate in a "Cognitive Exercise" that aims to facilitate social cognitive development. The cognitive exercises are highly integrative and focus on the use of multiple social cognitive abilities simultaneously, similar to the way these abilities must be integrated and applied in everyday life. All exercises are conducted center stage in front of the group and usually include two of the group members. "Condensed Message" is an example exercise that is conducted later in the course of the forty-five-week group curriculum that aims primarily to facilitate gistfulness, perspective taking, and social context appraisal. In this exercise, two of the group members are given a scenario that presents a social problem that requires the construction of a brief message by one of the persons in the scenario to another person in the scenario who is the intended recipient of the message. However, communication methods are limited, and a meaningful message must be constructed within a maximum number of words (ten or less) that takes the perspective of the recipient and provides enough information to get the recipient to act on the social problem. In one of the condensed message exercises, "The Airport," a son has dropped his father off at the airport. Soon before his father's flight is to depart, the son receives a telephone call from a restaurant at the airport letting him know that his father left his wallet there. The restaurant is willing to send a brief page over the airport PA system to the father to get him to retrieve his wallet, if the son can construct a message in ten words of less. After reading the details of this scenario, the two participants move to the front of the room and work on a white board to construct a meaningful message that takes into account the father's perspective and what he will need to hear to act quickly (e.g., that something important was left behind) and that gives enough detail so that an action can be taken (e.g., instructions to retrieve the important lost item at the specific restaurant immediately). In this particular example, the social context is also very important for group members to consider, as there could be serious consequences to announcing to the entire airport that a wallet is available at one of the restaurants. In this way, group members actively engage in working together to solve a social problem that requires the use of multiple social cognitive abilities in a highly social setting. Exercises are conducted with different scenarios over multiple group sessions so that all participants have the opportunity to participate.

After the completion of the cognitive exercise, "Feedback" is given to the participants about their performance, first by the other group members and then by the coaches in the group. This keeps the group members not completing the exercise actively involved in the group and presents its own exercise in social cognition to them. For example, group members are asked to give tactful feedback to the participants about how they handled the intellectual challenges of the task, the emotional demands of the task, and their ability to engage in teamwork. This requires them to not only attend to the participants in the exercise but also take their perspective on how they might be thinking or feeling during the task and foresee how the participants are likely to respond to their feedback, as well as to observe verbal and nonverbal emotional cues as the participants work to manage their emotions during the challenging exercises. The coaches then provide feedback to the participants to support their efforts and give suggestions for areas of improvement. When the feedback concludes, a coach then gives a brief "Psychoeducational Talk." The topic of these lectures is structured around the modules of the group, such that early topics focus on basic psychoeducation about schizophrenia. During the Social Cognition module, topics focus on a broad range of social cognitive abilities, including perspective taking, reading nonverbal cues, social context appraisal, using elaborated speech, and getting the social "gist." In the CET Applications module, topics explicitly cover applying social cognitive strategies and abilities learned in CET to everyday life. When the task concludes, a "Homework Assignment" is given that is to be completed during the week based upon the psychoeducational talk. The homework assignment is designed to get participants to think more deeply about the concepts presented and apply them outside of the group. In this manner, CET provides a uniquely comprehensive approach to social cognitive training that is designed to generalize beyond the group experience.

Effects of CET on Cognition, Behavior, and the Brain

The evidence base for CET is growing and now has one of the greater levels of empirical support of the cognitive remediation approaches that have been tested in patients with schizophrenia. With the support of the National Institute of Mental Health, two randomized controlled trials have been completed in 121 patients with chronic (Hogarty et al., 2004) and 58 patients with early course (Eack et al., 2009) schizophrenia. These trials randomized participants to receive two years of either CET or an active enriched supportive therapy (EST) control, which is an illness management and psychoeducation intervention based on the demonstrably effective Personal Therapy (Hogarty et al., 1997a; Hogarty et al., 1997b). Participants were assessed with a comprehensive battery of cognitive and behavioral measures prior to beginning treatment and then annually thereafter over the course of two years. Both trials demonstrated highly significant levels of improvement favoring CET for improving social and nonsocial cognition over the course of treatment (see Figure 15.1). Neurocognitive improvement was greater in chronic patients, primarily due to the greater pretreatment cognitive ability of early course patients. The social cognitive domains studied were highly diverse across both of the trials and ranged from significant improvement in foresight and perspective taking (Hogarty et al., 2004; Eack et al., 2009) to improved emotional intelligence (Eack, Hogarty, Greenwald, Hogarty, & Keshavan, 2007). Perhaps most important, these cognitive improvements translated into meaningful gains in social adjustment and functional outcome, including improved role adjustment, instrumental task performance, and vocational functioning (Hogarty et al., 2004; Eack, Hogarty, Greenwald, Hogarty, & Keshavan, 2011). Subsequent mediator analyses from both trials indicated that the cognitive improvement observed in CET patients significantly contributed to gains in functional outcome (Hogarty, Greenwald, & Eack, 2006; Eack, Pogue-Geile, Greenwald, Hogarty, & Keshavan, 2011). Furthermore, these improvements in functioning were highly durable and lasted for at least one year posttreatment in both the chronic (Hogarty, Greenwald, & Eack, 2006) and early course samples (Eack, Greenwald, Hogarty, & Keshavan, 2010). Taken together, such findings provided strong support for the efficacy of CET for improving cognition and functional outcome in diverse samples of patients with schizophrenia.

The early benefits of CET on cognition observed in chronic schizophrenia patients led to an interest in the possibility that when CET is applied as an early intervention approach, it might be able to capitalize on a presumed neuroplasticity reserve and alter core neurobiologic mechanisms to achieve its effects (Keshavan & Hogarty, 1999). As a consequence, the second trial of CET, which focused on early course schizophrenia patients, included pretreatment and annual repeated brain imaging assessments. Of the fifty-eight early course schizophrenia patients randomized to CET or EST, fifty-three had high-resolution structural neuroimaging data available for analysis (two participants were too large to fit into the scanner, one had a metal object embedded in his thigh, one could not complete the scanning procedure due to anxiety, and one withdrew consent before the collection of imaging data). The only observed difference between patients who completed magnetic resonance imaging (MRI) procedures and those who did not was that individuals with available MRI data tended to have higher levels of education. Voxel-based morphometry analyses employing linear mixed-effects models adjusting for potentially confounding demographic and medication effects were conducted to examine the differential effects of CET versus EST on brain structure over the course of the study. Dramatically, results revealed that patients who received CET demonstrated a protection against the commonly reported gray matter loss in early course schizophrenia (DeLisi, 2008), compared to those receiving EST. In particular,

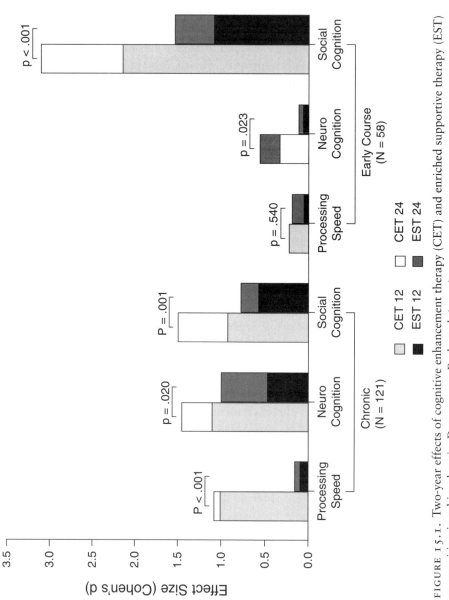

FIGURE 15.1. Two-year effects of cognitive enhancement therapy (CET) and enriched supportive therapy (EST) on cognition in schizophrenia. Data source: Eack et al. (2009).

significant neuroprotective effects were observed in medial-temporal areas of the brain that have been repeatedly implicated in social cognition, including the left amygdala, parahippocampal gyrus, and fusiform gyrus (see Plate 10) (Eack et al., 2010b). Trend-level effects were observed in the prefrontal cortex and right insula, but these did not withstand correction for multiple inference testing in confirmatory volumetric analyses. While the majority of the effects on social cognitive brain networks exhibited properties of neuroprotection (i.e., a maintenance of gray matter in CET patients compared to those receiving in EST), the left amygdala also demonstrated significant growth, suggesting potential neurogenesis in this region.

After observing the neuroprotective benefits of CET against gray matter loss in medial-temporal areas of the brain implicated in social cognition, linear mixed-effects growth models were used to examine the effects of these neuroplastic changes on cognitive improvement observed throughout the course of the trial. Results revealed that less gray matter loss in the left parahippocampal and fusiform gyrus and greater gray matter increases in the left amygdala were significantly related to improvements in social cognition. Further, these changes in gray matter volume partially mediated the differential effects of CET on social cognition, indicating that they were potential mechanisms of social cognitive improvement during the trial. Neuroprotection against gray matter loss in the left parahippocampal and fusiform gyrus also was significantly associated with two-year neurocognitive improvement and mediated the differential effects of CET on neurocognition, suggesting that the neural changes observed in these regions had cognitive benefits beyond social cognitive domains (Eack et al., 2010b). Taken together, these findings provide the first evidence of the neuroplastic effects of a social cognitive rehabilitation program in patients with schizophrenia, and the results of ongoing studies examining how these effects translate to changes in brain function are eagerly awaited.

Conclusions

The brain has now been shown to be more plastic than most early neuroscientists could have ever imagined, and its remarkable capacity to change and adapt to new cognitive demands extends beyond the basic domains of information processing and well into the realm of social cognition. The reality of neuroplasticity has begun to be harnessed to improve the social brain in a variety of conditions ranging from socially deprived Romanian orphans (Nelson et al., 2007) to patients with schizophrenia (Hogarty et al.,

2004). Schizophrenia is a disorder that is characterized by pervasive neu-robiologically based impairments in social cognition (Pinkham, Penn, Perkins, & Lieberman, 2003) that significantly limit functional recovery from the condition (Fett et al., 2011). Unfortunately, pharmacologic agents have had little impact on this important domain of functioning (Sergi et al., 2007), and few treatment approaches have been developed to remediate social cognitive deficits. CET (Hogarty & Greenwald, 2006) represents a unique, comprehensive approach designed to address impairments in both social and nonsocial cognition in schizophrenia by providing the enriched environmental and secondary socialization experiences needed to facilitate neuroplastic change and jump-start social cognitive development in the disorder. Based on a neurodevelopmental framework (Hogarty & Flesher, 1999a), CET integrates sixty hours of computer-based training in attention, memory, and problem solving, with forty-five social cognitive group sessions to provide and help individuals with schizophrenia shift from a reliance on concrete and rigid rules for behavior to a more gistful and spontaneous abstraction of social themes. Repeated evidence has documented the efficacy of CET for improving social cognition in schizophrenia (Hogarty et al., 2004; Eack et al., 2009), and now recent findings indicate that these improvements are indeed reflective of underlying changes in the social brain (Eack et al., 2010b). It is expected that the next generation of social cognitive rehabilitation studies in schizophrenia and other disorders will build upon this exciting evidence base to define with greater precision the boundaries of plasticity in the social brain and the methods that can be used to harness this plasticity for positive social and cognitive development.

References

Adolphs, R. (2003). Cognitive neuroscience of human social behaviour. *Nature Reviews Neuroscience, 4*(3), 165–178.

Allison, T., Puce, A., & McCarthy, G. (2000). Social perception from visual cues: Role of the STS region. *Trends in Cognitive Sciences, 4*(7), 267–278.

American Psychiatric Association. (2000). *Diagnostic and statistical manual of mental disorders* (4th ed., text rev.). Washington, DC: Author.

Baron-Cohen, S. (1990). Autism: A specific cognitive disorder of 'mind-blindness'. *International Review of Psychiatry, 2*(1), 81–90.

Ben-Yishay, Y., Piasetsky, E. B., & Rattok, J. (1985). A systematic method for ameliorating disorders in basic attention. In M. J. Meir, A. L. Benton, & L. Diller (Eds.), *Neuropsychological rehabilitation* (pp. 165–181). New York: Guilford.

Blakemore, S. J., & Choudhury, S. (2006). Development of the adolescent brain: Implications for executive function and social cognition. *Journal of Child Psychology and Psychiatry, 47*(3–4), 296–312.

Brackett, M. A., & Mayer, J. D. (2003). Convergent, discriminant, and incremental validity of competing measures of emotional intelligence. *Personality and Social Psychology Bulletin, 29*(9), 1147–1158.

Bracy, O. L. (1994). *PSSCogRehab* [computer software]. Indianapolis, IN: Psychological Software Services.

Branchi, I., D'Andrea, I., Fiore, M., Di Fausto, V., Aloe, L., & Alleva, E. (2006). Early social enrichment shapes social behavior and nerve growth factor and brain-derived neurotrophic factor levels in the adult mouse brain. *Biological Psychiatry, 60*(7), 690–696.

Braw, Y., Bloch, Y., Mendelovich, S., Ratzoni, G., Gal, G., Harari, H., Tripto, A., & Levkovitz, Y. (2008). Cognition in young schizophrenia outpatients: Comparison of first-episode with multiepisode patients. *Schizophrenia Bulletin, 34*(3), 544–554.

Bruel-Jungerman, E., Davis, S., & Laroche, S. (2007). Brain plasticity mechanisms and memory: A party of four. *Neuroscientist, 13*(5), 492–505.

Brune, M., Abdel-Hamid, M., Lehmkamper, C., & Sonntag, C. (2007). Mental state attribution, neurocognitive functioning, and psychopathology: What predicts poor social competence in schizophrenia best? *Schizophrenia Research, 92*(1–3), 151–159.

Corrigan, P. W. (1994). Social cue perception and intelligence in schizophrenia. *Schizophrenia Research, 13*(1), 73–79.

Couture, S. M., Penn, D. L., & Roberts, D. L. (2006). The functional significance of social cognition in schizophrenia: A review. *Schizophrenia Bulletin, 32*(Suppl. 1), S44–S63.

DeLisi, L. E. (2008). The concept of progressive brain change in schizophrenia: Implications for understanding schizophrenia. *Schizophrenia Bulletin, 34*(2), 312–321.

Eack, S. M., Hogarty, G. E., Greenwald, D. P., Hogarty, S. S., & Keshavan, M. S. (2007). Cognitive enhancement therapy improves emotional intelligence in early course schizophrenia: Preliminary effects. *Schizophrenia Research, 89*(1–3), 308–311.

Eack, S. M., & Newhill, C. E. (2007). Psychiatric symptoms and quality of life in schizophrenia: A meta-analysis. *Schizophrenia Bulletin, 33*(5), 1225–1237.

Eack, S. M., Greenwald, D. P., Hogarty, S. S., Cooley, S. J., DiBarry, A. L., Montrose, D. M., & Keshavan, M. S. (2009). Cognitive enhancement therapy for early-course schizophrenia: Effects of a two-year randomized controlled trial. *Psychiatric Services, 60*(11), 1468–1476.

Eack, S. M., Greenwald, D. P., Hogarty, S. S., & Keshavan, M. S. (2010). One-year durability of the effects of cognitive enhancement therapy on functional outcome in early schizophrenia. *Schizophrenia Research, 120*(1), 210–216.

Eack, S. M., Dworakowski, D., Montrose, D. M., Miewald, J., Gur, R. E., Gur, R. C., Sweeney, J. A., & Keshavan, M. S. (2010a). Social cognition deficits among individuals at familial high risk for schizophrenia. *Schizophrenia Bulletin, 36*(6), 1081–1088.

Eack, S. M., Hogarty, G. E., Cho, R. Y., Prasad, K. M. R., Greenwald, D. P., Hogarty, S. S., & Keshavan, M. S. (2010b). Neuroprotective effects of cognitive enhancement therapy against gray matter loss in early schizophrenia: Results from a two-year randomized controlled trial. *Archives of General Psychiatry,* 67(7), 674–682.

Eack, S. M., Hogarty, G. E., Greenwald, D. P., Hogarty, S. S., & Keshavan, M. S. (2011). Effects of cognitive enhancement therapy on employment outcomes in early schizophrenia: Results from a two-year randomized trial. *Research on Social Work Practice,* 21(3), 32–42.

Eack, S. M., Pogue-Geile, M. F., Greenwald, D. P., Hogarty, S. S., & Keshavan, M. S. (2011). Mechanisms of functional improvement in a 2-year trial of cognitive enhancement therapy for early schizophrenia. *Psychological Medicine,* 41(6), 1253–1261.

Ehring, T., Tuschen-Caffier, B., Schnülle, J., Fischer, S., & Gross, J. J. (2010). Emotion regulation and vulnerability to depression: Spontaneous versus instructed use of emotion suppression and reappraisal. *Emotion,* 10(4), 563–572.

Ekman, P. (1993). Facial expression and emotion. *American Psychologist,* 48(4), 384–392.

Elbert, T., Pantev, C., Wienbruch, C., Rockstroh, B., & Taub, E. (1995). Increased cortical representation of the fingers of the left hand in string players. *Science,* 270(5234), 305–307.

Eriksson, P. S., Perfilieva, E., Björk-Eriksson, T., Alborn, A. M., Nordborg, C., Peterson, D. A., & Gage, F. H. (1998). Neurogenesis in the adult human hippocampus. *Nature Medicine,* 4(11), 1313–1317.

Fett, A. K. J., Viechtbauer, W., Dominguez, M. G., Penn, D. L., Van Os, J., & Krabbendam, L. (2011). The relationship between neurocognition and social cognition with functional outcomes in schizophrenia: A meta-analysis. *Neuroscience & Biobehavioral Reviews,* 35(3), 573–588.

Flavell, J. H. (1976). Metacognitive aspects of problem solving. In B. Resnick (Ed.), *Nature of intelligence* (pp. 231–235). Hillsdale, NJ: Erlbaum.

Flavell, J. H. (1992). Perspectives on perspective-taking. In H. Beilin & P. B. Pufall (Eds.), *Piaget's theory: Prospects and possibilities. The Jean Piaget symposium series* (pp. 305–339). Hillsdale, NJ: Erlbaum.

Gladstone, T. R. G., & Kaslow, N. J. (1995). Depression and attributions in children and adolescents: A meta-analytic review. *Journal of Abnormal Child Psychology,* 23(5), 597–606.

Gogtay, N., Giedd, J. N., Lusk, L., Hayashi, K. M., Greenstein, D., Vaituzis, A. C., Nugent, T. F., Herman, D. H., Clasen, L. S., Toga, A. W., et al. (2004). Dynamic mapping of human cortical development during childhood through early adulthood. *Proceedings of the National Academy of Sciences of the United States of America,* 101(21), 8174–8179.

Green, M. F., Kern, R. S., Braff, D. L., & Mintz, J. (2000). Neurocognitive deficits and functional outcome in schizophrenia: Are we measuring the right stuff. *Schizophrenia Bulletin,* 26(1), 119–136.

Green, M. F., Nuechterlein, K. H., Gold, J. M., Barch, D. M., Cohen, J., Essock, S., Fenton, W. S., Frese, F., Goldberg, T. E., Heaton, R. K., et al. (2004). Approaching a consensus cognitive battery for clinical trials in schizophrenia: The NIMH-MATRICS conference to select cognitive domains and test criteria. *Biological Psychiatry,* 56(5), 301–307.

Green, M. F., Penn, D. L., Bentall, R., Carpenter, W. T., Gaebel, W., Gur, R. C., Kring, A. M., Park, S., Silverstein, S. M., & Heinssen, R. (2008). Social cognition in schizophrenia: An NIMH workshop on definitions, assessment, and research opportunities. *Schizophrenia Bulletin, 34*(6), 1211–1220.

Halperin, J. M., Marks, D. J., Bedard, A. C. V., Chacko, A., Curchack, J. T., Yoon, C. A., & Healey, D. M. (2013). Training executive, attention, and motor skills: A proof-of-concept study in preschool children with ADHD. *Journal of Attention Disorders, 17*(8), 711–721.

Harlow, H. F. (1958). The nature of love. *American Psychologist, 13*(12), 673–685.

Heinrichs, R. W., & Zakzanis, K. K. (1998). Neurocognitive deficit in schizophrenia: A quantitative review of the evidence. *Neuropsychology, 12*(3), 426–445.

Hogarty, G. E., Kornblith, S. J., Greenwald, D., Dibarry, A. L., Cooley, S., Ulrich, R. F., Carter, M., & Flesher, S. (1997a). Three-year trials of personal therapy among schizophrenic patients living with or independent of family: I. Description of study and effects of relapse rates. *American Journal of Psychiatry, 154*(11), 1504–1513.

Hogarty, G. E., Greenwald, D., Ulrich, R. F., Kornblith, S. J., Dibarry, A. L., Cooley, S., Carter, M., & Flesher, S. (1997b). Three-year trials of personal therapy among schizophrenic patients living with or independent of family: II. Effects on adjustment of patients. *American Journal of Psychiatry, 154*(11), 1514–1524.

Hogarty, G. E., & Flesher, S. (1999a). Developmental theory for a cognitive enhancement therapy of schizophrenia. *Schizophrenia Bulletin, 25*(4), 677–692.

Hogarty, G. E., & Flesher, S. (1999b). Practice principles of cognitive enhancement therapy for schizophrenia. *Schizophrenia Bulletin, 25*(4), 693–708.

Hogarty, G. E., Flesher, S., Ulrich, R., Carter, M., Greenwald, D., Pogue-Geile, M., Keshavan, M., Cooley, S., DiBarry, A. L., Garrett, A., et al. (2004). Cognitive enhancement therapy for schizophrenia: Effects of a 2-year randomized trial on cognition and behavior. *Archives of General Psychiatry, 61*(9), 866–876.

Hogarty, G. E., & Greenwald, D. P. (2006). *Cognitive enhancement therapy: The training manual.* Pittsburgh, PA: University of Pittsburgh Medical Center. Available through www.CognitiveEnhancementTherapy.com.

Hogarty, G. E., Greenwald, D. P., & Eack, S. M. (2006). Durability and mechanism of effects of cognitive enhancement therapy. *Psychiatric Services, 57*(12), 1751–1757.

Horan, W. P., Green, M. F., DeGroot, M., Fiske, A., Hellemann, G., Kee, K., Kern, R. S., Lee, J., Sergi, M. J., Subotnik, K. L., et al. (2012). Social cognition in schizophrenia, Part 2: 12-month stability and prediction of functional outcome in first-episode patients. *Schizophrenia Bulletin, 38*(4), 865–872.

Just, M. A., Cherkassky, V. L., Aryal, S., & Mitchell, T. M. (2010). A neurosemantic theory of concrete noun representation based on the underlying brain codes. *PLoS One, 5*(1), e8622.

Karni, A., Meyer, G., Jezzard, P., Adams, M. M., Turner, R., & Ungerleider, L. G. (1995). Functional MRI evidence for adult motor cortex plasticity during motor skill learning. *Nature, 377*(6545), 155–158.

Keefe, R. S. E., Bilder, R. M., Davis, S. M., Harvey, P. D., Palmer, B. W., Gold, J. M., Meltzer, H. Y., Green, M. F., Capuano, G., Stroup, T. S., et al.

(2007). Neurocognitive effects of antipsychotic medications in patients with chronic schizophrenia in the CATIE Trial. *Archives of General Psychiatry, 64*(6), 633–647.

Keshavan, M. S., & Hogarty, G. E. (1999). Brain maturational processes and delayed onset in schizophrenia. *Development and Psychopathology, 11*(3), 525–543.

Keshavan, M. S., Diwadkar, V. A., Montrose, D. M., Rajarethinam, R., & Sweeney, J. A. (2005). Premorbid indicators and risk for schizophrenia: A selective review and update. *Schizophrenia Research, 79*(1), 45–57.

Keshavan, M. S., Kulkarni, S., Bhojraj, T., Francis, A., Diwadkar, V., Montrose, D. M., Seidman, L. J., & Sweeney, J. (2009). Premorbid cognitive deficits in young relatives of schizophrenia patients. *Frontiers in Human Neuroscience, 3*(62), 1–14.

Kleim, J. A., Barbay, S., & Nudo, R. J. (1998). Functional reorganization of the rat motor cortex following motor skill learning. *Journal of Neurophysiology, 80*(6), 3321–3325.

Kohler, C. G., Walker, J. B., Martin, E. A., Healey, K. M., & Moberg, P. J. (2010). Facial emotion perception in schizophrenia: A meta-analytic review. *Schizophrenia Bulletin, 36*(5), 1009–1019.

Liepert, J., Miltner, W. H. R., Bauder, H., Sommer, M., Dettmers, C., Taub, E., & Weiller, C. (1998). Motor cortex plasticity during constraint-induced movement therapy in stroke patients. *Neuroscience Letters, 250*(1), 5–8.

Lopes, P. N., Salovey, P., & Straus, R. (2003). Emotional intelligence, personality, and the perceived quality of social relationships. *Personality and Individual Differences, 35*(3), 641–658.

Lopes, P. N., Grewal, D., Kadis, J., Gall, M., & Salovey, P. (2006). Evidence that emotional intelligence is related to job performance and affect and attitudes at work. *Psicothema, 18*, 132–138.

Lu, L., Bao, G., Chen, H., Xia, P., Fan, X., Zhang, J., Pei, G., & Ma, L. (2003). Modification of hippocampal neurogenesis and neuroplasticity by social environments. *Experimental Neurology, 183*(2), 600–609.

Marwaha, S., & Johnson, S. (2004). Schizophrenia and employment: A review. *Social Psychiatry and Psychiatric Epidemiology, 39*(5), 337–349.

McGurk, S. R., Twamley, E. W., Sitzer, D. I., McHugo, G. J., & Mueser, K. T. (2007). A meta-analysis of cognitive remediation in schizophrenia. *American Journal of Psychiatry, 164*(12), 1791–1802.

Milev, P., Ho, B., Arndt, S., & Andreasen, N. C. (2005). Predictive values of neurocognition and negative symptoms on functional outcome in schizophrenia: A longitudinal first-episode study with 7-year follow-up. *American Journal of Psychiatry, 162*(3), 495–506.

Mitchell, J. P., Banaji, M. R., & MacRae, C. N. (2005). The link between social cognition and self-referential thought in the medial prefrontal cortex. *Journal of Cognitive Neuroscience, 17*(8), 1306–1315.

Mueser, K. T., & Tarrier, N. (1998). *Handbook of social functioning in schizophrenia*. Boston, MA: Allyn & Bacon.

Nakato, E., Otsuka, Y., Kanazawa, S., Yamaguchi, M. K., Watanabe, S., & Kakigi, R. (2009). When do infants differentiate profile face from frontal face? A near-infrared spectroscopic study. *Human Brain Mapping, 30*(2), 462–472.

Nelson, C. A., Zeanah, C. H., Fox, N. A., Marshall, P. J., Smyke, A. T., & Guthrie, D. (2007). Cognitive recovery in socially deprived young children: The Bucharest Early Intervention Project. *Science, 318*(5858), 1937–1940.

Newman, L. S. (2001). What is social cognition? Four basic approaches and their implications for schizophrenia research. In P. W. Corrigan & D. L. Penn (Eds.), *Social cognition and schizophrenia* (pp. 41–72). Washington, DC: American Psychological Association.

Palmer, B. A., Pankratz, V. S., & Bostwick, J. M. (2005). The lifetime risk of suicide in schizophrenia: a reexamination. *Archives of General Psychiatry, 62*(3), 247–253.

Pantev, C., Oostenveld, R., Engelien, A., Ross, B., Roberts, L. E., & Hoke, M. (1998). Increased auditory cortical representation in musicians. *Nature, 392*(6678), 811–814.

Parsons, T., & Bales, R. (1956). *Family, Socialization and Interaction Process.* London: Routledge and Kegan Paul.

Penn, D. L., Corrigan, P. W., Bentall, R. P., Racenstein, J., & Newman, L. (1997). Social cognition in schizophrenia. *Psychological Bulletin, 121*(1), 114–132.

Pinkham, A. E., Penn, D. L., Perkins, D. O., & Lieberman, J. (2003). Implications for the neural basis of social cognition for the study of schizophrenia. *American Journal of Psychiatry, 160*(5), 815–824.

Robertson, I. H., & Murre, J. M. J. (1999). Rehabilitation of brain damage: Brain plasticity and principles of guided recovery. *Psychological Bulletin, 125*(5), 544–575.

Robinson, D. G., Woerner, M. G., Mcmeniman, M., Mendelowitz, A., & Bilder, R. M. (2004). Symptomatic and functional recovery from a first episode of schizophrenia or schizoaffective disorder. *American Journal of Psychiatry, 161*(3), 473–479.

Roy, N. S., Wang, S., Jiang, L., Kang, J., Benraiss, A., Harrison-Restelli, C., Fraser, R. A. R., Couldwell, W. T., Kawaguchi, A., Okano, H., et al. (2000). In vitro neurogenesis by progenitor cells isolated from the adult human hippocampus. *Nature Medicine, 6*(3), 271–277.

Salovey, P., & Mayer, J. D. (1990). Emotional intelligence. *Imagination, Cognition, and Personality, 9*(3), 185–221.

Sergi, M. J., Rassovsky, Y., Nuechterlein, K. H., & Green, M. F. (2006). Social perception as a mediator of the influence of early visual processing on functional status in schizophrenia. *American Journal of Psychiatry, 163*(3), 448–454.

Sergi, M. J., Green, M. F., Widmark, C., Reist, C., Erhart, S., Braff, D. L., Kee, K. S., Marder, S. R., & Mintz, J. (2007). Cognition and neurocognition: Effects of risperidone, olanzapine, and haloperidol. *American Journal of Psychiatry, 164*(10), 1585–1592.

Sitzer, D. I., Twamley, E. W., & Jeste, D. V. (2006). Cognitive training in Alzheimer's disease: A meta-analysis of the literature. *Acta Psychiatrica Scandinavica, 114*(2), 75–90.

Surguladze, S. A., Marshall, N., Schulze, K., Hall, M. H., Walshe, M., Bramon, E., Phillips, M. L., Murray, R. M., & McDonald, C. (2010). Exaggerated neural response to emotional faces in patients with bipolar disorder and their first-degree relatives. *Neuroimage, 53*(1), 58–64.

Swartz, M. S., Perkins, D. O., Stroup, T. S., Davis, S. M., Capuano, G., Rosen-heck, R. A., Reimherr, F., McGee, M. F., Keefe, R. S. E., McEvoy, J. P., et al. (2007). Effects of antipsychotic medications on psychosocial functioning in patients with chronic schizophrenia: Findings from the NIMH CATIE Study. *American Journal of Psychiatry, 164*(3), 428–436.

Talassi, E., Guerreschi, M., Feriani, M., Fedi, V., Bianchetti, A., & Trabucchi, M. (2007). Effectiveness of a cognitive rehabilitation program in mild dementia (MD) and mild cognitive impairment (MCI): A case control study. *Archives of Gerontology and Geriatrics, 44,* 391–399.

Tallal, P., Merzenich, M. M., Miller, S., & Jenkins, W. (1998). Language learning impairments: Integrating basic science, technology, and remediation. *Experimental Brain Research, 123*(1), 210–219.

Tamm, L., Hughes, C., Ames, L., Pickering, J., Silver, C. H., Stavinoha, P., Castillo, C. L., Rintelmann, J., Moore, J., Foxwell, A., et al. (2010). Attention training for school-aged children with ADHD: Results of an open trial. *Journal of Attention Disorders, 14*(1), 86–94.

Temple, E., Deutsch, G. K., Poldrack, R. A., Miller, S. L., Tallal, P., Merzenich, M. M., & Gabrieli, J. D. E. (2003). Neural deficits in children with dyslexia ameliorated by behavioral remediation: Evidence from functional MRI. *Proceedings of the National Academy of Sciences, 100*(5), 2860–2865.

Thorndike, E. L. (1920). Intelligence and its uses. *Harper's Magazine,* 140, 217–235.

Wyer, R. S., & Srull, T. K. (Eds.). (1994). *Handbook of social cognition. Vol. 1: Basic processes.* Hillside, NJ: Lawrence Erlbaum.

16.

Conclusions

Russell K. Schutt, Larry J. Seidman, and Matcheri S. Keshavan

S OCIAL NEUROSCIENCE did not emerge as a distinct field until the early 1990s, and thus it is not surprising that its potential for trans-disciplinary integration has not yet been fully realized (Cacioppo & Berntson, 1992). What is surprising is the rapid pace of discoveries in the ensuing two decades and the transformative potential they have demonstrated (Meyer-Lindenberg & Tost, 2012). From description of neuropeptides in the brain and their relationship to sociability to analysis of social networks in the community, our chapter authors have highlighted many recent discoveries in neuroscience and particularly salient connections between brain, mind, and society. From approaches to enhancing social cognition to psychological consequences of exposure to violence, our chapter authors have also identified implications of social neuroscience for treating mental illness and improving community life. As research in neurology, social psychology, social network analysis, and other areas identifies more cross-level interactions and as technological advances improve our investigative tools and our means for engaging with others, we are confident that the intellectual foundation for and practical implications of social neuroscience will continue to expand.

Already, our ability to develop an integrated foundation for psychiatry, psychology, and sociology stands in stark contrast to the barriers the founders of our disciplines confronted more than 100 years ago. Freud's shift away from neuroanatomy (Sulloway, 1992, p. 15), John B. Watson's and B. F. Skinner's behaviorist foundation for psychology, and Émile Durkheim's and Max Weber's rejection of possible links of sociology to biology and psychology each reflected in part the inability of early social scientists to investigate the brain and to identify neurological responses to or effects on social processes. The multilevel analyses that are essential to research in social neuroscience would have seemed neither possible nor prudent to earlier generations (Cacioppo & Berntson 1992). They are possible today.

The human brain's extraordinary complexity, with its one hundred billion neurons and one hundred trillion interneural connections, still defies complete description and comprehensive understanding with even the fastest supercomputers and the most refined neuroimaging. However, the Human Connectome Project, launched by the National Institutes of Health (NIH) in the fall of 2010; the BRAIN (Brain Research through Advancing Innovative Neurotechnologies) Initiative, launched by President Obama in April 2013; and the Human Brain Project, launched by the European Commission in the same year, ensure that description and understanding of brain functioning will continue to develop rapidly. Already, neural connections relevant to the surrounding social environment are being increasingly identified. The rapidly expanding body of research that has emerged from investigations like those reported in this volume has already revealed the profoundly social orientation of the human brain, suggested an evolutionary basis for human social propensities, and highlighted unceasing interaction between the social brain and the social world. The knowledge deficits that contributed to the simplicities of social Darwinism, the willful blindness of behaviorism, and the determined dualism of Durkheim's and Weber's theorizing have been replaced by new awareness of the multiple links between brain, mind, and society.

This chapter provides an opportunity for review, reconsideration, and extension. We review key findings from the preceding contributed chapters and reconsider objections to an interdisciplinary approach in light of these findings. We then highlight unresolved questions and new research directions. Our goal is to establish the value of a multilevel perspective on human behavior and orientations and identify directions for an integrated explanatory framework.

Review of Findings

Although we humans were "small, slow and weak" in comparison to many other animals on the African savanna, our species was able to decisively outcompete all others for resources over the course of tens of thousands of years (Zaki & Ochsner, 2012, p. 675). The research reviewed by Jonathan

Turner from both evolutionary biology and neurobiology points to human sociality as the key to our survival as the "fittest" and to the evolution of our brains as the basis of our unique social capacities (see also Massey, 2002).

Understanding how evolved human brain circuits enable social behavior and social cognition—the mental processes supporting sociality—has been a key contribution of social neuroscience (Keshavan, Chapter 2). Jonathan Turner (Chapter 3) specified links between particular neural structures and capacities for different aspects of interpersonal dynamics. Paul Nestor, Victoria Choate, and Ashley Shirai (Chapter 4) defined the "social brain" that resulted from this evolutionary history as a network of functionally and anatomically distinct cortical and subcortical regions modulated by particular neurotransmitters and closely linked to specific neuropeptides. Christine Hooker (Chapter 5) identified the networks of brain structures that are recruited to support the different dimensions of social cognition. Human sociality is thus deeply embedded in the brain's biology and, as a result, in both the conscious and unconscious operation of our minds.

The social impairments characteristic of schizophrenia may be characterized in part by abnormalities in the brain's social features. Nestor's research (Chapter 4) has identified abnormalities in fiber tracts connecting neural networks involved in higher-order cognition in schizophrenia as well as deficits in gray matter volume in brain regions that support social communication. The consequences include greater likelihood of both positive and negative symptoms as well as deficiencies in face processing, eye gaze movements, facial memory, and executive attention. Hooker's research (Chapter 5) points to volumetric and processing deficits in brain regions that are associated with an inability to recover from interpersonal conflicts, social anhedonia, and inadequate performance on "theory-of-mind" tasks.

The shift described by Larry Seidman (Chapter 6) in psychology's focus from explaining behavior to understanding cognition led in turn to recognition of the importance of cognitive abilities for maintaining social relations. Lee, Horan, and Green (Chapter 7) reviewed the various dimensions into which social cognition is currently divided and the evidence for impairments associated with schizophrenia. Empathic accuracy has been less studied than other aspects of social cognition but appears particularly impaired. Research reported by Addington and Barbato (Chapter 8) has identified many of these same deficits in individuals identified as at high risk for schizophrenia, defined either by family history of illness in close relatives or by subthreshold psychotic symptoms.

Matcheri Keshavan (Chapter 2) introduced the concepts of experience-expectant and experience-dependent neuroplasticity as a framework for understanding the lasting impact of the social environment encountered in

early as well as subsequent brain development. Jill Hooley (Chapter 9) identified an experience-dependent impact of high levels of expressed emotion in
the family environment. Critical or hostile talk by close relatives can over-
activate the amygdala and in turn raise the risk of depression and lead to
relapse in individuals with schizophrenia. The social world shapes development of minds and brains.

Russell Schutt (Chapter 10) highlighted sociologists' long-standing recognition of the importance of social ties for human functioning, despite lack
of awareness of the neurobiological basis of human sociality. Bernice Pescosolido's (Chapter 11) integrated framework for understanding suicide
shows how far sociology has come since Durkheim insisted that sociologists should focus only on "social facts," as does Jonathan Turner's
(Chapter 3) connection of brain functioning to human emotionality and
social psychological processes. Pescosolido's cross-level analysis of the propensity to commit suicide directly demonstrates how social neuroscience
allows sociologists to use biological factors to improve explanation of the
same behavior on which Durkheim focused.

Michael Behen and Harry Chugani (Chapter 12) provide dramatic evidence of the lasting harm caused by detrimental social environments experienced in early development. The children they studied who experienced
early, severe social deprivation in orphanages subsequently suffered from
neurocognitive impairment and behavioral difficulties. These problems in
turn reflected changes in neural growth and functioning that had enduring
effects. On a more positive note, though, Behen and Chugani present evidence that neural growth and more normal brain functioning can be re-
stored at least in part through positive changes in the social environment.
Sharkey and Sampson (Chapter 13) then present evidence of a cognitive
effect on children of social relations in the larger community. The implication is that the quality of social ties can affect neurobiology even among
people who are not direct participants in those social ties. All of these point
to a degree of plasticity or malleability in which cognitive function may be
influenced by social experience to some extent.

Allan Horwitz's focus on the consequences for depression of the experience of bereavement (Chapter 14) reinforces Pescosolido's (and Durkheim's)
emphasis on the importance of social ties as a deterrent to suicide. Yet by
questioning the link between the emotions associated with bereavement and
the diagnosis of depression, Horwitz also cautions us that the boundary
between biological and sociological explanation is fuzzy and that the extent
and duration of the social environment's impact on the human organism
is quite variable.

Eack and Keshavan (Chapter 15) extend our understanding of the variable impact of the social environment by demonstrating the "experience-

dependent neuroplasticity" of the brain (Keshavan, Chapter 2). While they focus only on how an enriched, supportive social environment can improve social cognition and social functioning among persons diagnosed with schizophrenia by stimulating neural connectivity, this causal mechanism is one that we believe can be generalized to a wide variety of social settings.

Our chapters have thus spanned the human experience from "neurons to neighborhoods"—in the language of Bernice Pescosolido—and illustrated the role of human sociality in the bidirectional relations between brain, mind, and society. The chapters by Behen and Chugani and by Sharkey and Sampson also illustrate the importance of understanding the potential long-term impact of social policy on human functioning: Social policies that encourage orphanages—particularly ones that attach little importance to human nurturance—and those that fail to stanch gun violence can result in declines in neurobiological functioning in those affected.

Reconsideration of Resistance to Integration of Biology and Social Science

The basis of social scientists' resistance throughout most of the twentieth century to incorporating biological processes in explanations of human behavior can be summarized in one sentence: *Homo sapiens* evolved capacities that liberated human behavior from neurobiological constraints—including emotional pressure—and ensured almost infinite malleability in response to environmental influence as well as the ability to socially construct that environment. Each of the four beliefs embedded in this statement (Schutt, Seidman, and Keshavan, Chapter 1)—evolutionary displacement, human malleability, societal rationalization, and social construction—must be reexamined in light of the evidence presented in this volume.

Evolutionary Displacement Reconsidered

The belief in evolutionary displacement—that the evolved capacity of the human brain freed the human mind from neurological constraints—is inconsistent with new insights about evolution and neurobiology. The human brain was sculpted by evolution to support social ties and improve group functioning in order to maximize the odds of survival. Enlargement of the frontal lobes and thus executive functioning and the capacity for planning and self-control was a critical step in creating human potential, but the consequences of this development can only be understood in relation to the ongoing importance of social cognition and emotional needs. From the ability of infants to read emotions to the rapid reactions of adults to emotionally charged stimuli, "the language of emotions . . . is still the primal and primary language of humans" (Turner, Chapter 3). When neural development or connections are impaired at birth or as a result of epigenetic effects of environmental stress, schizophrenia and other illnesses can result. Thus, the products of the human mind cannot be understood without taking account of the neurobiology of the human brain.

There are still sharp disagreements about the course of evolution of human sociality and so about its ultimate products. The theory of group-based selection and of culture playing a role in influencing group survival chances is still controversial (Pinker, 2012). Despite support by E. O. Wilson (2012) and many others (Sussman & Chapman, 2004) for multilevel selection theory, many evolutionary psychologists argue that natural selection occurs only at the level of individuals and their genetically related kin (Tooby & Cosmides, 1992). Herbert Gintis, Samuel Boyles, and others (Gintis et al., 2005) believe that evolution had to favor the emergence of a disposition to punish those who engaged in "free riding" in a group in order to reap the benefits of group membership without contributing to it (see also Christakis & Fowler, 2009, p. 217). This conclusion is consistent with social psychological experiments that identify a considerable minority (perhaps one-third) as noncontributors who "free ride" if they are not sanctioned (Fehr & Gintis, 2007, pp. 50, 57). Boyd et al. (2005) suggest that altruistic punishment can maintain cooperation in groups at relatively small cost. And in this volume and elsewhere, Jonathan Turner (2007) has argued that humans evolved from low-sociality apes and have retained emotions that do not enhance sociality.

Despite these uncertainties about the evolutionary imprint on human sociality, the evolutionary origins and biological foundations of human sociality have become indisputable. Social connection is a primary human need that is a part of our biology, and social behavior cannot be understood apart from that context.

Human Malleability Reconsidered

The discoveries of modern neuroscience and human genetics have enhanced, rather than diminished, appreciation for the malleability of humans in response to their environment (National Institutes of Health, 2013). Both brain plasticity and epigenetic modifiability are evolved mechanisms for ensuring adaptability in response to environmental pressure. This adaptability was essential for the survival of early humans in response to a changing environment, and a high degree of adaptability continues to ensure that our most potent experiences leave a lasting impression on our bodies. But the recognition that biology does not mean destiny is cause simultaneously for consternation as well as celebration: environmental stress can have toxic and enduring effects on the brain, just as environmental enrichment can result in lasting gains in neural functioning. And the necessity of social engagement for human development and functioning profoundly limits human malleability.

Further research is needed to determine the range of environmental variation that has lasting neurobiological effects. Behen and Chugani (Chapter 12) and Hooley (Chapter 9) have highlighted the detrimental effects on the brain of extremely stressful interpersonal social environments, while Sharkey and Sampson (Chapter 13) found that exposure to violence in the surrounding community may have detrimental neurological effects on children. By contrast, Eack and Keshavan (Chapter 15) indicated that a highly enriched social environment can have lasting neurological benefits, while Behen and Chugani (Chapter 12) showed that adoption into a stable home could diminish some of the detrimental effects of early social deprivation. Between these negative and positive extremes, further research is needed about the type of variation in the social environment that can have significant and lasting neurobiological effects. These are difficult studies to carry out, but one example is instructive. Tienari et al. (2004) showed that the frequency of development of schizophrenia was reduced significantly among high-risk children (those with a biological parent with schizophrenia) by being brought up in adoptive families with healthy family interaction compared to those with dysfunctional interactions. Thus, a disorder with distinct genetic susceptibilities such as schizophrenia (Schizophrenia Working Group, 2014) may not manifest itself if a protective environment is present.

As neuroscientists are able to investigate neural processes at increasingly basic levels, we expect that the evidence of environmental influence will increase proportionately (cf. Schutt, 2011). We anticipate that the final result will be identification of a continuum of environmental influence, with more extreme environmental conditions producing more pronounced and lasting neurological effects.

Societal Rationalization Reconsidered

Jonathan Turner (Chapter 3) has brought to our book the understanding emerging from modern evolutionary biology that human emotions are an evolved mechanism to facilitate social ties. Much neurobiological and neuro-psychological research has confirmed that what may seem to be decision making on purely rational grounds is in fact shaped by emotions (Damasio, 1994). Because the belief that reasoned action can be separated from emotional motives is no longer tenable, the expectation that society can be constructed on a purely legal-rational basis is deficient (Massey, 2002, pp. 20–21). Although the frontal lobes do provide important control over emotional expression that in turn maintains group solidarity and societal cohesion (Kahneman, 2011), the ubiquity of human emotion creates strains that cannot be eliminated.

There is broad agreement among social neuroscientists and other specialists on the evolved importance of emotions for maintaining and shaping social bonds, but they differ in the emotions they view as primary. Most psychologists focus on the four primary emotions discussed by Nestor, Choate, and Shirai (Chapter 4)—happiness, fear, sadness, anger—but Jonathan Turner (Chapter 3) has emphasized the many variants on this theme. Sociologist Thomas Scheff (1990) argued that just one emotion, shame, is a master emotion that in turn shapes human social experience. More research on the impact of emotions on social interaction will help to clarify their relative importance, but the ubiquity and necessity of emotions in human thought and action is already widely accepted.

Social Construction Reconsidered

Social construction is a claim that is made all too easily about psychiatric maladies whose root causes and mechanisms of effect are not readily apparent. Social constructivists term schizophrenia a "social construction" in part because disordered thoughts could have other interpretations in other cultures, such as shamanism (Lysaker et al., 2005 Szasz, 1993). Indeed, research demonstrating that some individuals may have psychotic symptoms without psychotic illness (Van Os et al., 2009), especially if certain predisposing environmental factors do not occur, supports the idea that illnesses like schizophrenia are activated by environmental influence. But arguments that these illnesses are purely socially constructed become hard to maintain in the face of neurobiological and genetic evidence of diseases and their associated deficits in brain volume, neural circuits, and neurochemistry (Nestor, Choate, and Shirai, Chapter 4, this volume; also see Schizophrenia Working Group, 2014). Such arguments are also hard to maintain in the face of evidence that human sociality is made possible by subcortical structures whose evolution preceded the development of human culture (Turner, Chapter 3).

Gene-environment interactions add complexity to understanding neurobiological influences. Gene-environment interactions have been identified across a wide range of health conditions, including the risk of psychosis in response to environmental stress (Keshavan, Chapter 2), and the risk of depression in response to a stressful family environment (Hooley, Chapter 9) (and see Tooby & Cosmides, 1992, p. 84). Differential responsiveness to the social environment would in turn result in differences in how people think about, and hence mentally "construct," that environment. What the brain experiences in the social world and how the mind interprets that experience inevitably influence each other and necessarily vary in their influence between individuals.

The Value of an Integrated Framework

An integrated explanatory framework like Jonathan Turner's thus allows us to return to the vision of the earliest founders of psychiatry, psychology, and sociology but with a more sophisticated understanding of neurobiological processes and their origins that was not possible a century ago. Understanding that evolution wrote sociality into the human genome, recognizing that neuroplasticity and epigenetics both create bidirectional links between the environment and the brain, tracing the neural pathways that process social stimuli, and identifying the long-term harm of a deficient social environment and the salubrious effects of enriched social stimuli each support an integrated framework that permits more complete explanations of human behavior and orientations and better treatments for psychiatric illness.

This new transdisciplinary foundation for the social and clinical sciences is certainly not complete. New discoveries about connections between brain, mind, and society have been so rapid in the past two decades that the most ambitious claim we can make is to have taken stock of what has been accomplished with sufficient clarity and breadth to identify important next steps. The Connectome Project (NIH, 2009), the Obama BRAIN Initiative (Collins & Prabhakar, 2013), and the European Union's Brain Project ("Head Start," 2013) will accelerate in the next decade the foundation of neuroscientific knowledge on which our transdisciplinary effort builds. Nonetheless, it is no longer tenable to greet every effort to investigate biological influences on human behavior with a charge of "reductionism." Since both human neurons and the human genome are designed to respond to environmental influence, failing to take account of human biology is equivalent to refusing to consider the mechanism by which the environment influences behavior or to admit that biological changes induced by the environment in turn affect individuals' subsequent reactions to and ability to influence the environment.

Developing an integrated transdisciplinary framework for the explanation of human behavior and orientations also requires acknowledging the importance of group processes and societal influence. Yet many biologists continue to ignore the macro level of human experience when studying determinants of human behavior (Duster, 2006, pp. 3–6). Recently, the National Science Foundation's Advisory Board for funding evolutionary research, the National Evolutionary Synthesis Center (NESCent), included not a single social scientist (NESCent, 2013). Transdisciplinarity thus requires more attention in each of the relevant disciplines.

We also anticipate increased innovations in mental health treatment as research continues to improve understanding of connections between the brain, mind, and society (Collins & Prabhakar, 2013; NIH, 2013). Although no drugs have yet been developed that improve deficits in the neural circuits underlying social cognition, recent findings identify possible targets for pharmacological intervention. White matter and glial cells respond to social isolation and social stimulation (Makinodan et al., 2012). Mirror neurons appear to be disturbed in autism (Rizzolatti, 2005), and specific genetic variants are related to the risk of autism and schizophrenia (Lee et al., 2013).

But we have also highlighted the potential for improving the prevention of and response to mental illness through interventions directed at social experience. Interventions to alleviate abnormal expressed emotion in families can reduce the likelihood of subsequent depression, as identified by Hooley (Chapter 9), while heightened and directed social interaction can restore some of the social functioning that is deficient in schizophrenia (Eack and Keshavan, Chapter 10). Reducing rates of premature births is a macro-level change that could help to reduce the subsequent prevalence of psychiatric illness (Nosarti et al., 2012), while reducing the rate of child abuse can in turn diminish the likelihood of harmful, enduring genetic changes (McGowan, 2012). Many more such connections have been identified in recent decades, and their number will certainly multiply in the next few decades.

Sociality is a key part of humans as biological beings, so understanding individuals in their social environment must rest on recognizing bidirectional influences between neurobiology and the social environment. The social world is in our brains and it shapes our minds, while at the same time it is with our brains and minds that we construct our society. A trans-disciplinary social neuroscience allows us to understand ourselves and our society, and thus improve both.

References

Boyd, R., Gintis, H., Bowles, S., & Richerson, P. J. (2005). The evolution of altruistic punishment. In H. Gintis, S. Bowles, R. Boyd, & E. Fehr (Eds.), *Moral sentiments and material interests: The foundations of cooperation in economic life* (pp. 215–227). Cambridge, MA: MIT Press.

Cacioppo, J. T., & Berntson, G. G. (1992). Social psychological contributions to the decade of the brain: Doctrine of multilevel analysis. *The American Psychologist, 47,* 1019–1028.

Christakis, N. A., & Fowler, J. H. (2009). *Connected: The surprising power of our social networks and how they shape our lives.* Boston: Little, Brown.

Collins, F., & Prabhakar, A. (2013, April 2). BRAIN initiative challenges researchers to unlock mysteries of human mind. The White House Blog. www.whitehouse.gov/blog/2013/04/02/brain-initiative-challenges-researchers-unlock-mysteries-human-mind.

Damasio, A. (1994). *Descartes' error: Emotion, reason, and the human brain.* New York: Putnam.

Duster, T. (2006). Comparative perspectives and competing explanations: Taking on the newly configured reductionist challenge to sociology. *American Sociological Review, 71,* 1–15.

Fehr, E., & Gintis, H. (2007). Human motivation and social cooperation: Experimental and analytical foundations. *Annual Review of Sociology, 33,* 43–64.

Gintis, H., Bowles, S., Boyd, R., & Fehr, E. (2005). *Moral sentiments and material interests: The foundations of cooperation in economic life.* Cambridge, MA: MIT Press.

Head start: Europe's mega-project to simulate the human brain has much to offer neuroscience research—whether or not it delivers on its central promise. (2013, November 7). *Nature, 503.* www.nature.com/news/head-start-1.14091. https://www.humanbrainproject.eu/.

Kahneman, D. (2011). *Thinking, fast and slow.* New York: Farrar, Straus and Giroux.

Lee, S. H., Ripke, S., Neale, B. M., Faraone, S. V., Purcell, S. M., Perlis, R. H., . . . Wray, N. R. (2013). Identification of risk loci with shared effects on five major psychiatric disorders: A genome-wide analysis. *Lancet, 381*(9875), 1371–1379.

Lysaker, P. H., France, C. M., Hunter, N. L., & Davis, L. W. (2005). Personal narratives of illness in schizophrenia: Associations with neurocognition and symptoms. *Psychiatry, 68*(2), 140–151.

Makinodan, M., Rosen, K. M., Ito, S., & Corfas, G. (2012). A critical period for social experience-dependent oligodendrocyte maturation and myelination. *Science, 337*, 1357–1360.

Massey, D. S. (2002). A brief history of human society: The origin and role of emotion in social life. 2001 Presidential Address, American Sociological Association. *American Sociological Review, 67*, 1–29.

McGowan, P. O. (2012). Epigenetic clues to the biological embedding of early life adversity. *Biological Psychiatry, 72*(1), 4–5.

Meyer-Lindenberg, A., & Tost, H. (2012). Neural mechanisms of social risk for psychiatric disorders. *Nature Neuroscience, 15*, 663–668.

National Evolutionary Synthesis Center (NESCent). (2013). www.nescent.org/.

National Institutes of Health (NIH). (2009). *NIH launches the Human Connectome Project to unravel the brain's connections.* Bethesda, MD: National Institutes of Health. www.nih.gov/news/health/jul2009/ninds-15.htm.

———. (2013). The Human Connectome Project. http://www.neuroscienceblue print.nih.gov/connectome/.

Nosarti, C., Reichenberg, A., Murray, R. M., Cnattingius, S., Lambe, M. P., Yin, L., . . . Hultman, C. M. (2012). Preterm birth and psychiatric disorders in young adult life. *Archives of General Psychiatry, 69*(6), E1–E8.

Pinker, S. (June 2012). The false allure of group selection: An Edge original essay. *Edge.* http://edge.org/conversation/the-false-allure-of-group-selection

Rizzolatti, G. (2005). The mirror neuron system and its function in humans. *Anatomy and Embryology (Berlin), 210*, 419–421.

Scheff, T. J. (1990). *Microsociology: Discourse, emotion, and social structure.* Chicago: University of Chicago Press.

Schizophrenia Working Group of the Psychiatric Genomics Consortium. (2014). Biological insights from 108 schizophrenia-associated genetic loci. *Nature, 511*, 421–427.

Schutt, R. K. (with Goldfinger, S. M.). (2011). *Homelessness, housing, and mental illness.* Cambridge, MA: Harvard University Press.

Sulloway, F. J. (1992). *Freud, biologist of the mind: Beyond the psychoanalytic legend.* Cambridge, MA: Harvard University Press.

Sussman, R. W., & Chapman, A. R. (Eds.). (2004). *The origins and nature of sociality.* New York: Aldine de Gruyter.

Szasz, T. (1993). Crazy talk: Thought disorder or psychiatric arrogance? *British Journal of Medical Psychology, 66*(Pt. 1), 61–67.

Tienari, P., Wynne, L. C., Sorri, A., Lahti, I., Lalsy, K., Moring, J., . . . Wahlberg, K. E. (2004). Genotype-environment interaction in schizophrenia-spectrum disorder: Long-term follow-up study of Finnish adoptees. *British Journal of Psychiatry, 184*, 216–222.

Tooby, J., & Cosmides, L. (1992). The psychological foundations of culture. In J. H. Barkow, L. Cosmides, & J. Tooby (Eds.), *The adapted mind: Evolutionary psychology and the generation of culture* (pp. 19–136). New York: Oxford University Press.

Turner, J. H. (2007). *Human emotions: A sociological theory.* Oxford, UK: Routledge.

Van Os, J., Linscott, R. J., Myin-Germeys, I., Delespaul, P., & Krabbendam, L. (2009). A systematic review and meta-analysis of the psychosis continuum: Evidence for a psychosis proneness–persistence–impairment model of psychotic disorder. *Psychological Medicine, 39,* 179–195.

Wilson, E. O. (2012). *The social conquest of Earth.* New York: Liveright.

Zaki, J., & Ochsner, K. N. (2012). The neuroscience of empathy: Progress, pitfalls and promise. *Nature Neuroscience, 15,* 675–680.

Glossary

Affect recognition. The ability to identify and discriminate affect in others.

Amygdala. Almond-shaped set of neurons located deep in the brain's medial temporal lobe; one of the structures of the limbic system, the amygdala is thought to be involved in the processing of emotions. The amygdala is a part of the limbic system and plays a primary role in initiating response to threat, including social threat.

Anterior cingulate cortex (ACC). A brain area that is involved in conflict detection and decision making and that has connections with other brain areas involved in executive functioning.

Apoptosis. Programmed cell death.

Arcuate fasciculus. A white matter pathway that reciprocally projects to the frontal, parietal, and temporal cortices; the arcuate fasciculus connects the classical (Broca's, Wernicke's) language areas.

Attributional style. How one explains the causes for positive and negative events of their lives.

Biological embedding. Term coined by Clyde Herzmann to describe how factors of the social environment affect biological processes, or how "society gets under the skin."

Bioprogrammers. Bioprogrammers, or genetically driven behavioral features hardwired in the brain circuits during evolution.

Blockface. One side of a street between two consecutive intersections. For example, a blockface can be one side of a city block.

Brain plasticity. Brain's capacity to change as a result of experience or injury. It is also called neuroplasticity.

Cingulate bundle. A white matter fiber pathway in the brain, considered the most prominent white matter pathway in the limbic system. It furnishes both input and output to the dopaminergic-rich anterior cingulate cortex and lateral and ventral medial prefrontal sites, including the orbital frontal cortex, as well as to the amygdala, nucleus accumbens, and medial dorsal thalamus.

Cladistic analysis. The reconstruction of the likely behaviors and patterns of social organization of the last common ancestor to humans and present-day great apes.

Clinical high risk. Individuals who appear to be putatively prodromal for developing psychosis due to the presence of specific subthreshold psychotic symptoms.

Cognitive enhancement therapy. Cognitive rehabilitation intervention for schizophrenia designed to improve social and nonsocial cognition through the integration of computer-based neurocognitive training with group-based social cognitive treatment.

Cognitive functioning. The capacity to absorb and learn information, maintain attention and focus, and use knowledge and reasoning effectively.

Cognitive rehabilitation. An approach to cognitive treatment designed to improve information processing and brain function using systematic exercises targeting specific cognitive abilities.

Cognitive remediation. See *cognitive rehabilitation*.

Collective efficacy. Social cohesion among neighbors combined with their willingness to intervene on behalf of the common good.

Comparative neuroanatomy. Comparing the structures of the great ape and human brains to note differences and similarities, with differences revealing the route that natural selection took to make hominins and then humans more social through the dramatic increase in the size and connectivity of emotion centers of the brain and their connection to the neocortex.

Corticospinal tract. Descending fiber bundles (motor pathways) that arise in the primary motor cortex descend to the brainstem and cross at the level of the medulla; important for voluntary motor control.

Culture. The use of cognitive capacities of the neocortex or newer parts of the mammalian brain to create systems of meanings through the use of artificial symbols, such as language—a capacity that only evolved late in hominin evolution.

Defense mechanisms. Those tendencies of humans to push to the subconscious negative feelings where they are out of conscious awareness but where they begin to generate new kinds of negative emotions and dysfunctional behaviors that impede human happiness and well-being.

Deprivation-specific pattern. Behavioral patterns that are strongly associated with institution rearing and associated deprivation. These patterns rarely are observed in samples of children not exposed to institution rearing. Patterns include quasi-autism, disinhibited attachment, cognitive impairment, and an inattentive-overactive phenotype.

Diffusion tensor imaging (DTI). A Mmagnetic Rresonance Iimaging (MRI) technique which that uses magnets to allow the mapping of white matter tracts in the brain via detection of water molecules in the brain which that are diffused across these tracts. It can be used to detect connectivity of certain brain regions to other brain regions.

Dorsolateral prefrontal cortex (DLPFC). A brain area that plays an important role in executive functioning and in cognitive control.

Double dissociation. To demonstrate a double dissociation, a researcher must show that two separate independent variables or experimental conditions exert two distinct effects on two unique dependent variables (one manipulation affects X but not Y, while the other affects Y but not X). Double dissociation provides arguably the strongest neuropsychological evidence for linking specific cognitive functions to discrete brain regions.

DSM. *Diagnostic and Statistical Manual of Mental Disorders.* Manual developed by the American Psychiatric Association to standardize criteria for diagnosis of mental disorders.

Electroencephalogram (EEG). Recording of the brain's electrical activity; EEG measures voltage fluctuations within the neurons of the brain; commonly used in research and clinical applications (i.e., diagnosis of seizure activity).

Emotional overinvolvement (EOI). Reflects dramatic, exaggerated, overprotective, or devoted attitudes or behaviors toward a family-member patient by a family relative.

Emotional processing. The ability to perceive and utilize emotion to facilitate adaptive functioning.

Empathy. The ability to share and understand the unique emotional experiences of other people.

Epigenome/epigenetics. The markings on the genome (e.g., methyl group, histones) that do not change the DNA itself but are crucial to "turning on" or "turning off" genetic features of inheritance and are due primarily to environmental influence.

Event-related potential (ERP). A quantified electrophysiological brain response; used to study the physiological correlates of a sensory, cognitive, or motor event.

Experience-dependent neuroplasticity. Refers to the ability of the brain to change its function and structure in relation to new experience.

Experience-expectant. Describes neural growth that requires a certain kind of environmental stimulation that is almost certain to occur in the experience of most members of a species; an example is the development of the visual system that requires exposure to light in order to occur.

Expressed emotion. A measure of negative aspects of the family environment, EE reflects the extent to which a relative of a psychiatric patient speaks about that patient in a critical, hostile, or emotionally overinvolved way.

Eye gaze. Eye gaze plays an important role in social signaling that governs our basic evolved behavioral tendencies of approach and avoidance and is also involved in joint attention, which is a vital building block for the evolution of cooperation and collaboration.

Family high risk. Individuals who have a first-degree relative with a specific mental illness (e.g., psychosis).

Fiber tractography. Technique used to visually represent and quantify diffusion properties of white matter tracts using data collected via diffusion tensor imaging.

Fitness. The capacity of a species of life to reproduce itself in a given environment.

Fractional anisotropy. A metric that describes the degree of anisotropy of a diffusion process; its directionality. A value of 1 means that diffusion occurs along one axis (in one direction) and is fully restricted along all other directions. FA is commonly used as a measure derived from diffusion imaging, where it is thought to represent the microstructural integrity of white matter.

Frontostriatal pathways. Neural pathways that reciprocally project to the frontal cortical regions and the basal ganglia.

Functional magnetic resonance imaging (fMRI). A magnetic resonance imaging technique that measures brain activity by quantifying blood flow change. The sequence detects changes in blood oxygenation that occurs in response to neural activity.

Fusiform gyrus (FG). The FG is located bilaterally in the ventral lateral portion of the temporal lobe of the brain. This region has been shown to be heavily involved in the detection, perception, and processing of human faces. Once known as the "Fusiform Face Area," this region is now understood to have a specialty for recognizing human faces as well as defining features of a stimulus as a unique individual (e.g., bird faces, specific cars).

Gistfulness. Summarizing of details into main, abstract points.

Great apes. The closest remaining ancestors of humans in the primate order, consisting of gorillas (two subspecies), chimpanzees (two subspecies), and orangutans.

Hippocampus. Brain region located in the medial temporal lobe; a limbic structure known to be involved in the consolidation of new information into declarative memory and spatial navigation.

Hominin (or hominid). Those ape-line species on or near the line of evolution to humans.

Inattentive-overactive phenotype. Behavioral phenotype characterized by caregiver-reported inattention and overactivity frequently observed in children with histories of early social deprivation.

Inhibition of return. IOR is a fundamental mechanism of human perception that biases attentional orienting to novel locations in the environment. Behaviorally, IOR reflects slower reaction time (RT) to stimuli presented in previously cued locations. Under certain circumstances, IOR is disrupted in individuals with schizophrenia.

Interoceptive awareness. Sensitivity to stimuli originating within the body.

Iowa Gambling Task. Card selection game that incorporates risk, punishment, reward, and uncertainty. This neuropsychological task is intended to simulate real-life decisions and is thought to detect decision-making impairments.

Last common ancestor. The last ancestor before the human ancestral lines separated from the great apes line some eight million years ago.

Limbic system. A complex set of structures that lies on both sides of the thalamus, just under the cerebrum. It includes the hypothalamus, the hippocampus, the amygdala, and several other brain regions. It is thought to be involved in emotions and memory functions.

MACH-IV scale. Standardized self-report measure used to assess individual differences in Machiavellianism, a personal style that involves prioritizing self-interest above those of the group and lying and/or manipulating others for personal gain.

Mean diffusivity. A measure of overall magnitude of water diffusion independent of anisotropy. The metric is thought to reflect the maturity of white matter or brain injury.

Mental state attribution. The ability to infer intentions, dispositions, and beliefs of others.

Mirror neurons. Mirror neurons were first discovered in the inferior frontal cortex and inferior parietal cortex in macaque monkeys and are hypothesized to be responsive to both motor actions executed by the animal and the same motor action when observed in other animals. Models of mirror neurons have not yet been confirmed in humans but are hypothesized to underlie the "mirror system," which subserves the social function of grasping the intentions of others.

Natural selection. Those processes whereby features of the phenotype (body) and underlying genotype are selected upon by the environment when they increase fitness or the capacity of an animal (or plant) to reproduce.

Networks and complex science. A relatively new branch of science that focuses on the multiple levels of connections that affect natural and social phenomena.

Neural pruning. Neurodevelopmental process by which neural structure becomes more differentiated and efficient via the elimination of unused or unneeded neural processes.

Neurocognition. Nonsocial aspects of information processing, including attention, memory, and problem solving.

Neuropeptides. Any peptide (protein-like molecules) found in brain tissue, used for intercellular communication among neurons. Neuropeptides are polymorphic in their function, acting as extrinsic neurotransmitter modulators within synapses or as neurohormones altering receptors far from the point of their release.

Orbital frontal cortex (OFC). A region of the frontal cortex thought to be heavily involved in social norm compliance and social functioning (note the case of Phineas Gage). The OFC is also thought to be sensitive to reward processing and receives multiple sensory inputs from cortical and subcortical regions of the brain.

Oxytocin. A neuropeptide that has been identified as a key neuromodulator of social cognition and behavior related to pair bonding, attachment, peer recognition, and social memory. It is thought to be involved in mother-offspring interactions and trust.

Perceived criticism (PC). A measure of a person's subjective impression of how critical someone close to them is, assessed using a 1 to 10 scale.

Perspective-taking. The ability to understand the thoughts, feelings, and intentions of others and use this to guide behavior.

PET. Positron emission tomography is an imaging technique for assessing brain function and chemistry. 2-Deoxy-2(18F)fluoro-D-glucose (FDG-PET) is a radiopharmaceutical used in positron emission tomography; allows the evaluation of glucose metabolism in the body, including the brain.

Prediction error learning. A mechanism of learning via reward, subserved by dopaminergic signaling in the brain. We generate and maintain expectancies about real-world contingencies based on past experiences; when our expectancies are unmet, called "prediction errors," we learn to adjust our actions and thoughts accordingly.

Psychoeducation. Education focused on understanding mental illness and ways to promote mental health.

Reward circuits. Networks in the brain that include distinct brain regions and transmission of dopaminergic neurotransmitters and are sensitive to the detection of rewarding or reinforcing stimuli. These widely distributed reward circuits begin in midbrain dopamine neurons, extending to the ventral striatum and spanning throughout the brain with key sites of the nucleus accumbens, amygdala, orbital frontal cortex, and anterior cingulate cortex. These circuits are responsible for the rewarding stimulus value of basic biological necessities (food, water, reproductive processes), as well as rewards from drugs that activate the system.

Sensitive period. Term that refers to a time-limited period during neural development, during which the effects of experience on the brain are especially strong.

Social brain. The social brain is hypothesized as a dominant model for understanding the evolution of cognition in primates and the attendant massive expansion in their neocortex volume. The organizing theoretical principle is that the selective pressures driving the evolution and development of the primate brain are social rather than ecological. Principal regions involved are the amygdala, orbital and medial frontal cortices, and temporal cortex.

Social cognition. The ability to process and interpret socioemotional information in oneself and others. Social cognition is the study of how humans process and utilize social information and how they apply it to social situations and interactions. It is defined as a complex set of representations of internal bodily states, knowledge of self, perceptions of others, and interpersonal motivations.

Social context appraisal. The ability to understand the appropriate rules and norms for behavior based on observations of others and the social setting.

Social embeddedness. Term most closely associated with Mark Granovetter that describes the many ways that individuals are attached to other individuals and institutions through social network ties.

Social knowledge. The awareness of rules, goals, and the roles that characterize social situations in order to identify social cues.

Social networks. Ties between and among individuals that tie them to or isolate them from their families, schools, workplaces, communities, countries, and other social groups and institutions. Social networks can have varying qualities—weak or strong, dense or sparse, frequent or infrequent, positive or negative, and so on.

Social perception. The ability to judge social cues and understand roles, rules, and goals that typically characterize different types of social situations or social relationships.

Social Symbiome. A framework to facilitate understanding of how natural, biological, and social forces at multiple levels work together or in opposition to shape what happens, from the molecular to the global level.

Spandrels. Spandrel is a phenotypic characteristic, such as language, that may have resulted an indirect by-product of some other characteristic during evolution.

Statistical Parametric Mapping. Software program that allows the construction and assessment of spatially extended statistical processes used to test hypotheses about functional and structural imaging data.

Stroop test. Color-naming task in which an individual is presented with the names of colors printed in colored ink incongruent to the word itself. The objective of the task is to serially identify the words' print color (e.g., say the word "blue" in response to the word "red" printed in *blue* ink). This task is commonly used to measure sustained attention and executive functioning.

Superior temporal gyrus (STG). The STG is a relatively large, long expanse of the cortex, located along the Sylvian fissure dorsally and the superior temporal sulcus ventrally, and consists of the primary and association auditory cortex (Brodmann's areas 41, 42, 22). The STG is involved in language comprehension, and research findings have demonstrated STG involvement when we correctly attribute the source of auditory stimuli, such as internal speech to our "inner voice" rather than to an external force.

Teratogen. Any agent or factor (i.e., drug, virus) that interferes with the normal development of an organism.

Theory of mind (ToM). Also known as "mentalizing," ToM allows humans to "read" the mental state of others. Theories on theory of mind suggest that certain brain regions are activated in social situations in which an observer is asked to hypothesize the intentions or motivations of another person's behavior.

Tract-based spatial statistics (TBSS). Automated groupwise observer-independent whole-brain analytic approach that aligns images from groups of subjects to allow statistical comparisons of imaging data (such as diffusion tensor imaging) without the need for subjectively defined regions or features of interest.

Uncinate fasciculus. A limbic pathway connecting medial temporal structures with the orbital frontal gyrus; thought to be involved in socioemotional and memory functions.

Urban stratification. The unequal distribution of resources, populations, institutions, and physical and social phenomena across city neighborhoods.

Vasopressin. A neuropeptide that has been identified as a key neuromodulator of social cognition and behavior related to pair bonding, attachment, peer recognition, and social memory. Thought to be involved in bonding.

Acknowledgments

We acknowledge first our gratitude to Michael Fisher, Harvard University Press's senior editor in biomedical sciences. It was Michael Fisher's enthusiasm, support, and occasional forbearance that allowed us to bring this effort to fruition. We are also grateful to Harvard's Radcliffe Institute for Advanced Study for funding our exploratory seminar, *Connecting the Social Brain to the Social World,* and to Phyllis Strimling, who managed the seminar and encouraged us to achieve fully its potential. We also thank our seminar note takers, Camila Mejia and Anne Remington from the Graduate Program in Applied Sociology at the University of Massachusetts Boston, and Jessica Agnew-Blais of the Harvard School of Public Health. University of Massachusetts Boston's Provost and Vice-Chancellor for Academic Affairs, Winston Langley, provided much-appreciated additional financial support and opening remarks at our seminar. We must also acknowledge the productive and collegial environment provided for our work by the Massachusetts Mental Health Center Public Psychiatry Division of the Beth Israel Deaconess Medical Center, of the Harvard Medical School, and the support of the additional institutions where we teach and conduct related research: the University of Massachusetts Boston (Schutt), the Massachusetts Department of Mental Health (Seidman), the Massachusetts General Hospital (Seidman), and the University of Pittsburgh (Keshavan). We are grateful to our families for their support and for all they have taught us about human sociality.

Contributors

Jean Addington, PhD, Department of Psychiatry, University of Calgary, Calgary, Canada

Mariapaola Barbato, PhD, Department of Psychiatry, University of Calgary, Calgary, Canada

Michael E. Behen, PhD, Children's Hospital of Michigan, Detroit Medical Center, Wayne State University School of Medicine, Detroit, Michigan

Victoria Choate, Department of Psychology, University of Massachusetts Boston, Boston, Massachusetts

Harry T. Chugani, MD, Children's Hospital of Michigan, Detroit Medical Center, Wayne State University School of Medicine, Detroit, Michigan

Shaun M. Eack, PhD, School of Social Work and Department of Psychiatry, University of Pittsburgh, Pittsburgh, Pennsylvania

Michael F. Green, PhD, Department of Psychiatry and Biobehavioral Sciences, University of California, Los Angeles, Los Angeles, California

Christine I. Hooker, PhD, Department of Psychology, Harvard University, Cambridge, Massachusetts

Jill M. Hooley, PhD, Department of Psychology, Harvard University, Cambridge, Massachusetts

William P. Horan, PhD, Department of Psychiatry and Biobehavioral Sciences, University of California, Los Angeles, Los Angeles, California

Allan V. Horwitz, PhD, School of Arts and Sciences, Rutgers University, New Brunswick, New Jersey

Matcheri S. Keshavan, MD, Department of Psychiatry, Harvard Medical School, Beth Israel Deaconess Medical Center, Boston, Massachusetts

Junghee Lee, PhD, Department of Psychiatry and Biobehavioral Sciences. University of California, Los Angeles, Los Angeles, California

Paul G. Nestor, PhD, Department of Psychology, University of Massachusetts Boston, Boston, Massachusetts, Department of Psychiatry, Harvard Medical School, Veteran Affairs (VA), Boston Healthcare System-Brockton Division, Brockton, Massachusetts

Bernice A. Pescosolido, PhD, Department of Sociology, Indiana University, Schuessler Institute for Social Research, Bloomington, Indiana

Robert J. Sampson, PhD, Department of Sociology, Harvard University, Cambridge, Massachusetts

Russell K. Schutt, PhD, Department of Sociology, University of Massachusetts Boston, Department of Psychiatry, Harvard Medical School, Beth Israel Deaconess Medical Center, Boston, Massachusetts

Larry J. Seidman, PhD, Department of Psychiatry, Harvard Medical School, Beth Israel Deaconess Medical Center, Boston, Massachusetts

Patrick Sharkey, PhD, Department of Sociology, New York University, New York, New York

Ashley Shirai, Department of Psychology, University of Massachusetts Boston, Boston, Massachusetts

Jonathan H. Turner, PhD, Department of Sociology, University of California, Riverside, Murrieta, California

Figure Credits

Figure 7.1

Green, M. F., Hellemann, G., Horan, W. P., Lee, J. & Wynn, J. K. From perception to functional outcome in schizophrenia: modeling the role of ability and motivation. *Archives of General Psychiatry* (Now *JAMA Psychiatry*), 69, 1216–1224. Copyright © 2012 American Medical Association. Adapted and reprinted with permission from the American Medical Association.

Figure 11.1

Pescosolido, B. A., & Levy, J. A. The role of social networks in health, illness, disease and healing: The accepting present, the forgotten past, and the dangerous potential for a complacent future. *Social Networks & Health*, 8, 3–25. Copyright © 2002 Emerald Group Publishing Limited. Adapted and reprinted with permission from Emerald Group Publishing Limited.

Figure 11.2

Adapted and reprinted by permission from "Organizing the Sociological Landscape for the Next Decades of Health and Health Care Research: The Network Episode Model IIIR as Cartographic Subfield Guide" by Bernice A. Pescosolido in Handbook of the Sociology of Health, Illness, and Healing: A Blueprint for the 21st Century, edited by Bernice A. Pescosolido, Jack K. Martin, Jane D. McLeod, and Anne Rogers, Figure 3.2, p. 47. Copyright © Springer Science+Business Media, LLC 2011.

Figure 13.1

Burdick-Will, Julia, Jens Ludwig, Stephen W. Raudenbush, Robert J. Sampson, Lisa Sanbonmatsu, and Patrick Sharkey. Figure 12.1 "Summary of Effects of Different Studies on Children's Verbal Test Scores" In *Whither Opportunity*, edited by Greg J. Duncan and Richard J. Murnane. Copyright © 2011 Russell Sage Foundation, 112 East 64th Street, New York, NY 10065. Reprinted with Permission from the Russell Sage Foundation.

Figure 13.2

Burdick-Will, Julia, Jens Ludwig, Stephen W. Raudenbush, Robert J. Sampson, Lisa Sanbonmatsu, and Patrick Sharkey. Figure 12.3 "Relationship Between Beat-Level Violent Crime and Children's Reading and Math Test Scores in MTO Demonstration and Randomized Mobility Groups" In *Whither Opportunity*, edited by Greg J. Duncan and Richard J. Murnane. Copyright © 2011 Russell Sage Foundation, 112 East 64th Street, New York, NY 10065. Reprinted with Permission from the Russell Sage Foundation.

Plate 1

Hooker, C. I., Germine L. T., Knight, R. T., & D'Esposito, M. Amygdala response to facial expressions reflects emotional learning. *Journal of Neuroscience*, 26, 8915–22. Copyright © 2006 Society for Neuroscience. Reprinted with permission from the Society for Neuroscience.

Plate 2

Hooker, C. I., Verosky, S. C., Miyakawa, A., Knight, R. T., & D'Esposito, M. The influence of personality on neural mechanisms of observational fear and reward learning. *Neuropsychologia*, 46, 2709–2724. Copyright © 2008 Elsevier Ltd. Reprinted with permission from Elsevier.

Plate 3

Hooker, C. I., Verosky, S. C., Miyakawa, A., Knight, R. T., & D'Esposito, M. The influence of personality on neural mechanisms of observational fear and reward learning. *Neuropsychologia*, 46, 2709–2724. Copyright © 2008 Elsevier Ltd. Reprinted with permission from Elsevier.

Plate 4

Hooker, C. I., Gyurak, A., Verosky, S. C., Miyakawa, A., & Ayduk, O. Neural activity to a partner's facial expression predicts self-regulation after conflict. *Biological Psychiatry*, 67, 406–413. Copyright © 2009 Society of Biological Psychiatry. Published by Elsevier, Inc. Reprinted with permission from Elsevier.

Plate 5

Hooker, C. I., Bruce, L., Lincoln, S. H., Fisher, M., & Vinogradov, S. Theory of Mind Skills Are Related to Gray Matter Volume in the Ventromedial Prefrontal Cortex in Schizophrenia. *Biological Psychiatry*, 70, 1169–1178. Copyright © 2011 Society of Biological Psychiatry. Published by Elsevier, Inc. Reprinted with permission from Elsevier.

Plate 6

Chugani H. T., Behen M. E., Muzik O., Juhasz C., Nagy F., Chugani D. C. Local brain functional activity following early deprivation: A study of postinstitutionalized Romanian orphans. *NeuroImage*. 2001; 14: 1290–1301. Copyright © 2001 by Academic Press. Reprinted by permission of Elsevier.

Plate 9

Ben-Yishay, Y., Piasetsky, E. B., & Rattok, J. Orientation Remediation Module. A systematic method for ameliorating disorders in basic attention. In M. J. Meir, A. L. Benton, & L. Diller (Eds.), *Neuropsychological Rehabilitation* (pp. 165–181). New York: Guilford, 1985. Reprinted with permission from Yehuda Ben-Yishay.

Plate 10

Eack, S. M., Hogarty, G. E., Cho, R. Y., Prasad, K. M. R., Greenwald, D. P., Hogarty, S. S., & Keshavan, M. S. Neuroprotective effects of Cognitive Enhancement Therapy against gray matter loss in early schizophrenia: Results from a two-year randomized controlled trial. *Archives of General Psychiatry* (Now *JAMA Psychiatry*), 679. Copyright © 2010 American Medical Association. Reprinted with permission from the American Medical Association.

Index

Page references in *italics* refer to figures